NURSING
RESEARCH

A Quantitative and Qualitative Approach

CAROL A. ROBERTS, R.N., M.S.
SHARON OGDEN BURKE, R.N., Ph.D.

School of Nursing
Queen's University
Kingston, Ontario

JONES AND BARTLETT PUBLISHERS
Boston   •   Portola Valley

Production: Technical Texts, Inc.
Text Design: Sylvia Dovner
Cover Design: Rafael Millán
Typesetting: Polyglot, Pte, Ltd.

Editorial, Sales, and Customer Service Offices
Jones and Bartlett Publishers
20 Park Plaza
Boston, MA 02116

Printed in the United States of America
10 9 8 7 6 5 4 3 2 1

ISBN: 0-86720-415-X

Library of Congress Cataloging-in-Publication Data
Roberts, Carol A.
 Nursing research.

 Includes bibliographies and index.
 1. Nursing—Research—Methodology. I. Burke, Sharon Ogden. II. Title. [DNLM: 1. Nursing. 2. Research—methods. WY 20.5 R639n]
RT81.5.R63 1989   610.73′072   88-32867
ISBN 0-86720-415-X

We gratefully dedicate this book to
our parents and families.

≡ Contents ≡

_____ CHAPTER 5

Reviewing the Literature: An Essential Skill   110

_____ CHAPTER 10
Data Analysis: Understanding Principles and Evaluating Strategies   272

Preface

Our purpose in writing this text is to provide a basis for understanding and evaluating findings of nursing research and for using research findings in clinical practice. In order to build a sound knowledge base for nursing practice, nurses must be able to evaluate and use nursing research reports as a first step to research-based practice.

The text emphasizes using and applying nursing research, and it provides conceptual and nontechnical descriptions of the methods used by researchers. This understanding of research methods is necessary to critique nursing research for scientific adequacy and clinical application. The text not only covers the steps of the research process but also explains what a researcher does and provides a guide to evaluating each of these steps as reported in written research studies. The steps of the research process are illustrated with examples from research reports.

In this text we discuss the components of the research process chapter by chapter. An overview of the research process is presented early in the text and a flowchart of the process accompanies most chapters in order to place each step in relation to the overall process. In each chapter both scientific adequacy and the clinical applicability issues are addressed. While the central issue throughout the text is the applicability of specific research findings to practice, Chapter 3 focuses on this issue in detail. In Chapter 4 we describe the formation and critique of clinical nursing research problems. In Chapter 5 we discuss how research consumers and research team members review the nursing literature. Chapter 6 describes how studies are designed and how to assess the appropriateness of the designs and methods used to answer the research question. Chapter 7 is an exploration of the ethical issues related to conducting a research study and to applying research findings. Chapter 8 is an examination of sampling (the selection of the persons to be studied) in some detail. In Chapter 9 we describe how data (the information gathered by researchers) are collected and how data collection affects the applicability of the study results. In Chapter 10 we explore the process of data analysis and try to demystify most of the statistical language found in research articles. Chapter 11 is a description of the use of the computer throughout the entire nursing research process, with emphasis on making maximal use of this tool. We also identify particular types of errors that computers can introduce into a study and how a research consumer can use the computer to evaluate research findings. In the final chapter we examine the meaning of research findings from the broader viewpoint of the consumer and reexamine the various components of the research study by focusing on the applicability of research findings to clinical settings.

Today, the increasing emphasis on the use of qualitative methods to study nursing phenomena has lead us to integrate this theme with quantitative approaches throughout the text. We present the most common methods used in qualitative studies and illustrate them with many examples taken from qualitative research literature.

Exercises accompany most chapters to provide the opportunity to practice the skills and knowledge presented. Many of the examples used in the exercises were developed by our baccalaureate students. We are indebted to them for allowing us to share their ideas. In addition, all methods chapters contain guidelines for critiquing the scientific adequacy of the specific component of the research process under discussion. The appendix to Chapter 3 contains the complete guidelines for critique of research reports. An extensive glossary includes both qualitative and quantitative research terminology, which can assist the reader when evaluating research reports and studying new terms for each chapter.

Acknowledgments: This book has evolved over many years of teaching nursing research to undergraduate students and conducting research in the United States and Canada. We wish to thank our students who have helped us refine our teaching of nursing research over the years. Our thanks to our typist, Laurie Balderson, and our local editor, Donna Pothaar; both have been unfailingly cheerful and hard working in the production of the manuscript despite our many deadlines, three word processing languages, two computer systems, and two authors whose work styles are vastly different. Jim Keating, our executive editor at Jones and Bartlett, has been very patient and encouraging in explaining the publishing process for this first book. His enthusiasm for the project helped immeasurably. We also wish to thank the faculty at Queen's University School of Nursing for their support and encouragement, as well as their critiques of parts of the manuscript. A special thank you to Dr. Lisa Marchette and her Ph.D. students at the University of Miami School of Nursing, who tested and commented on the critique guidelines. Thanks to Betty O'Bryant and others at Technical Texts, Inc., for this fine production.

Most importantly, we thank Carol's husband, Fred, Sharon's husband, John, and her daughters for their cheer, the comic relief they provided, and their support for what must have seemed to be a never ending project.

We hope that the book will provide the background and guidelines needed to critique and judiciously use the vast array of published nursing research, a major step in developing research-based professional practice.

Carol A. Roberts
Sharon Ogden Burke

NURSING
RESEARCH

1

Developing a Research Consumer's Attitude: Past, Present, and Future Trends

INTRODUCTION

This chapter will provide you with some background for beginning the study of clinical nursing research. It introduces the idea that understanding nursing research is more than learning a method of inquiry; it requires an inquisitive attitude and a sound understanding of process for the implementation and application of clinical research in practice settings. Emphasis is placed on the critical role of research in creating positive change in client care and in developing nursing as a mature profession. The last sections of the chapter outline the major historical events in the evolution of nursing research and provide an overview of national and international trends that are emerging.

OBJECTIVES

After reading this chapter, you will be able to

1. Appreciate the reasons for conducting nursing research and using clinical nursing research findings in practice.
2. Identify the relationship between research and the professionalization of nursing.
3. Articulate the relationships between basic, applied, and clinical nursing research.
4. Relate historical and current trends to future developments in nursing research.
5. Appreciate the national and international movements to promote research-based practice in nursing.

NEW TERMS

Authority

Autonomy

Accountability

Basic research

Applied research

Clinical research

KEYS TO SUCCESS IN USING _____
NURSING RESEARCH

Nursing research is a systematic process of problem investigation conducted by nurses that aims to uncover new knowledge for the improvement of the care that nurses provide to clients. This process of inquiry involves three important components:

— An understanding of research methods
— The motivation to read and use research
— A knowledge about current nursing practices.

An examination of the literature on nursing research reveals a wide variety of related terms and definitions, such as applied research, basic research, clinical research, quantitative research, and, more recently, qualitative research. Basically, these terms reflect the range of methods, philosophies, and objectives for nursing research. In the next two chapters you will begin to sort out these various terms, and you will see that the different approaches are not separate and unique entities, but are integral components of the broader research process in nursing.

At the beginning of each chapter is a list of the new terms used in that chapter. The first time each new term is used it will be **boldfaced**. A brief definition will be given in the text, and more information, including synonyms, will be found in the Glossary at the end of this book.

The methods used to study problems in nursing are similar in many ways to those used by other disciplines. The nursing research process draws heavily upon the scientific and qualitative methods used in both the pure and behavioral sciences to collect and analyze information about nursing problems. With guided study and practice the beginner will have little difficulty in acquiring the basic skills necessary to become an intelligent consumer and neophyte nursing research team member. However, without a strong motivation to use these skills as an essential component of practice, this knowledge will remain an academic ideal.

To develop this motivation, nurses need to consider the purpose and place of research in professional practice and be convinced that nursing research does provide sound information on which to base changes for the improvement of client care. This text aims to spark your enthusiasm as well as enhance your ability to question and think critically and creatively about events in the clinical setting and about published nursing research.

IMPORTANCE OF NURSING RESEARCH: A PROFESSIONAL MANDATE

Let's begin our discussion by examining the relationship between research and being a professional. Many of us in nursing simply accept our professional status based upon tradition. However, an examination of the literature reviewing professionalization of occupations leads one to the conclusion that nursing must continue to grow to meet the professional ideal. In the late 1950s, Ernest Greenwood (1957) proposed a model to evaluate the degree of professionalization an occupation has attained. He used this model to analyze his own field—social work—and believes it can be useful in examining other occupations as well. Greenwood maintains that five elements are essential to an ideal profession and that all occupations in society fall on a continuum of professionalization accordingly.

The five elements proposed by Greenwood are

1. Professional practice is based upon a systematic body of theoretical knowledge.
2. Professional authority is recognized by clients.
3. Professional authority has a broad community sanction.
4. Professional relations are regulated by a code of ethics.
5. Professional culture is maintained through formal professional organizations.

In addition to these five elements the concepts of career and service are seen as central to being a professional.

In light of these criteria, one can easily place nursing high on the professional continuum in terms of service, culture, and ethics. However, the criteria for both theory and authority are less convincing.

Knowledge, Theory, and Nursing Research

Traditionally, the theoretical or knowledge base for nursing practice has been derived from a variety of pure and social sciences. However, there is little evidence that these fragments of knowledge provide a sound rationale for nursing practice. Nursing has become increasingly concerned about its knowledge base for practice, and the literature abounds with strategies for building a "nursing science" (Abdella & Levine, 1979; Downs & Fleming, 1979; Jacox, 1984; Johnson, 1959; Chinn & Jacobs, 1983). Although considerable controversy exists as to what elements should comprise the scientific body of nursing knowledge, most nursing leaders agree that the creation of this critical body of knowledge can only take place with the aid of nursing research. Donna Diers (1979) maintains that much of the questioning surrounding the status of nursing may be related to the lack of nursing research; she poses this thought-provoking question: "How can one successfully agree that nursing makes a difference without the data?" (p. 5).

How far has nursing come in its search for a scientific knowledge base? An examination of the research literature can provide us with some evidence. A recent review of published nursing research conducted by three nurse researchers—Brown, Tanner, and Padrick (1984)—covering the past thirty years reveals some interesting trends. The analysis focused on four questions considered essential for the development of a scientific knowledge base for nursing.

- To what extent have nurses responded to the call to conduct research?
- Has the focus of nursing research shifted toward issues of clinical practice?
- Has research become more theory-oriented?
- What methods have been employed in nursing research, and how have they changed over the past three decades?

The results of this study indicate that nursing research has steadily increased in volume, that the focus is on clinical problems, that a strong theory base is developing, and that problems in nursing are being studied through more sophisticated research methods. These authors conclude, however, that nursing has not achieved a systematic scientific knowledge base for practice largely because research efforts tend to be scattered singular attempts rather than those cumulative works that are necessary to build a body of knowledge valuable to a wide variety of clients and nursing practice settings. To produce this desired outcome, nurse researchers must continue to find and use sound research methods. These authors suggest that nursing research studies in the future should be guided by these considerations in order to bring nursing closer to its goal of scientific based practice. A study by O'Connell (1983), reviewing the progress of nursing practice research in the 1970s, yielded similar results. In addition, this study noted an increase in the number of funded research studies as well as more collaboration between nurses and non-nurses in doing nursing research toward the end of the decade.

In summary, nursing has not been idle in the attempt to build a theoretical base for practice but it is steadily moving upward on the continuum of professionalization in this respect. Nonetheless, several important factors need reemphasis. Nurses must unify and solidify their efforts in doing and applying nursing research. The majority of those who conduct nursing research are educationally prepared at the masters and doctoral levels—and indeed much of graduate study is focused on research. Does this mean that only nurses prepared at this level need be concerned about nursing research? In reality most of these nurses are academics and have less direct contact with client care than most other nurses. If nursing research is to become the basis for client care, there must be direct involvement of nurses at all levels of preparation and experience. Bridging the gap will take considerable work, collaboration, and time.

This text is guided by the basic philosophy that recognizes the need for collaboration between researchers in service or educational settings and front-line practitioners. All practicing nurses require a sound knowledge base in methods and skills to interpret and evaluate research findings for consideration of application into practice. Further, all nurses must be prepared to participate as team members in the testing and replication of research studies in the practice situation, and they must be able to question objectively nursing interventions and to generate researchable clinical nursing questions. Needless to say, greater collaboration and involvement between nurse researchers and practicing nurses are critical ingredients.

The solution to this problem is causing growing concern among nursing leaders. In 1981 the American Nurses' Association, Commission on Nursing Research, outlined *Guidelines for the Investigative Function of Nurses.* This document clearly outlines a research role for all four levels of professional preparation with an emphasis on the consumer and application roles in research at the undergraduate levels, a heavier emphasis on the investigative role at the masters level, and leadership roles in nursing research at the doctoral level. In Canada, the Canadian Nurses' Association has recently issued a position statement that aims to integrate nursing research into the practice setting by the year 2000 (CNA, 1984).

Concerted efforts are being made in both the United States and Canada to prepare the undergraduate student and the practicing nurse to become effective consumers of and participants in nursing research. The National League for Nursing surveys conducted in the United States (Spruck, 1980; Thomas & Price, 1980) indicate that most accredited baccalaureate nursing programs require students to study a research component as part of the undergraduate program. In Canada, the Canadian Association of University Schools of Nursing, which

proposes criteria for the accreditation of Canadian programs, recognizes that research is an important component for baccalaureate
education for undergraduates (ORCAUSN, 1983).

In addition, considerable attention is being focused on practicing
nurses who have not received a research background as part of their
basic preparation. The CURN project (1983), sponsored by the Michigan
Nurses' Association, developed a landmark strategy for ongoing development of staff nurses to evaluate research findings and apply them into
practice. Another model, from Massachusetts General Hospital, guides
staff development for the clinical application of nursing research
(Stetler, 1984). A few basic textbooks are now aimed at the consumer
rather than the investigator in nursing research. Reflecting institutional awareness, many service agencies are employing doctorally
prepared nurse researchers to assist in the development of nursing
research within their organizations.

Authority, Autonomy, Accountability, and Nursing Research

A second professional characteristic that is of great concern
to nursing is **authority** recognized by the client. One definition of
authority is a right conferred upon an individual to make decisions,
command resources, issue orders, or impose sanctions (Gilles, 1982). This
issue has been the subject of much discussion by nursing leaders over the
past two decades, and numerous factors have been identified that can be
shown to diminish authority for nursing:

— Nursing's dependent role in the nurse-physician relationship
— Problems associated with societal views of women's traditional role
— The largely female composition of the nursing profession
— The variety of levels of education received by nurses entering practice

These factors have all been cited as deterrents to the recognition of
nursing's professional authority. It is beyond the scope of this text to
examine these issues except to create an awareness of their existence
as factors contributing to a problem of greater underlying cause. The
authority problem relates back to our earlier discussion concerning
nursing's questionable knowledge base and the need to build that base

through sound nursing research. As you progress through this text you will gradually observe and understand the relationship between research and knowledge and how it can increase your authority as a nurse.

How can research-generated knowledge promote greater recognition of nursing's authority by society? Recognized sources of authority include the law, position or status, and knowledge. Nursing derives its basic authority through its licensing bodies and nurse practice acts. Although nurse practice acts have greatly expanded the scope of nursing practice over the past ten years or so (Bullough, 1983), nursing's position in the health care system still is viewed by society largely as one of employees practicing according to the rules and regulations established by bureaucratic organizations, under the supervision of physicians.

This perceived lack of nursing authority is closely tied to the issue of **autonomy** in nursing, or the freedom for nursing to define, control, and monitor its own practice. Nurses need not only the right to act, but the freedom to do so. Traditionally, nursing has not encouraged its practitioners to pursue this freedom. In recent years more autonomous models for nursing practice have emerged through primary nursing and independent nursing practice roles. Although these roles are important steps in raising the status of nursing to one of authority and autonomy in the eyes of the public, the crucial issue remains that many nurses in these roles, along with the nursing majority, are unable to define what elements of practice are uniquely nursing. They are, therefore, unable to provide clients with the evidence that nursing really does make a difference.

Building nursing's knowledge base through research is essential if nursing is to develop as a mature profession over the next few decades. If individual nurses can clearly articulate what nursing is and provide sound nursing research data for decisions, then nurses as a group will become more accountable to their clients for care given. **Accountability** is considered a hallmark of well-developed professions (Passos, 1973). It not only embodies responsibility for care given but involves professionals being answerable and liable to the client for the "what" and "why" of care. Through nursing research, nurses can become primarily accountable to society and be recognized as a learned and autonomous profession, working interdependently with other health care professionals.

Figure 1.1 depicts the central relationship of nursing research within the nursing profession, and its connection to knowledge and accountability for care to the client. Authority and autonomy are seen as components of accountability.

_____ Figure 1.1 _____

NURSING RESEARCH AND PROFESSIONAL PRACTICE

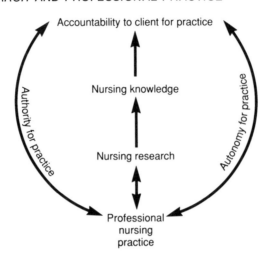

CLASSIFYING NURSING RESEARCH FOR APPLICABILITY TO PRACTICE

Earlier in this chapter we discussed the ultimate purpose of nursing research—building a science of nursing through the discovery of new knowledge to enhance the quality of client care. This process of discovery involves several types or classifications of nursing research, which can be roughly grouped into basic research and applied research. **Basic research** is often referred to as theoretical research, the major purpose of which is to solve a problem that expands knowledge without immediate concern for direct application into practice. **Applied research,** on the other hand, seeks to solve a problem that has direct and immediate implications for practice. Consider Examples 1.1 and 1.2 from the nursing research literature.

Both studies in Examples 1.1 and 1.2 primarily aim to uncover knowledge; taken alone, neither would have immediate or direct implications for change in maternal-child nursing practice. The Raff study is dramatically removed from the clinical situation and studies animal rather than human subjects under very controlled laboratory conditions. Its ultimate purpose is to demonstrate the relationship between exercise in pregnancy and the postnatal physical development and weight gain in offspring. Certainly, this line of research would contribute to knowledge that could eventually have significance for

Example 1.1

PRENATAL EXERCISE FOR RATS

Raff (1977) conducted a laboratory experiment to determine the effect of planned prenatal exercise in the last week of pregnancy on measures of development and body weight in the offspring of albino rats. She rationalized that as the fetus increased in size its ability to move, stimulate itself, and receive oxygen from the maternal blood supply was diminished. By providing exercise to the mother rats in advanced pregnancy, she predicted the flow of oxygen to the fetus would be enhanced and body weight and developmental rate would be increased postnatally in offspring whose mother had received the experimental exercise program.

See Raff, B. S. (1977). The relationship of planned prenatal exercise to postnatal growth and development in offspring of albino rats. In F. Downs & M. Newman (Eds.), _A source book of nursing research,_ 2nd ed. Philadelphia: F. A. Davis.

Example 1.2

ANXIETY AMONG PREGNANT WOMEN

Glazer (1980) conducted a study to examine expressed concerns and anxieties among pregnant women and to determine if there is a relationship between the level of anxiety and number of concerns expressed, selected demographic characteristics, weight gain, and trimester of pregnancy. The researcher rationalized that identification of concerns expressed most frequently by pregnant women and their levels of anxiety could serve to reduce anxiety indirectly through nursing intervention.

See Glazer, G. (1980). Anxiety levels and concerns among pregnant women. _Research in Nursing and Health, 3,_ 107–113.

humans and implications for client teaching and counseling in maternal-child nursing. However, considerably more research needs to be done at the laboratory level before conducting such studies with human subjects, and only after careful testing can we consider incorporating this knowledge into practice.

The Glazer study is less removed from the clinical setting and deals with human subjects. The reduction of anxiety and identification of concerns are central issues to nursing, particularly when the well-being of mother and child is at stake. This study served to uncover considerable knowledge about concerns expressed by pregnant women and levels of anxiety experienced by these women according to age, income, and a number of other sociodemographic indices. However, much more theoretical research is needed to provide further knowledge about the precise relationship between expressed concerns and anxiety. For example, practicing nurses need to know whether clients expressing high concern will evidence high levels of anxiety or vice versa, and what is an effective nursing approach to reduce or prevent anxiety and concern in these clients. This study does provide the practicing nurse with some insight regarding anxiety levels and concerns of pregnant women in certain age and socioeconomic groups. Nursing interventions, however, were not studied.

The studies in Examples 1.1 and 1.2 are clearly closer to basic research than to applied research in that they aim to build knowledge, even though the Glazer study has much more immediate clinical relevance than the Raff study. Example 1.3 is an example from the nursing literature that can be considered applied research. The Rettig and Southby study depicts a specific nursing problem that may hold some immediate and direct implications for change in practice.

Example 1.3

INJECTION DISCOMFORT AND MUSCLE RELAXATION

Rettig and Southby (1982) conducted a study in which they rationalized that giving an intramuscular injection into a relaxed muscle resulted in less client discomfort. Sixty clients receiving preoperative medication reported on their discomfort under one of four controlled treatment conditions. The researchers concluded that clients receiving a dorsogluteal injection into a relaxed muscle, through internally rotating the femur, reported decreased discomfort from the injection.

See Rettig, F. M., & Southby, J. R. (1982). Using different body positions to reduce discomfort from dorsogluteal injections. *Nursing Research, 31,* 219–221.

The Basic/Applied Continuum

You can observe from Examples 1.1, 1.2, and 1.3 that it is difficult to classify research in nursing as simply applied or basic as there is often much overlap between the two. Downs (1979) proposes that nursing research be classified along a basic/applied continuum and that the critical difference is the purpose of the study. The following five categories of nursing research studies were modified from Gage's *Handbook of Research on Teaching* (1963) and were applied to nursing by Downs.

— Category 1: Basic science content—not directly relevant to practice
— Category 2: Basic science content—relevant to practice
— Category 3: Descriptions of practically oriented nursing problems
— Category 4: Experiments involving problems of practice in controlled situations
— Category 5: Clinical trials of a nursing intervention

The continuum begins with the purest form of basic research and progresses to those types of studies that can be translated most readily into practice. If we examine the foregoing examples from the literature, most likely we can place the Raff study (Example 1.1) at the top of the continuum, the Glazer study (Example 1.2) at the second level, with the Rettig and Southby study (Example 1.3) at about level four. You will be returning to examine this continuum in more detail in Chapter 3, which discusses the application of nursing research to practice.

Clinical Research: Basic, Applied, or Both?

Another scheme for classifying studies in nursing research is determining whether or not it is **clinical research.** Some writers consider as clinical research only that research that has obvious direct application to practice, as in Downs' categories 3–5. Downs does not share this view, arguing that basic research uses the same methods as applied research and is often conducted in clinical settings. Much basic nursing research holds some relevance for individual practice and cuts across the basic/applied continuum. For example, the Glazer study (Example 1.2) could be classified in category 2 as basic research with some relevance to nursing.

Another way to view the likely clinical applicability of a study is to examine its place on two intersecting continua. These continua are

_____ Figure 1.2 _____

ZONES OF CLINICAL APPLICABILITY: THE INTERFACE BETWEEN THE
BASIC/APPLIED CONTINUUM AND RELEVANCE OF THE STUDY TO A
PARTICULAR TYPE OF NURSING PRACTICE

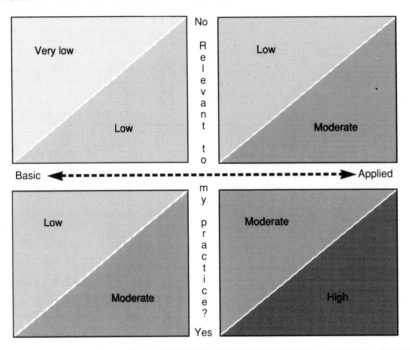

the basic/applied continuum and the continuum showing the degree of
direct relevance of the problem to current clinical practice. In Figure 1.2
you can see this diagrammed. Here the Glazer study (Example 1.2) would
be classed as basic research (left side of Figure 1.2). Whether or not the
findings had clinical relevance would depend on your own clinical area.
Thus, for someone who teaches prenatal classes the study would be
relevant with moderate applicability (lower left); for someone in another
setting the clinical applicability might be low or very low (upper left).

_____ *HISTORICAL PERSPECTIVES AND* _____
           CURRENT TRENDS

Research is not a new concept in nursing. Most writers recognize
Florence Nightingale as the first nurse to engage in systematic inquiry
into nursing care as she recorded detailed observations of conditions

and the care provided soldiers during the Crimean War. However, it is well into the twentieth century before we find evidence of organized efforts to pursue nursing research within the discipline. The earliest formal studies focused on nursing education and nursing service, which began in the early 1920s and dominated nursing research well into the 1960s. The present trend toward clinical nursing research does not become predominant in the literature until the late 1960s. The following discussion presents some important highlights in the development of nursing research on an international level from these earlier times to the 1980s.

United States

Recognizing significant research contributions to the body of nursing knowledge will provide some perspective on the roots of nursing research as we look toward the future. Abdella (1970) and Abdella and Levine (1979) provide a good outline of important milestones in the development of nursing research in the United States from its beginnings in the early 1900s through the 1970s. Another overview is presented by Gortner and Nahm (1977). Our discussion here draws upon information detailed in both of these excellent sources.

In 1923 an important study into nursing education was conducted by Josephine Goldmark, sponsored by the Committee for the Study of Nursing Education. This study was perhaps the first representative survey of the role of nurses in public health, teaching, and administration. Recommendations in this report included separate support for the maintenance of nursing education programs in hospitals and better preparation for nurses in the roles of teacher, administrator, and public health nurse. The 1920s were when baccalaureate education took a firm hold in the United States, reflecting a recognition of the need for more advanced preparation of nurses to scientifically study nursing education and service. Yale University School of Nursing was established in 1923, and Vanderbilt University School of Nursing, in 1925.

Throughout the 1930s and 1940s a number of studies examined the supply and demand for qualified nurses and the economics of nursing service and nursing education. Three projects were conducted from 1926 to 1934 by the Committee on Grading of Nursing Schools. These surveys uncovered much valuable information about nurses and nursing in the United States and provided a base for the establishment of the National Nursing Accrediting Service in 1950, which accredits nursing education programs (Abdella & Levine, 1979).

In 1948 the Brown Report, a scholarly document prepared for the National Nursing Council, outlined a number of recommendations that initiated many nursing research studies in the 1950s. Some examples include studies in inservice education, nursing functions, roles, and attitudes as well as hospital environments and nurse-patient relationships. In that same year (1948) the United States Public Health Service, Division of Nursing, conducted state-wide nursing surveys and developed manuals for the conduct of nursing research (Abdella, 1952).

The 1950s and 1960s represented years of rapid growth for nursing research in the United States. In 1952, *Nursing Research,* the official journal of the American Nurses' Association (ANA) for reporting nursing research studies, was first published. The Institute of Research and Service in Nursing Education was established at Teacher's College, Columbia University, in 1953. This institute was the first within a university system to firmly establish a structure for nursing research. The major goal was to enhance nursing education through research. In 1955, the American Nurses' Foundation was formed. The foundation is heavily supported by the ANA and plays a major role in consulting, administering, and providing grants for research as well as conducting nursing research. That same year a further funding mechanism for nursing research was established through the Division of Nursing, United States Public Health Service (Abdella & Levine, 1979).

Two important developments occurred in 1957. First, a department of nursing was formed in the Walter Reed Army Institute of Research to concentrate on client care research and prepare a small specialized group of nurse practitioners-researchers. This was the first such institute to promote Nursing research. Second, the Western Council on Higher Education in Nursing sponsored the Western Interstate Commission for Higher Education (WICHE) to augment the quality of higher education for nurses, especially in preparation for conducting nursing research and communication of research findings (Abdella & Levine). The council has sponsored several nursing research conferences and in the 1970s carried out a large survey to identify important priorities for nursing research (WICHE, 1974).

A significant report influencing nursing research was issued in 1963 by The Surgeon General's Consultant Group on Nursing. This report recognized the great potential for nursing research to improve client care and recommended increased federal funding for the conduct of nursing research by universities and health care agencies as well as support for preparation of nurse researchers. In 1965 the ANA began to sponsor a series of nursing research conferences for the dissemination of nursing research and discussion of related issues. Dissemination of findings was further facilitated by the establishment of the *International Nursing Index* in 1966.

By 1970, a definite increase in clinical nursing studies had occurred. Brown, Tanner, and Padrick (1984) note this trend in their analysis of nursing research literature over a thirty-year period. Clinical practice studies increased from 29% of total published studies in 1952 to 40% in 1970. Studies in education decreased from 50% in 1952 to 33% in 1970. This trend continued into the 1980s with 63% of studies in 1980 focusing on clinical practice and 21% focusing on nursing education. The Lysaught report (1970), sponsored by the National Commission for the Study of Nursing, recommended increased support for research into nursing practice as well as education.

In the 1970s, reflecting the growth and support for nursing research, a number of new journals emerged. Among these journals devoted to the publication of nursing research studies are *Research in Nursing and Health, Advances in Nursing Science,* and *The Western Journal of Nursing Research*, which complement the earlier established *Nursing Research*.

In 1970 also the ANA Commission on Nursing Research was established and issued position statements on the protection of human rights in conducting nursing research (1974), recommended undergraduate preparation for research (1976), and outlined priorities for nursing research in the 1980s. These priorities include research directed toward the development of new knowledge to enhance practice in the following areas (ANA, 1981):

— Promotion of health for all age groups as well as competency for personal care

— Prevention of health problems that endanger productivity, abilities to cope, and life satisfaction

— Reduction of the impact of health problems on individuals and families

— Ensurance that the care needs of vulnerable groups are met

— Development of cost-effective health care systems for the delivery of nursing care

In 1985, the American Nurses' Association, Cabinet on Nursing Research, produced an important paper entitled *Directions for Nursing Research: Toward the Twenty-first Century*. This document outlines a

_____ Figure 1.3 _____

PRIORITIES FOR NURSING RESEARCH

1. Promote health, well-being, and ability to care for oneself among all age, social, and cultural groups.
2. Minimize or prevent behaviorally and environmentally induced health problems that compromise the quality of life and reduce productivity.
3. Minimize the negative effects of new health technologies on the adaptive abilities of individuals and families experiencing acute or chronic health problems.
4. Ensure that the care needs of particularly vulnerable groups, such as the elderly, children with congenital health problems, individuals from diverse cultures, the mentally ill, and the poor, are met in effective and acceptable ways.
5. Classify nursing practice phenomena.
6. Ensure that principles of ethics guide nursing research.
7. Develop instruments to measure nursing outcomes.
8. Develop integrative methodologies for the holistic study of human beings as they relate to their families and lifestyle.
9. Design and evaluate alternative models for delivering health care and for administering health care systems so that nurses will be able to balance high quality and cost-effectiveness in meeting the nursing needs of identified populations.
10. Evaluate the effectiveness of alternative approaches to nursing education for the kind of practice that requires broad knowledge and a wide repertoire of skills and for the kind of practice that requires specialized knowledge and a focused set of skills.
11. Identify and analyze historical and contemporary factors that influence the shaping of nursing professionals' involvement in national health policy development.

_____

Source: American Nurses' Association, Cabinet on Nursing Research (1985). *Directions for Nursing Research: Toward the Twenty-First Century.* Kansas City, Mo.: American Nurses' Association. Used with permission.

_____

number of predictions for the year 2000 concerning health care systems, consumers, and the nursing profession. These predictions provide the basis for a set of eleven priorities for conducting future nursing research, as outlined in Figure 1.3.

Also in 1985, a National Center for Nursing Research was created under the direction of the ANA. The center represents tremendous political effort on the part of the association and is a significant step toward promoting professional conduct, dissemination of findings, and support for clinical and basic nursing research (Bauknecht, 1986). It is believed the center will provide nurse researchers with better opportunities for interaction among themselves and with researchers from other disciplines; this will further the development of a professional scientific base for practice (Bauknecht).

In summary, these events taken together point to the 1980s and 1990s as a time to narrow the gap between research and practice.

Canada

The focus of nursing research in Canada parallels that in the United States, although growth progressed at a slower pace until the early 1970s. The development of nursing research in Canada is less well documented than that in the United States. Writings by Stinson (1977, 1986) and Cahoon (1985, 1986), two Canadian leaders in nursing research, provide the most comprehensive overviews. Cahoon (1986) reports that, beginning in the late 1920s, educational studies were predominant, continuing until the late 1960s with very few clinical studies evident. Stinson (1986) describes the real "birth" of Canadian nursing research in 1971 when over 300 nurses gathered for the first national research conference in Ottawa. However, rapid progress is observed in the 1970s and 1980s.

Stinson cites a number of factors contributing to the development of nursing research in Canada. Two of these factors are a shortage of nurse researchers and few funded nurse researcher positions. The lack of nursing researchers is indeed a significant factor. As we have observed, the growth of nursing research in the United States has been influenced by the evolution of university programs for nursing and prepared nurse researchers at the graduate level. Recent surveys indicate that Canada has relatively fewer nurses educated at advanced levels who could conduct research. Stinson notes that over 80% of nurses are educated at the diploma level in hospital and community college programs (most common), where nursing research courses are not introduced. It is only since the early 1970s that research and statistics courses have been a part of the baccalaureate curriculum. Of Canada's over 200,000 registered nurses, approximately 2,000 possess master's degrees and less than 200 are prepared at the doctoral level. However, indications are that these numbers are growing in spite of funding difficulties for university programs. Masters programs grew in number (10 programs presently exist nationwide) and expanded considerably in the 1970s. These programs provide sound research preparation for graduates. Ph.D. programs in nursing are not yet in place but appear imminent at two or three universities.

Few nurses are employed in full-time research in Canada. The first classified full-time Canadian nurse researcher was Pamela Poole, who was employed as a consultant by the federal government, department of health (NHRDP), in 1965. Stinson estimates this number increased to 20 full-time nurse researchers by 1984. However, these numbers do not reflect the much larger group of nurses who conduct research as a portion of their professional role. To date, the majority of clinical nursing research studies have represented joint collaboration between university nursing faculties and nursing departments of major teaching hospitals. Cahoon (1986) describes two collaborative examples. In the late 1960s a project to implement and evaluate the system for patient-centered care was initiated through Margaret Allemany of the School of Nursing, University of Toronto, on a unit at Sunnybrook Medical Centre, Toronto, which led to a full-scale joint project in 1980. In the early 1970s, Dr. Moyra Allen of McGill University School of Nursing in Montreal, with NHRDP funding and in collaboration with community agencies, developed a research center, which conducted a number of important clinical studies.

Stinson views organization and collaboration at the national, provincial, and local levels as key factors in the development of Canadian nursing research. The Canadian Nurses' Association (CNA) first developed a plan for nursing research in 1951 to promote studies in the areas of professional organization, nursing service, and nursing education (Cahoon, 1985). In 1971 a Special Committee on Nursing Research was established and became a standing committee in 1976 (Stinson, 1977). The CNA has provided the leadership over the last ten years or so in organizing for nursing research at the national and provincial level. This program has benefited from strong support of the Canadian Association of University Schools of Nursing (CAUSN) and the Canadian Nurses' Foundation (CNF). The latter provides funding for graduate education for nurses (Stinson, 1986). The close collaboration of these three organizations has been extremely effective in facilitating development of nursing research throughout the country.

A number of significant developments to promote nursing research have taken place at provincial, regional, and local levels. Most provincial nursing associations have some form of committee structure to advance nursing research in the area. The close collaboration among university schools of nursing and provincial associations has resulted in several national and one international nursing research conference since 1971. These events have been crucial in disseminating Canadian nursing research on a national and international level. Although Canadian nursing research regularly appears in international journals, Canadian nurse researchers have few vehicles for publication within the country. *Nursing Papers,* devoted mainly to research, is published by McGill University School of Nursing and has a small circulation. The national nursing journal, *Canadian Nurse,* a CNA publication, is not subject to peer review.

The movement toward clinical nursing research in Canada echoes that of the United States; however, there is still a long road to research-based practice. Cahoon (1986) emphasizes the importance of "chains or clusters of related research studies in clinical settings to produce cumulative results" and stresses that "practice research requires partnership between practitioners and researchers" (p. 200).

United Kingdom and Continental Europe

The evolution of nursing research in the United Kingdom is well advanced on several fronts, particularly in its highly organized structure. The most interesting development involves the growth of nursing research units or centers for the concentration of nursing research activities.

According to Dr. Lisbeth Hockey (1986), who founded the first research unit at the University of Edinburgh in 1971, the seven existing centers are financed by private or government funds and provide nurses with the opportunity to conduct studies in a specific area of nursing education, practice, or administration. Each center focuses on a different area of nursing, which facilitates the conduct of nursing research and the dissemination of findings. The units are both university and community or hospital based, and provide research education through "learning while doing" for university as well as some nonuniversity associated nurses.

Nursing research in continental Europe also appears to be growing. A recent analysis of nursing research content in the international literature by Ivo Abraham (1986) indicates recent trends in nursing research and theory development in West Germany, France, and Switzerland as well as Great Britain. Although Great Britain, and to some extent Switzerland, surpassed other European countries in output of nursing research literature over a five-year period, there are definite trends indicating a recognition of nursing as a practice profession with a theoretical foundation.

Abraham argues that this evolution will yield positive results. Unlike the early United States trend, which produced much nursing research without notable application to practice, the European approach begins with a sound theoretical foundation. Indeed, much work has been done and is in progress in Europe to promote nursing re-search and the concurrent building of theory through the organized efforts of the World Health Organization (WHO), the International Council of Nurses (ICN), and the Workgroup of European Nurse Researchers. We can look forward to a major increase in published clinical nursing research studies from all European countries within the next decade.

_____ *SUMMARY* _____

Research development over the twentieth century has been one of gradual acceleration. More collaborative research on concentrated clinical themes, with active utilization and testing of findings by nurses in practice, is necessary to reach the ideal of research-based practice. Experience in both Europe and North America suggests that the most fruitful strategies for producing clinically useable results are collaboration with clinical facilities, concurrent theoretical development, adequate funding for researcher training, and financial support for the conduct of clinically relevant nursing research studies. Nursing research is a powerful tool in creating positive change for client care. Furthermore, it is a professional necessity to build a sound knowledge base for nursing practice and to establish favorable social recognition of nursing.

_____ *REFERENCES* _____

Abdella, F. G. (1952). State nursing surveys and community action. *Public Health Report, 67,* 544–560.

———— (1970). Overview of nursing research. *Nursing Research,* 6–17, 151–162, 239–252.

Abdella, F. G., and Levine, E. (1979). *Better patient care through nursing research.* New York: Macmillan.

Abraham, I. L. (1986). Chronological analysis of nursing research content in an international context. In S. M. Stinson & J. C. Kerr (Eds.), *International issues in nursing research.* London: Croom Helm.

American Nurses' Association, Cabinet on Nursing Research. (1985). *Directions for nursing research: Toward the twenty-first century.* Kansas City, Mo.: American Nurses' Association.

———— Commission on Nursing Research. (1981a). *Guidelines for the investigative function of nurses.* Kansas City, Mo.: American Nurses' Association.

———— Commission on Nursing Research. (1981b). *Research priorities for the 1980s.* Kansas City, Mo.: American Nurses' Association.

Bauknecht, V. L. (1986). Congress overrides veto, nursing gets center for research. *American Nurse, 18*(1), 24.

Brown, J. S.; Tanner, C. A.; & Padrick, K. P. (1984). Nursing's search for scientific knowledge. *Nursing Research, 33,* 26–32.

Bullough, B. (1983). The relationship of nurse practice acts to the professionalization of nursing. In N. L. Chaska (Ed.), *The nursing profession: A time to speak.* New York: McGraw-Hill.

Cahoon, M. C. (1985). Development of the knowledge base. In M. Stewart, J. Innis, S. Searl, & C. Smillie (Eds.), *Community health nursing in Canada.* Toronto: Gage Publishing.

———— (1986). Research development in clinical settings: A Canadian perspective. In S. M. Stinson & J. C. Kerr (Eds.), *International issues in nursing research.* London: Croom Helm.

Canadian Nurses' Association. (1984). The research imperative for nursing in Canada: A 5-year plan towards year 2000. Task Force Report.

Chinn, P. L., & Jacobs, M. K. (1983). *Theory and nursing: A systematic approach.* St. Louis: C. V. Mosby.

CURN (1981). *Using research to improve nursing practice.* New York: Grune & Stratton.

Diers, D. (1979). *Research in nursing practice.* New York: Lippincott.

Downs, F. S. (1979). Clinical and theoretical research. In F. S. Downs and J. W. Fleming (Eds.), *Issues in nursing research.* New York: Appleton-Century-Crofts.

Downs, F. S., & Fleming, J. W. (Eds.). (1979). *Issues in nursing research.* New York: Appleton-Century-Crofts.

Gage, N. L. (1963). Paradigms for research on teaching. In N. L. Gage (Ed.), *Handbook of research on teaching.* Chicago: Rand McNally.

Gilles, D. A. (1982). *Nursing management: A systems approach.* Philadelphia: W. B. Saunders.

Glazer, G. (1980). Anxiety levels and concerns among pregnant women. *Research in Nursing and Health, 3,* 107–113.

Goldmark, J. (1923). *Nursing and nursing education in the United States.* Report of the committee for the study of nursing education and report of a survey by Josephine Goldmark. New York: Macmillan.

Gortner, S. R., & Nahm, H. (1977). An overview of nursing research in the United States. *Nursing Research, 26,* 10–33.

Greenwood, E. (1957). Attributes of a profession. *Social Work, 2.*

Hockey, L. (1986). Nursing research in the United Kingdom: The state of the art. In S. M. Stinson & J. C. Kerr (Eds.), *International issues in nursing research.* London: Croom Helm.

Jacox, A. (1984). Toward the development of a science of nursing. In M. Kravitz & J. Laurin (Eds.), *Nursing papers (Special supplement). Nursing research: A base for practice.* Proceedings of the 9th National Conference (pp. 15–25). Montreal: McGill University, School of Nursing.

Johnson, D. E. (1959). The nature of a science of nursing. *Nursing Outlook, 7,* 292.

Kelly, L. Y. (1985). *Dimensions of professional nursing* (5th ed.). New York: Macmillan.

Lysaught, J. P. (1970). *An abstract for action.* New York: McGraw-Hill.

O'Connell, K. A. (1983). Nursing practice: A decade of research. In N. L. Chaska (Ed.), *The nursing profession: A time to speak.* New York: McGraw-Hill.

ORCAUSN (1983). *Documents for the accreditation process.* Ottawa: Canadian Association of University Schools of Nursing, Ontario Region.

Passos, J. (1973). Accountability: Myth or mandate. *Journal of Nursing Administration, 3,* 16–21.

Raff, B. S. (1977). The relationship of planned prenatal exercise to postnatal growth and development in offspring of albino rats. In F. Downs & M. Newman (Eds.), *A source book of nursing research,* 2nd. ed. Philadelphia: F. A. Davis.

Rettig, F. M., & Southby, J. R. (1982). Using different body positions to reduce discomfort from dorsogluteal injections. *Nursing Research, 31,* 219–221.

Spruck, M. (1980). Teaching research at the undergraduate level. *Nursing Research, 29,* 257–259.

Stetler, C. B. (1984). *Nursing research in a service setting.* Massachusetts General Hospital, Department of Nursing. Reston, Va.: Reston Publishing.

Stinson, S. M. (1977). Central issues in Canadian nursing research. In B. LaSor and M. R. Eilliot (Eds.), *Issues in Canadian nursing.* Scarborough, Ontario: Prentice-Hall of Canada.

(1986). Nursing research in Canada. In S. M. Stinson & J. C. Kerr (Eds.), *International issues in nursing research.* London: Croom Helm.

The Surgeon General's Consultant Group on Nursing. (1963). *Toward quality in nursing: Needs and goals.* U.S. Public Health Service Pub. 992. Washington, D.C.: Government Printing Office.

Thomas, B., & Price, M. (1980). Research preparation in baccalaureate education. *Nursing Research, 29,* 259–261.

University of Alberta. (1986). *New frontiers in nursing research.* Proceedings of International Nursing Research Conference. Edmonton, Alberta: University of Alberta, Faculty of Nursing, May.

Vollmer, H. M., & Mills, D. L. (Eds.). (1966). *Professionalization.* Englewood Cliffs, N. J.: Prentice-Hall.

Watson, J. (1981). Nursing's scientific quest. *Nursing Outlook,* 413–416.

WICHE (1974). *Delphi survey of clinical research priorities.* Boulder, Col.: Western Interstate Commission for Higher Education.

2

The
Research Process
and Nursing Practice

INTRODUCTION

This chapter provides an overview of the activities undertaken by nurse
research consumers when reading and evaluating research findings, and
by nurse researchers when conducting research studies. A basic knowledge of these activities is important for nurses who plan to use research
as a basis for practice since the process of application requires
evaluating research activities as well as scientifically testing researched
interventions in one's own clinical situations. Similarly, given present
trends, many nurses in clinical settings will become active research team
members conducting various aspects of a research study.

In nursing research, as in all disciplines, similar ideas often appear
under several names. Research terms often have more specific meanings
than those in general use. For example, researchers have a more complex
but narrower definition of the term *problem* than the general public. This
chapter and the Glossary identify and define such terms and clarify
nursing research meanings.

OUTLINE

Overview of the Research
  Process

People Involved in Research-
  Based Practice

Problem Solving in Nursing
  Research and Practice

Ways of Knowing in Research
  and Practice

Ways of Thinking in Research
  and Practice

OBJECTIVES

After reading this chapter, you will be able to

1. Identify differences and similarities between the processes used in nursing research and in nursing practice.
2. Become aware of a nurse's roles as a nursing research consumer and research team participant.
3. Identify various ways of expanding knowledge in both practice and research.
4. Use the Glossary as a tool for better understanding the language of research.

NEW TERMS

Qualitative research

Quantitative research

Research team

Research consumer

Principal investigator

Delphi method

Inductive reasoning

Deductive reasoning

Scientific method

Causality

Association

Time priority

Nonspurious relationships

Rationale

Figure 2.1

RESEARCH PROCESS FLOWCHART

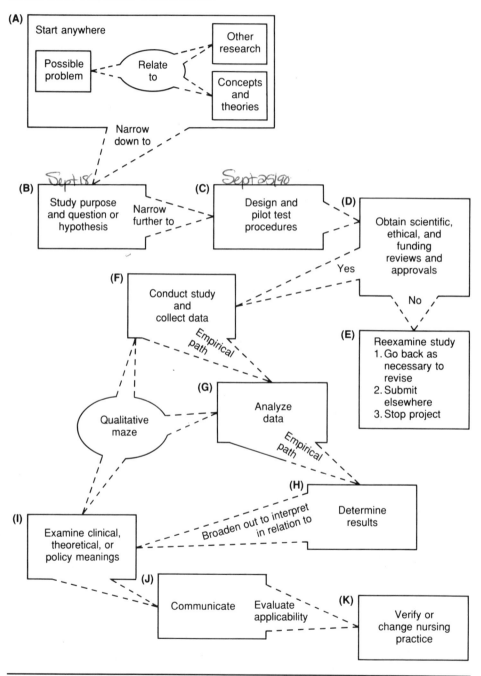

OVERVIEW OF THE RESEARCH PROCESS

The nursing research process consists of the interactive steps taken to apply scientific methods to nursing problem solving. It is interactive because the process rarely follows simply from one step to another. It is a process because it is not static but has continuous action. For example, when you read a research article in a nursing journal, the process may seem to have come to an end, but it has not because the researcher and you probably will take further action and do more thinking on the topic. The nursing research process is a specialized application and thus a modification of scientific methods for the specific use of the nursing profession.

The clinical nursing research process is diagrammed in Figure 2.1. The same diagram appears in other chapters of the book, and the particular aspects of the process under discussion in each chapter are highlighted.

Most nursing research textbooks contain a similar outline of the process (see Polit & Hungler, 1987; Seaman, 1987; Shelley, 1984). However, the path that a researcher eventually takes is usually not as straightforward as most texts and research articles seem to imply. Thus, the diagram shows some of this flow back and forth. This diagram also merges some aspects of the **qualitative research** approaches, which move from specific subjective observations to general concepts or theories, with **quantitative research** approaches, which move from more general concepts or problems to specific observations or testing. In contrast, the steps in qualitative research are less encapsulated, but they flow in the same directions (Chenitz & Swanson, 1986; Field & Morse, 1985). These two approaches are increasingly seen as complementary rather than oppositional (Chinn, 1986). Both are dealt with in this text.

This diagram outlines the activities of the **research team** in the course of conducting a research study. Nurse researchers often direct such teams, while nurses are often research team members. The role of a team member can involve contributing to most or only a few of the steps along the way. For example, a team member might collect and review related research reports while the project is at step A or participate in the collection of the *data* (information collected to answer the *research question*) for step B.

Perhaps less obvious is the role of the nursing **research consumer.** Table 2.1 shows the many parallels between the researcher's process and the research consumer's process. For example, a researcher might write an article for a nursing journal in order to communicate the team's *findings,* and the consumer might tell colleagues or present the

_____ Table 2.1 _____

EXAMPLES OF PROBLEM SOLVING IN NURSING PRACTICE AND RESEARCH

Nursing Process: Optimal Client Care	Researcher's Process: Development of Nursing Knowledge and Theory	Research Consumer's Process: Improved Nursing Practice
Assess	Examine problem area for researchable questions	Evaluate rationale for logic and applicability of study to this or other clinical questions
	Determine purpose	
	Check other research	Look for similar findings in other studies
	Check concepts and theories	
	Ensure relevance to nursing theory and practice	Evaluate relevance of this question to your practice
Diagnosis	Write question	

Plan	Design study
	  Locate subjects
	  and ensure rights
	  Select data
	  collection tools
	  Plan data analysis
		Evaluate likelihood that design will yield meaningful results for clinical use

	Determine limitations	Evaluate relevance of design for clinical use

Intervene	Conduct study
	  Collect data
	  Analyze data
		Evaluate appropriateness and thoroughness of data collection and analysis

	Write up results	
Evaluate	Interpret results regarding problem area, other research, theory, and practice	Evaluate quality relevant to practice
	State conclusions and recommendations	Determine other conclusions or recommendations

findings in the hospital newsletter for step J. The consumer examines the clinical, theoretical, and policy implications of the study for a particular practice setting. The research team might have done the same thing, but focused on implications for further research or reached somewhat different clinical *conclusions* for step I.

Throughout this text we will discuss components of the research process chapter by chapter. In each chapter the issues of both scientific adequacy and clinical applicability will be addressed. The central issue, applicability of specific research findings to practice, is indicated at the bottom of Figure 2.1 and is discussed in detail in the next chapter. The formation and critique of clinical nursing research problems (steps A and B) are described in Chapter 4. In Chapter 5 we discuss how research consumers and research team members review the nursing literature (this takes place most intensively at steps A, I, and J). Chapter 6 describes how studies are designed and how to assess the appropriateness of designs (step C). Ethical issues related to doing a research study and applying research findings (steps D and E) are explored in Chapter 7. Sampling is examined in some detail in Chapter 8 (this is planned in step C and done in step F). How the collection of data is done (step F) and how this will affect the applicability of the study results, is described in Chapter 9. The process of analysis (step G) is explored in Chapter 10. There will be enough information in that chapter and the Glossary to demystify most of the statistical language you will find in research articles. The use of the computer throughout the entire nursing research process, Chapter 11, emphasizes the maximal use of this tool and the identification of the particular types of errors that computers can introduce to a study. How a research consumer can use the computer to evaluate findings in light of other research is also included. The final chapter focuses on step I, an examination of the meaning of the findings. However, a broader view is presented for the consumer in that the overall critique of the various components of the research study is reexamined in the light of the rest of the text. The focus is on the applicability of the findings to your own clinical setting.

PEOPLE INVOLVED IN RESEARCH-BASED PRACTICE

The Clinical Research Consumer

Who is a clinical research consumer? Any nurse who has used research findings or a study's data collection tools or the conceptual models developed for a study is a consumer of nursing research. The term *consumer* also encompasses the nurse who sees a clinical problem and thinks that it should be researched or considers looking for published research about the problem.

As emphasized in Chapter 1, there is a clear mandate for the professional nurse to be a research consumer. You have probably discovered already that this is a complex and challenging role. In this text, we will present a path to follow.

Not surprisingly, the process for the nursing research consumer has many parallels with the nursing research process. Furthermore, both the nursing research and the research consumer's processes have many parallels with the nursing process used in day-to-day practice. Table 2.1 represents an abbreviated example of these processes and their logical similarity to one another. However, take particular note of the differences in the aims and the examples of activities involved. All these processes have a deceptively simple surface structure, but are, in fact, very complex when one attempts to apply them. Much has been written about the nursing process and the research process. Our focus is on the nursing research consumer's process.

Specialization within nursing has led to increased expertise, but the focus of individual practice is often narrow. Whereas practicing nurse clinicians are often expert in the application of the nursing process for clients with particular nursing diagnoses, the nurse researcher is often skilled in a narrower range of clinical practice, but is more expert in the use of the nursing research process. The research consumer's process brings together the work of the nurse clinician and nurse researcher for improved patient care.

The Nurse Research Team Member

Have you participated in a research project? No? Think again. Have you ever helped to identify likely clients for a study, or been responsible for having them sign a consent form for participation in a study, or filled in a questionnaire yourself, or told a researcher what you thought should be studied next, or collected library materials for a professor, or sat on an ethics review committee? If the answer to any of these questions is "yes," then you probably have been involved in a research project. You were a research team member.

Understanding the whole nursing research process will help you to fit your piece of the puzzle into the picture. If you have participated and are only now realizing it or if you wondered at the time how your contribution fit into the total picture, then you will find this chapter illuminating.

Each participant in a research project has rights and responsibilities. From the **principal investigator** who directs the project, the head nurse on the ward where a study is being conducted, and the nurse who does interviews with clients (data collector) to the person being studied, each person needs an understanding of the project as a whole.

Nurse researchers and nurse clinicians work together to enhance one another's knowledge and skill. Participating in a research project is an excellent way to learn more about the research process and thus become a better consumer of nursing research. Successful research projects need the help of knowledgeable team members, skilled nurses who add their particular expertise. One of the most important contributions nurse team members make to a study is to ensure its clinical relevance. The best study results come from teams with both research and clinical expertise.

PROBLEM SOLVING IN NURSING RESEARCH AND PRACTICE

Problem solving is the underlying process for the clinical research consumer as well as the clinical nurse and the nurse researcher. The processes involved in nursing, nursing research, and the use of research in practice (Table 2.1) all demand systematic ways of knowing in order to reach valid conclusions. However, the aims of each are different, and thus the activities of the nurse involved in a problem-solving process with a client can seem very different from the activities of the nurse researcher or from the research consumer's process. Table 2.1 gives examples of the types of activities involved in each of these processes.

Stated in a global and simplified manner, the aim of the nursing process is to provide the best possible care for a client. The aim of nursing research is to develop or test theory that involves knowledge of relationships between elements, causes of events or states, and ways to observe these elements. The aim of the research consumer's process is to improve nursing practice by the application of the knowledge and theory developed in nursing research.

To become a skilled consumer of nursing research you will need to learn about the nursing research process and also the consumer's process. Underlying each are various ways of thinking and knowing or coming to believe that something is true.

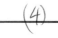 ## WAYS OF KNOWING IN RESEARCH
AND PRACTICE

Human beings come to believe in information or actions as true or effective by several methods. The more common sources of nursing knowledge are discussed below along with their place in the research and consumer processes. There are other methods of knowing such as meditation or empathy, but because they are less well structured and understood—not because they are necessarily of less value—they are not often used in research that has clinical applicability. In addition to the ways of knowing presented in this section is the scientific method. It is one of the most powerful ways of knowing and is presented separately later in the chapter since it is of particular importance to the nursing research process.

sci method → later in chapter

 ### Tradition

Tradition encompasses knowledge that is often repeated and held to be true by a large proportion of nurses. The phrases "tried and true" and "because we have always done it that way" typify thinking based on this way of knowing. Examples are some of our "standard procedures," such as taking q4 hr temperatures, a policy that all breach birth babies must be in an isolette for 24 hours, and the belief that the wearing of rings will increase the chance of infection for patients. (The last example has been researched: for a researcher's approach and answer to this belief see Jacobson, et al., 1985.)

Researchers often discount this knowledge because there is seldom any scientific evidence to justify it. However, traditional beliefs tend to be rigidly adhered to and therefore there is often a great deal of resistance if a researcher suggests a scientific examination of the validity of the traditional belief. Nevertheless, traditions are a rich source of research questions.

As a research consumer, your view of traditional knowledge will focus on distinguishing the traditions that can, or cannot, be supported by research evidence from those traditions for which there is no research evidence one way or the other. The examination of traditional knowledge in nursing can be frustrating for two reasons: first, other nurses who hold strongly to the traditional view will be very resistant to change even in the face of overwhelming research evidence; second, the body of research-generated knowledge about the myriad traditional beliefs embedded in nursing practice is still relatively scant. Nevertheless, as a research consumer, you will regularly review and question traditional nursing knowledge.

 ### *Authority*

Nursing knowledge often becomes believable because of the written words of experts. In our culture the written word carries authority by virtue of being printed in black and white. It is often not questioned and yet, many times experts may disagree with one another.

Researchers rely on authorities and experts at many steps in the research process and as a double check for their findings (see Figure 2.1, steps A and I). In some types of research, the data upon which the researcher bases final conclusions are the rank-ordered and carefully analysed opinions of many experts. An example of this is in studies that use a technique called the **Delphi method,** in which many experts are polled and repolled in an attempt to get consensus on an issue. However, a researcher is not apt to rely exclusively on the opinions of one or even a few experts or authorities, particularly if their opinions do not seem to be logically consistent or are not based on their own research.

A research consumer makes a distinction between expert opinion and data-based facts provided by experts. The research consumer checks with several different experts and makes a critical assessment of the likely validity of the consensus.

In practice, it sometimes happens that one authority becomes ensconced in an ivory tower, and any questioning of that expert can be difficult. For example, some agencies have adopted a singular nursing theory as a basis for nursing practice in their setting. In these situations two opposing camps can develop—those unquestioningly in favor and those strongly opposed to the theory. Using the research consumer's approach, one can systematically question a theory and offer alternate ideas based on research findings. Ultimately, the research consumer's approach goes beyond the unquestioning acceptance of an authority. It allows you to distinguish between what is valid or invalid, applicable or inapplicable, in the theories or opinions of authorities.

The researcher directing a project or the author of a research article can easily become an unquestioned authority figure. As a research consumer, and also as a participant in research projects, it is wise to guard against this. Be skeptical of the researcher who asks you to collect data, but does not have the time to explain how and why the data will be used. The best research comes from teams that include not only an expert researcher, but also inquisitive and well-informed team members.

Trial and Error Experience

The trial and error method of coming to know a fact, or of finding the best way to proceed, is very common in clinical nursing practice. In the trial and error approach there may be a problem, such as a lengthy admission procedure that is resulting in patient complaints. The problem is addressed by radically altering the procedures. If the new method works well, it is retained; otherwise, the search for a solution continues until the problem is solved, and then the trials stop.

There is a parallel in some nursing research methods if checks and balances are not built into the process. For example, when using an analysis procedure called content analysis (see Chapter 10), the researcher is searching for the meanings and categories contained in tape-recorded interview data. If the researcher completes the analysis based only on the first set of categories to be found, or if the researcher fails to verify the findings by omitting to check other sources of data, then the analysis will lack logic and also be incomplete.

For researchers, the trial and error process does not result in knowledge that is completely believable for several reasons. While the notion of trials of alternate methods is attractive, the conclusion of the trials before all likely alternates are tested can lead to less than optimal new ideas or practices. The lack of a systematic and thorough analysis of the problem or data to elicit all the factors involved can result in "throwing out the baby with the bath water." For example, if a piece of equipment is frequently breaking down, it could be that only small adjustments are called for rather than replacement, even though replacement will also solve the problem. Unless all possible explanations or solutions are systematically examined, the researcher will remain skeptical of the conclusions. Finally, unless the development of the alternate procedures involves a careful analysis of the possible causes or factors behind the problems, many errors are apt to be made in the trial and error process.

Research consumers do not rely on methods of trial and error to solve a clinical problem. They make a critical analysis of the problem and examine several solutions before selecting their final choice. When necessary, a research consumer will propose a full search of the literature of research-based solutions, or initiate a formal study of the possible options. The relative merits of the two approaches have to be weighed. Clearly, not all problems are serious enough or complex enough to require a full research study. However, some problems, which involve patient safety or extensive use of nurse time, could benefit from the more thorough and systematic research or research consumer's approach. The clinician is often in a better position to make such a decision than the relatively removed nursing research expert.

(2) WAYS OF THINKING IN RESEARCH AND PRACTICE

The development of ideas and the organization of these ideas into meaningful structures takes place in different parts of your brain. The left hemisphere generates the logical linear processes, while the right hemisphere is involved with patterns and their manipulation. Hence, there are two ways of thinking—intuition and logical reasoning.

Intuition —good at beginning & end of research
—documented better in qual studies but also used in quant

Intuition is at work when something occurs to you suddenly and in a nearly complete form. It is a fundamental part of creativity. It is what happens when you are studying some small detail in your lecture notes and have an unsolicited insight that makes the whole point of the course become clear.

Researchers use intuitive thinking throughout the research process, but particularly at the onset and at the end. Intuitive and creative thinking are essential when trying to sharpen the focus of the problem to be studied, when trying to create the best design to answer the questions, and, at the end of the study, when trying to understand the alternate interpretations of the findings.

In quantitative studies, which are based on a positivist philosophical perspective, these intuitive aspects will not be well documented since there is a bias among these researchers to discuss their findings in more logical and orderly ways. In Example 2.1 you can see that Levin (1982) probably used intuitive thinking in coming to conclusions that fell outside of the initial study question—the effect of patient choice and locus of control on the perceptions of pain. The unexpected finding that the patients' perception of pain was closely related to the background and experience of the nurse must have involved some intuitive thinking. Although the thinking behind the original questions is dealt with in considerable logical detail, the intuitive supposition is presented in its final form and is merely supported with data.

_____ Example 2.1 _____

WAYS OF THINKING IN QUANTITATIVE RESEARCH

Levin's (1982) study question was whether or not a client's participation in the choice of the site of an injection and the client's locus of control affected her or his perception of pain with the injection. The theoretical framework out of which the hypotheses grew was based on the concepts of cognitive dissonance and locus of control. Levin hypothesized that choice and internal locus of control would be associated with lower perceptions of injection pain. The study methods included a convenience sample of 138 preoperative adults who were randomly assigned to the choice–no choice groups. Data for locus of control were collected the night before and ratings of pain immediately after the injection. The statistical analysis did not support the hypotheses.

The researcher also reported on findings which were not directly related to her hypotheses. She reported that past experience, age and sex, and the nurse who gave the injections were factors in the perceptions of pain.

_____

See Levin, R. F. (1982). Choice of injection site, locus of control, and the perception of momentary pain. *Image, 14,* 26–32.

In contrast with quantitative studies, qualitative studies, such as Example 2.2, that are based on a phenomenological perspective, tend to be more explicit about the use of this type of thinking. Hutchinson's study (1984, 1986) of nurses' stress in a neonatal intensive care unit clearly reports her intuitive strategies: "With time and by working with an understanding the data . . . ." She used questions such as "what is going on in the data?" to force what she refers to as theoretical thinking.

The validity and utility of these types of intuition-based conclusions are hotly argued in the research literature (see Eisner [1981] for the pros and Downs [1977] for the cons).

While valuing the contributions of intuitive thought, research consumers expect the insight to be supported by concrete evidence. In addition, researchers who use this method are expected to document their procedures.

_____ Example 2.2 _____

WAYS OF THINKING IN QUALITATIVE RESEARCH

Hutchinson (1984, 1986) undertook this study to generate a theory that could explain the well-known stress inherent in neonatal intensive care nursing. A review of the literature confirmed the presence of such stress and the need for a theoretical linkage. The researcher was a participant-observer* in an NICU where she watched, talked with, and interviewed the nurses. The method used was grounded theory,* which is a systematic way of collecting and handling subjective information in order to produce explanatory theory. Three hundred pages of typed notes were systematically reviewed and contemplated by the researcher and this led to the identification of categories within the data. From these categories the researcher constructed her perceptions of what these theoretical meanings signified to the NICU nurses. The results of the study showed how these meanings were put together in a conceptual model to explain how the nurses confronted the horror of their work by creating meaning in an emotional, technical, or rational way. The reports are rich with examples of how the nurses did this, which lends credibility to the categorizations. It was concluded that the creation of such meanings will reduce the stress of working with these babies in the NICU setting, and implied that nurses should be informed of this process and aided in developing innovative methods for creating such meanings.

* These terms are explained in more detail in the data collection and data analysis chapters.
See Hutchinson, S. A. (1984). Creating meaning out of horror. *Nursing Outlook, 32,* 86–90,   (1986). Creating meaning: A grounded theory of NICU nurses. In C. Chenitz & J. M. Swanson (Eds.), *From practice to grounded theory: Qualitative research in nursing* (pp. 191–204). Menlo Park, Calif.: Addison-Wesley.

Logical Thinking

There are two major types of logical reasoning—inductive and deductive. Figure 2.2 illustrates these patterns and gives some examples.

Inductive Inductive reasoning involves moving from the specific to the general. In Hutchinson's study (Example 2.2), she repeatedly observed the stress of the nurses in one NICU and was able to document an apparent method some used to give events personal meaning; she associated this with reduction in work-related stress. All of these aspects are specific pieces of the puzzle that can be said to be true of those nurses at that time and in that place. Then, she used inductive reasoning to conclude that in a NICU culture the ability to create such meanings could decrease staff turnover, improve morale, and reduce stress.

The central risk in inductive thinking is taking the specifics too far with the generalization. In Hutchinson's study, the specifics were true for those nurses at that time in that place, but the generalization seems too broad given the evidence presented. You cannot be sure that it

_____ *Figure 2.2* _____

THE INDUCTIVE AND THE DEDUCTIVE FLOW OF LOGIC

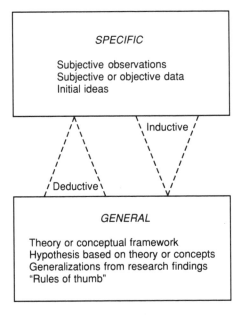

would apply to your NICU. You still might want to test it in your setting to discover if her conclusions have some utility there.

Deductive   Conversely, deductive reasoning involves moving from the general to the specific. In Levin's study (Example 2.1) there was a generalization—stated as a theoretical relationship between locus of control, choice of injection sites, and perceptions of pain—that was tested in the specific instance of the adult preoperative patient. Levin found no relationships. If she had used only deductive reasoning and accepted the generalization about control and perceptions of pain, she would have concluded that the preoperative patients with the most control would have perceived the least pain. However, using the scientific method in a research study, she found no relationships between control and perceptions of pain.

The primary problem in the use of deduction in nursing is the relative lack of tested theory. Where there is no theory, it is clear that no specifics can be deduced. The more general the theory and the more specific the conclusion, the more likely the conclusion is to be false. Practicing nurses and researchers alike need to recognize that unproven theories lead to false specific conclusions.

The Scientific Method and Causality

The scientific method is a way of knowing that incorporates both inductive and deductive thinking with checks and balances to avoid the fallacies that can emerge with either method used alone. The **scientific method** is the most complex, well-developed, and well-documented approach available for quantitative research. It was developed for use in the pure sciences, but has been adapted by all the behavioral sciences including nursing. It is the basis for most of the nursing research process, the nursing process, and the nursing research consumer's process. Some qualitative researchers disagree with its philosophic basis (logical positivism) and argue that more intuitive, naturalistic approaches are better suited to nursing research. The stance taken in this text is that the contributions made by both approaches—research based on the scientific method and research based on the phenomenological approach—complement each other. Briefly stated, the steps in the scientific method are

STEP 1   State the problem.

STEP 2   Collect and organize all currently available related facts.

STEP 3   State a hypothesis.

STEP 4 Devise an experiment to test the hypothesis.

STEP 5 Accept or reject the hypothesis.

STEP 6 Check the conclusions against other related facts and by further experiments.

Several important characteristics of the scientific method are embedded in the steps above. The method is systematic, controlled, empirical, and critical (Kerlinger, 1973). In summary, the scientific method is conducted in such a way that other scientists will have confidence in its conclusions. The method is the basis for most quantitative research. Although qualitative researchers tend to reject the philosophical basis of the scientific method's orderly steps, many recent qualitative studies and texts use a significant portion of the scientific method as well as its terminology. For example, the Field and Morse (1985) description of a qualitative research proposal reflects most of the elements of the scientific method.

The aim for a nurse who uses the scientific method is to determine causes and thereby control factors for the benefit of clients. Thus, the concept of **causality** is central to the research process wherein one predicts in order to gain control. Scientists attribute cause to events under the following four circumstances (Labovitz & Hagedorn, 1981):

- —**Association:** two or more variables are consistently and greatly associated with one another
- —**Time priority:** the causal event or situation occurs or changes *before* the expected outcome
- —**Nonspurious relationships:** the association cannot be explained by a third factor
- —**Rationale:** the relationships between the cause and the effect are theoretically logical or meaningful

These circumstances are neither necessary nor sufficient in themselves to prove cause. The most clinically applicable nursing research is implicitly or explicitly aimed at demonstrating causality by developing rationales or theories, manipulating or observing changes in the supposed causes, and observing for the resultant effect.

The Scientific Method and Nursing Research

Nursing faces problems in the strict application of the scientific method. The problems revolve around the primary subject of our studies—people. They simply do not behave in the more consistent ways that chemicals do, for instance. Furthermore, ethical considerations do not allow the range of experimentation on people that is possible with inanimate objects or even animals. A plant can be dissected to determine the effect of a chemical on its system. A person cannot. The most elegant research studies are the ones that have found simple ways to test for causality within the complexity of the human client and within complex medical and social settings.

The nursing research process as it is presented here relies heavily on the scientific method with its logical positivist philosophy, quantitative methods, objective outlook, and deductive logic. These quantitative methods are well developed and have been used extensively and effectively in nursing research for many years. Nevertheless, at the other end of the continuum, the phenomenological, qualitative, subjective, and inductive approaches are also applicable to nursing practice and research. Though newer to nursing, these latter methods are better suited to some of the problems facing nursing today.

Whatever methods are used, they should be carried out with the utmost care and skill. In the following chapters we describe how to determine whether or not the research is well done and, by extension, whether or not the findings should be applied to the clinical setting.

SUMMARY

This chapter presents an overview of the nursing research process, compares this process as used by different researchers, and discusses various methods of problem solving and their *application* to nursing research. The parallels between the nursing research process and the nursing process are made explicit. The roles of the researcher and the consumer in the provision of research-based nursing practice are described and contrasted. Finally, ways of knowing and thinking that are used in both nursing practice and nursing research are examined.

EXERCISES

1. Look at the introduction to this chapter. Note the term *problem*. As a nurse, how would you define this term? As a patient, how would you define it? How would it be defined by a lay person? Check the Glossary in this text for the research-specific use of this term.

2. Look at the article by Tulman (1986) in the Appendix. Note terms that might have research-specific definitions and look them up in the Glossary. For example, look up method, sample, *t, df, p,* M, and SD. The Glossary will help you to read previously obscure sections of research articles and reports.

3. Find a research article in any journal of interest to you in your current work and use the Glossary in this text to clarify any terms that are unknown to you or that you suspect might have research-specific meanings.

REFERENCES

Chenitz, C., & Swanson, J. M. (1986). *From practice to grounded theory: Qualitative nursing research.* Menlo Park, Calif.: Addison-Wesley.

Chinn, P. L. (1986). *Nursing research methodology: Issues and implementation.* Rockville, Md.: Aspen Systems.

Downs, F. S. (1977). Elements of a research critique. In F. S. Downs, & M. A. Newman (Eds.). *A source book of nursing research* (pp. xi–xvi). Philadelphia: F. A. Davis.

Eisner, E. (1981). On the differences between scientific and artistic approaches to qualitative research. *Educational Research, 10,* 5–9.

Field, P. A., & Morse, J. M. (1985). *Nursing research: The application of qualitative approaches.* Rockville, Md.: Aspen Systems.

Hutchinson, S. A. (1984). Creating meaning out of horror. *Nursing Outlook, 32,* 86–90.

———— (1986). Creating meaning: A grounded theory of NICU nurses. In C. Chenitz & J. M. Swanson (Eds.). *From practice to grounded theory: Qualitative research in nursing* (pp. 191–204). Menlo Park, Calif.: Addison-Wesley.

Jacobson, G.; Thiele, J. E.; McCune, J. H.; & Farrell, L. D. (1985). Handwashing: Ring-wearing and number of microorganisms. *Nursing Research, 34,* 186–190.

Kerlinger, F. N. (1973). *Foundations of behavioral research.* New York: Holt, Rinehart and Winston.

Labovitz, W., & Hagedorn, R. (1981). *Introduction to social research,* 3rd ed. New York: McGraw-Hill.

Levin, R. F. (1982). Choice of injection site, locus of control, and the perception of momentary pain. *Image, 14,* 26–32.

Oskins, S. (1979). Identification of situational stressor and coping methods by intensive care nurses. *Heart and Lung, 8,* 953–960.

Polit, D. F., & Hungler, B. P. (1987). *Nursing research: Principles and methods,* 3rd ed. Philadelphia: J. B. Lippincott.

Seaman, C. H. C. (1987). *Research methods: Principles, practice and theory for nursing,* 3rd. ed. Norwalk, Conn.: Appleton and Lange.

Shelley, S. I. (1984). *Research methods in nursing and health.* Boston: Little, Brown.

3

Using Nursing Research in Clinical Practice

INTRODUCTION

This chapter focuses on the process of using nursing research findings in nursing practice. It will introduce some guidelines that you can draw upon in evaluating research for both its scientific value and its clinical application.

The chapter includes a discussion of the critical factors involved in integrating research and practice, as well as a review of several approaches for research utilization. This chapter also provides a model for research consumers—nurses who may want to apply research to their practice.

OUTLINE

Research-Based Practice: Three
  Complementary Efforts
Factors in the Use of Research
  in Practice

Strategies for Research-Based
  Practice
Research Consumers in Action

OBJECTIVES

After reading this chapter, you will be able to

1. Appreciate factors that aid or inhibit the use of research findings in practice.
2. Consider the applicability of nursing research studies to clinical situations.
3. Identify strategies to aid you in incorporating research findings into your practice.

NEW TERMS

Report selection
Validation
Comparative evaluation
Decision making

Outcome evaluation
Direct application
Cognitive application

_____ RESEARCH-BASED PRACTICE: THREE _____ COMPLEMENTARY EFFORTS

Research utilization, using the methods and products of research, involves two activities (Horsley, 1985). The first is the use of nursing research findings to test or generate theory in the design of new research studies. This is a central goal of the nurse theorist and researcher. The second set of activities involves using research findings to "verify" or "change" nursing practice, which is the principal concern of the professional practitioner. We would add a third set of activities— administrative support—for without a supportive research environment nurses may lack motivation to create research-based practice.

Chapter 1 emphasized the necessity for all professional nurses to engage in some aspect of nursing research if research-based practice is to be realized. The American Nurses' Association issues a clear expectation that nurses of all levels of preparation will participate in nursing research. Table 3.1 presents activities in which nurses can participate. These activities are outlined in detail in _Guidelines for the Investigative Function of Nurses_ (ANA, 1981). Although the roles of the nurse researcher and research consumer differ in emphasis and immediate purpose, the overall goal of building a sound scientific knowledge base for practice requires a complementary effort.

_____ FACTORS IN THE USE OF RESEARCH _____ IN PRACTICE

The question of factors that promote or inhibit the use of research has been the focus of considerable discussion in recent research literature because the process of integrating nursing research findings into practice has been a slow one, and nursing is still a considerable distance from fully realizing this goal. Numerous writers have addressed and investigated the factors that may serve as barriers to the use of research findings by practitioners (Horsley, Crane, Bingle, 1978; Horsley, Crane, Crabtree, Wood, 1983; Horsley, 1985; Fawcett, 1984; Stetler, Marram, 1976; Stetler, 1984, to name a few). Those factors include the need for

—More institutional support for the conduct and use of research
—Better understanding of the language of research and research methods
—Ways to facilitate access to research findings and application of findings to practice

Supportive Research Environments

If service organizations do not value research and do not reward nurses for the conduct and use of research in the clinical area, motivation of nurses toward creating research-based practice is diminished. Nurses require administrative support to identify nursing research that is relevant to clinical practice, to evaluate nursing research for scientific merit, and to develop and implement strategies to apply findings into practice.

Hefferin, Horsley, and Ventura (1982) conducted a random survey of 56 of the largest hospitals in the United States (V.A. and non-V.A.) to determine the present state of research utilization by nurses in these organizations. The data were collected from nurse researchers and administrators. Nursing administrators were viewed as most important in promoting the use of new practices, while head nurses were key persons in implementing practice changes. The findings indicated that administrators valued and accepted research participation by practicing nurses. However, factors such as heavy workloads, lack of material rewards for research involvement, and nurses' inability to understand research findings and therefore apply those findings into practice were perceived to be the barriers most detrimental to nurses involved in research-related activities.

Administrative support is needed to remove such barriers, heighten the value of research-based practice, and motivate change. This requires practical strategies to create a positive research environment and overcome deterrents. Planned programs for the dissemination of research findings and encouragement to establish research interest groups and journal clubs to evaluate relevant research reports are just two of the approaches that may assist the practicing nurse to develop an interest in understanding and using research.

Understanding Research Language
and Research Methods

Prior to the 1970s, little instruction in research methods was conducted in the basic educational preparation of nurses. In fact, it has become prevalent in baccalaureate programs only over the past ten years. The vast majority of practicing nurses are still diploma prepared; they have not benefited from an undergraduate course in research methodology and have not had the opportunity to appreciate the significance of using research in practice. Thus, it is not surprising that many practicing nurses show little interest in research and are not

Table 3.1

NURSES' CONTRIBUTIONS TO RESEARCH-BASED PRACTICE

Associate Degree in Nursing*	Baccalaureate in Nursing*	Master's Degree in Nursing	Doctoral Degree in Nursing or a Related Discipline
1. Demonstrates awareness of the value or relevance of research in nursing. 2. Assists in identifying problem areas in nursing practice. 3. Assists in collection of data within an established structured format.	1. Reads, interprets, and evaluates research for applicability to nursing practice. 2. Identifies nursing problems that need to be investigated and participates in the implementation of scientific studies. 3. Uses nursing practice as a means of gathering data for refining and extending practice. 4. Applies established findings of nursing and other health-related research to nursing practice. 5. Shares research findings with colleagues.	1. Analyzes and reformulates nursing practice problems so that scientific knowledge and scientific methods can be used to find solutions. 2. Enhances the quality and clinical relevance of nursing research by providing expertise in clinical problems and by providing knowledge about the way in which these clinical services are delivered. 3. Facilitates investigations of problems in clinical settings through such activities as contributing to a climate supportive of investigative activities, collaborating with others in investigations and enhancing nursing's access to clients and data.	A. Graduate of a practice-oriented doctoral program 1. Provides leadership for the integration of scientific knowledge with other sources of knowledge for the advancement of practice. 2. Conducts investigations to evaluate the contribution of nursing activities to the well-being of clients. 3. Develops methods to monitor the quality of the practice of nursing in a clinical setting and to evaluate contributions of nursing activities to the well-being of clients.

4. Conducts investigations for the purpose of monitoring the quality of the practice of nursing in a clinical setting.	B. Graduate of a research-oriented doctoral program
	1. Develops theoretical explanations of phenomena relevant to nursing by empirical research and analytical processes.
5. Assists others to apply scientific knowledge in nursing practice.	2. Uses analytical and empirical methods to discover ways to modify or extend existing scientific knowledge so that it is relevant to nursing.
	3. Develops methods for scientific inquiry of phenomena relevant to nursing.

* This language was developed as part of the work of the ANA Commission on Nursing Education and was included in the report of that commission to the 1980 ANA House of Delegates.

Source: Reprinted with permission from Guidelines for the Investigative Function of Nurses, published in 1981 by the American Nurses' Association, 2420 Pershing Road, Kansas City, Missouri 64018.

motivated to use nursing research findings in practice. The task of reading an article filled with research language and statistical jargon can be ominous.

Dealing with this problem is not an easy one and requires considerable effort on the part of individual nurses as well as service organizations. Workshops to develop skilled nurse research consumers are a start; other strategies include ongoing in-service education programs that provide nurses with the opportunity to practice the skills of identifying actual nursing problems in day-to-day practice, finding and reading relevant research literature associated with the problems identified, and evaluating the applicability of research to the problem situations.

Another step in making research more meaningful to the practicing nurse is actual exposure to the conduct of nursing research. Most practicing nurses view the nurse researcher as far removed from practice and the research process as highly objective in contrast with the individualized nursing process. Nurses who are provided the opportunity to work on a research project can gain practical first-hand knowledge of the research process and a better understanding of the complementary roles of consumer and researcher.

Many service institutions now employ professional nurse researchers to conduct clinical research and stimulate involvement of practicing nurses in research activity. The recent Nursing Studies Program developed at Massachusetts General Hospital for the integration of nursing research into day-to-day practice is an excellent example of a concerted attempt to involve all levels of nurses into utilization of and participation in nursing research (Stetler, 1984).

Clinical Access and Application of Findings

Many practicing nurses complain that they have little access to published nursing research findings. In reality, most practicing nurses subscribe to practice-oriented journals rather than the theoretical, scholarly publications where nursing research reports most frequently appear. If nursing research has not been integrated as part of the basic educational preparation, many graduates may not be aware of the existence of specialized research journals. Although more practice-oriented journals are publishing reports of clinical nursing research, the majority of reports remain in scholarly journals that are not frequently read by practicing nurses.

The problem of access is combined with the lack of skills to evaluate findings for clinical application. In addition to helping nurses understand the scientific and clinical value of nursing research, better methods of communicating available findings are necessary in the clinical setting. In the survey conducted by Hefferin et al. (1982) several methods were ranked high by administrators and researchers as being effective measures for disseminating research findings in the practice situation. These include

—Research conferences on clinical topics

—Research newsletters

—Use of research indexes on clinical nursing research

—Journal clubs

—Integration of research findings into inservice education sessions

—Referring specific research articles to nurses in the clinical setting

The last strategy was reported to be the most effective method used in the organizations surveyed.

If research findings can be effectively communicated and understood, there is the further problem of evaluating the applicability of findings to a particular clinical problem. For example, as pointed out in Chapter 1, many nursing research studies are singular attempts to answer problems rather than cumulative efforts to build a well-tested base of knowledge for clinical application. Therefore, it would be risky and irresponsible to change practice based on the results of one study conducted in one setting. In terms of the basic/applied continuum (see Figure 3.1), clinical research problems require rigorous clinical testing before the final step, dissemination of findings for application into practice (Downs, 1979). The applied end of the continuum involves retesting the interventions examined in previous research in the context of actual and representative client-care situations in order to establish practice significance. Practicing nurses need to be able to identify where a nursing research study falls on the basic/applied continuum. Only then can they begin to make an informed decision as to its suitability for adoption into practice. If it can be shown that the findings of a research study are based upon a sound theoretical background and have been adequately tested in real client situations with positive outcomes, then strategies for action are needed if this knowledge is to become a part of practice.

_____ Figure 3.1 _____

ZONES OF CLINICAL APPLICABILITY: THE INTERFACE BETWEEN THE
BASIC/APPLIED CONTINUUM AND THE RELEVANCE OF THE STUDY TO A
PARTICULAR TYPE OF NURSING PRACTICE

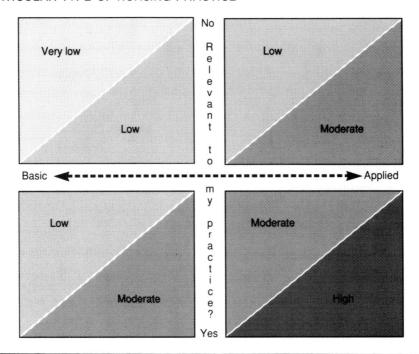

_____ STRATEGIES FOR RESEARCH-BASED _____
PRACTICE

The problem of integrating nursing research and practice is not an easy one. The factors described in the preceding section indicate that much work needs to be done by administrators, educators, researchers, and clinicians in the practice setting before the goal of research-based practice is reached. Several approaches to research utilization, which are aimed primarily at organizations rather than individual nurses, have been reported in the literature, and have met with some success in several areas of the United States. One example involves Conduct and Utilization of Research in Nursing (CURN), the famous project sponsored by the Michigan Nurses Association (Horsley, Crane, Crabtree, & Wood, 1983). The CURN Project is an example of or-

_____ *Figure 3.2* _____

CURN PROTOCOLS

1. Structured Preoperative Teaching
2. Reducing Diarrhea in Tube-Fed Patients
3. Preoperative Sensory Preparation to Promote Recovery
4. Preventing Decubitus Ulcers
5. Intravenous Cannula Change
6. Closed Urinary Drainage Systems
7. Distress Reduction through Sensory Preparation
8. Mutual Goal Setting in Patient Care
9. Clean Intermittent Catheterization
10. Pain: Deliberative Nursing Interventions

_____

Source: Horsley, J. A., Crane, J., Crabtree, M. K., & Wood, D. J. (1983). *Using research to improve nursing practice: A guide* (CURN Project). New York: Grune & Stratton. Used with permission.

ganizational efforts toward utilization that recognizes the need for organizational change, staff development, and additional resources, that are often beyond the direct control of individual nurses. It is recognized, however, that individual nurses are most important to the success of such programs.

The five-year CURN Project involved thirty-two nursing departments in the identification of client care problems and the use of research literature to develop clinical research-based solutions or protocols to deal with identified problems. The protocols were then tested clinically, using the research process. These protocols or solutions are an excellent reference for research-based practice that can be tested in other settings. The investigators (Horsley, et al.) have published a volume on the development of each of the protocols in addition to one volume describing the entire project, which we describe here briefly and you may wish to consult in more detail. The ten protocols developed through the CURN project are listed in Figure 3.2.

Although in this text we recognize the key role of organizational support in using nursing research, our emphasis is on assisting the individual to develop skills in evaluating the applicability of findings to the practice setting. Therefore, the balance of this chapter will focus in more detail on strategies that can be initiated more easily by the individual nurse. The application model proposed by Stetler and Marram (1976) and by Stetler (1983) will serve as a framework for the following discussion.

_____ RESEARCH CONSUMERS IN ACTION _____

The model developed by Stetler and Marram (1976) has three phases: validation, comparative evaluation, and decision making (see Figure 3.3). We extended their model by adding a preliminary and a final step: report selection and outcome evaluation. (Roberts, C., & Burke, S. O. (1986). These five steps are

STEP 1 **Report selection,** which requires reviewing the research literature for reports that are appropriate to clinical application

STEP 2 **Validation,** which requires a piece of nursing research be subjected to a rigorous critique of its scientific merit

STEP 3 **Comparative evaluation,** which includes evaluating the study in light of similar published research, evaluating the similarity of the research setting to the clinical setting where the study may be implemented, and evaluating the feasibility of making the clinical change

STEP 4 **Decision making,** which centers on deciding whether or not to adopt the change into practice

STEP 5 **Outcome evaluation,** which centers on evaluating the results of a change in clinical practice

These steps represent a problem solving process and as such parallel the nursing process and the research process as seen in Table 2.1.

Report Selection

Several factors will likely influence your selection of a research report for potential application into practice. For example, in the course of doing update reading in a professional journal you might run across a nursing study that appears to have findings that seem relevant to your clinical practice; or, in response to a particular clinical problem you might actively look for research that may provide some possible clues. Whatever the starting point, you will need to be able to locate easily nursing research studies. This involves knowing how to use library sources to find research literature pertaining to your topic of interest. Chapter 5 shows you how to use library indexes and computer searches, two valuable resources that will assist you in finding nursing research reports.

Once you have a study in hand, you will need to decide where it falls within the zones of clinical applicability according to the basic/applied continuum (see Figure 3.1). Studies that test an interven-

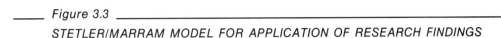

_____ *Figure 3.3* _____

STETLER/MARRAM MODEL FOR APPLICATION OF RESEARCH FINDINGS

PHASE I VALIDATION   PHASE II COMPARATIVE EVALUATION   PHASE III DECISION MAKING

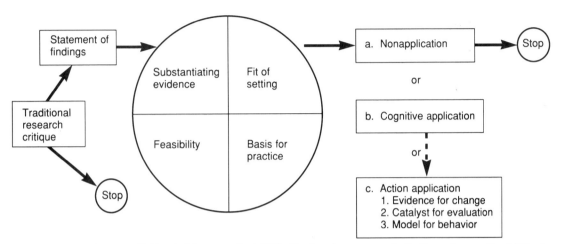

Source: Stetler, C. B., & Marram, G. (1976). Evaluating research findings for applicability in practice. *Nursing Outlook, 24*(9), 560. Copyright 1976 American Journal of Nursing Company. Used with permission. All rights reserved.

tion with real clients in clinical situations in light of a well-developed knowledge base fall higher toward the applied end of the continuum and have more direct applicability to practice. Basic research conducted in clinical settings may have implications for practice in that it contributes knowledge to help you examine existing practice, but it requires more applied testing before it can become a basis for change in practice. In selecting a study with some potential for clinical applicability, your efforts should focus on studies that fall within moderate or high zones on the continuum.

Scientific Validation

Before any piece of research can be used to change or modify existing practice, the research consumer must be convinced that the study

—Has been conducted in a scientific manner

—Is significant to nursing practice

—Has findings that can be applied to settings and groups beyond the research situation

This validation involves reading the study carefully and conducting a critique of how well the researcher has carried out each step of the research process (see Figure 2.1). Most research reports are divided into sections that roughly correspond to the steps taken by the researcher, and you will need a set of criteria for critiquing each of these sections. The remainder of this text discusses each step of the research process as it is used by the researcher and evaluated by the consumer. A set of criteria for the critique of each step of the research process follows the discussion in each chapter. The Appendix to this chapter presents an overview of the entire set of critique criteria, the implications for clinical application, the critical concepts underlying the criteria, and the chapters where they are discussed in the text. You can use this table now as you read research reports. After you understand the concepts explained in later chapters, these criteria and principles will be even more useful because you will be able to use them more skillfully. When you wish to critique portions of a research report in more depth, the elaborated tables for each portion of the research process in the following chapters will provide more detailed direction.

Making the final decision about the scientific validity of nursing research findings is not an easy one. The bulk of this text focuses on this one step. Most research studies have some limitations, especially since applied nursing research requires the study of clients in real-life situations where conditions may be beyond the total influence of the researcher. As a potential user of the findings, you must carefully weigh the strengths and weaknesses of the study to determine if limitations are serious enough to invalidate the use of findings in your clinical situation. If you decide that a study has sufficient scientific strength to warrant its use in practice, then you can proceed to the next phase—comparative evaluation.

Comparative Evaluation

This step involves evaluating the clinical relevance of the study and the feasibility of implementing findings into the clinical setting. This is a refinement of your preliminary judgment made in Step 1. Stetler and Marram (1976) divide this phase into four areas for evaluation:

—Substantiating evidence to support the findings of the critiqued study
—Evaluation of the study setting, subjects, and variables

compared to those involved in the prospective clinical
application area

— Consideration of factors affecting feasibility of application
in the proposed setting

— Examination of one's own practice in light of its knowledge
base and that of the critiqued study

Earlier in this chapter we suggested the possible risk surrounding
the use of findings of only one research study to change practice.
Similarly, the lack of replicated studies was seen as a factor in the slow
growth of a sound knowledge base for practice. Before deciding to
simply adopt findings of one study into your practice, it is crucial to do
a thorough search of the research literature to uncover similar or
replicated studies dealing with the problem. Findings may be conflicting,
or they may provide further support for the findings of your study at
hand.

The search for further studies can begin by noting studies quoted
in the literature review of the critiqued study. You will also need to
search library indexes for studies that may have been missed by the
researcher or published after the study was completed. This group of
studies should also be critiqued for scientific validity and findings
compared with those of the original study. You may find it helpful to
tabulate or summarize on paper the strengths and weaknesses as well
as the similarities and differences of all the studies reviewed. If
little evidence exists in the literature to support the findings of the
study selected, further testing is necessary before clinically implementing the findings. At this point you might consider plans to replicate the study in your own setting with the help of an experienced
nurse researcher.

A very important aspect to consider in making your decision to
proceed is the potential risk to clients and the legal implications for
your practice. This is a priority consideration in both conducting and
applying research findings. Chapter 7 provides a broad discussion on the
protection of human rights and ethics in nursing research. A proposed
new intervention must be rigorously screened for any possible physical,
social, or emotional risk or discomfort that might logically result to
clients. If the intervention has potential risk and has not been adequately tested through research, it should not be applied in practice
without further investigation under controlled research conditions.
A frequently cited example of the inappropriate adoption of nursing

research findings into practice, which exposed clients to real risk, is a study involving the use of topical insulin in the treatment of pressure sores (Van Ort & Gerber, 1976; Gerber & Van Ort, 1981). In spite of questionable findings, this intervention was integrated into nursing literature and practice and resulted in client complications such as hypoglycemia and coma (Kirchhoff, 1983).

If you are satisfied that the available evidence secured from the literature review indicates you are dealing with reasonably valid findings that can be safely adopted into practice, you will then need to compare and evaluate aspects of the study with your own clinical situation. Stetler and Marram (1976) and Stetler (1983) suggest a careful examination of similarities between the research setting, subjects, and variables and those in the clinical setting. For example, a study that involves testing an intervention with clients in an outpatient clinic may not be appropriate for adoption into an acute care hospital setting without additional research in the new setting.

A further step in the comparative evaluation phase of the Stetler and Marram model (1976) directs the nurse to examine his or her own practice in light of its theoretical foundation and that of the new research. Chapter 2 presented a variety of reasons why nurses adopt interventions, ranging from tradition to research-generated knowledge. Before adopting a new intervention, you should explore the origins of your current intervention and evaluate its effectiveness in meeting outcomes for practice. New interventions are not necessarily better. If you can show that what you are already doing has a sound theory base that has been tested through research with positive findings, a change may not be necessary at present. On the other hand, if you find that your intervention is not firmly secure in its theory base, a change or enrichment of your intervention through use of a research-tested intervention may enhance practice. The evaluation of theory underlying an intervention is a complex task. Chapters 4 and 5 discuss the processes wherein researchers review the literature and formulate research problems in the context of theory. These chapters should assist you in developing an ability to identify and evaluate your basis for practice.

A final practical consideration that affects the feasibility of implementing findings in the clinical setting includes the availability of resources. A new intervention that involves the purchase of expensive equipment, or a change in staffing arrangements, has budget implications for the organization. You will need to be convinced that your setting has the available resources to support the new intervention before the decision to implement it is made. This usually means gaining the cooperation of administrators directly involved with policy making and budget control.

Decision Making and Outcome Evaluation

The decision-making phase of the Stetler/Marram model (1976) is the final one in determining whether or not to apply findings into the clinical situation. If the evidence suggests that the study is valid and feasible for your practice setting, you may decide to apply the findings directly (direct application) or use them indirectly (cognitive application) as a base for current problem solving or as a step toward promoting future change.

Direct application often requires cooperation and support from peers and administration since new interventions must be tested and evaluated in one's own setting (Stetler and Marram, 1976; Stetler, 1983). There is no absolute certainty that the research findings of any one study are directly applicable to all settings. Many large service institutions have nursing practice committees as well as access to experienced nurse researchers who may assist in setting up a small project to replicate the study on your unit. This approach is particularly important if the proposed change in practice is complex, differs considerably from present interventions, and poses any question of risk to client outcomes.

If the change is a relatively simple one that can be easily incorporated into daily practice, you may decide to try it out on your own with the support of your unit. Evaluation of the outcome is similarly an integral activity in this type of application, and data concerning client responses must be systematically collected and recorded.

Both of these approaches will supply data about the applicability of the research findings in your setting. Coupled with your evidence derived from the literature review, you may have a sound rationale to motivate change in your practice behaviors as well as in others. Through having the data on hand, understanding their significance, and communicating them effectively to administrators and peers, you will be serving as a role model. These are important steps for individual practicing nurses to take in promoting the use of research-based interventions.

Unfortunately, you may often decide that the evidence derived from the comparative evaluation is not strong enough to use findings directly in practice. Perhaps more research is indicated or the proposed new intervention is not feasible within your setting without further resources, modification, or testing. Stetler and Marram (1976) discuss the importance of using **cognitive application** of findings as an alternative to direct applications. This approach involves using the findings conceptually to assist the practicing nurse in day-to-day problem solving.

For example, this step can have important implications for changing how you think about the care you and others provide clients. Many nursing studies that require more investigation at the applied end of the basic/applied continuum do contain some theoretical background that is excellent in approaching clinical problems. This background knowledge can be invaluable in broadening your scope in performing each phase of the nursing process, assisting you to rethink the rationale for current interventions, and serving as a starting point in generating clinical research questions from your practice.

SUMMARY

This chapter introduces some strategies for applying research findings to the practice setting as a central part of research-based practice. Emphasis is placed on the need for a collaborative effort between nurse researchers, administrators, educators, and practicing nurses in accomplishing this task. Although the role of administration is recognized as crucial in providing support, guidance, and organization in bringing about widespread change, the chapter focuses on ways individual nurses can contribute to the process. The CURN Project (Horsley et al, 1983) is discussed briefly in presenting an organizational approach, and the Stetler/Marram model (1976) serves as a framework for discussing how the research consumer may apply research findings to practice. Reading nursing research reports and understanding the scientific and clinical significance of findings are seen as the first steps toward responsible utilization. Guidelines are presented for use in conducting a research critique. These guidelines, elaborated on in the following chapters, help the consumer evaluate each phase of the research process and its relative contribution to the scientific and clinical significance of the overall findings of a report.

APPENDIX: GUIDELINES FOR EVALUATING SCIENTIFIC ADEQUACY AND CLINICAL APPLICABILITY OF NURSING RESEARCH REPORTS

Elements of Research	Scientific Adequacy		Implications for Clinical Applicability	Concepts for Review
	Quantitative Research Criteria	Qualitative Research Criteria		
Problem area or phenomenon (circumstances to be investigated)	1. Begins with a discussion of the general problem area or phenomenon 2. Presents sufficient background information 3. Discusses problem or phenomenon in relation to nursing	Criteria 1–3, with more emphasis on a phenomenon	Is enough information given to convince reader of clinical significance of the problem or phenomenon and the feasibility of researching the problem in a clinical setting?	Feasibility of research problems Researchability of research problems (Chapter 4)
Specific problem or research question	1. Identifies specific problem(s) by end of introduction	Criteria 1–4 usually not applicable at onset of study	Does the specific problem statement help reader begin to	Data Variables (a) independent

(continues)

Elements of Research	Scientific Adequacy		Implications for Clinical Applicability	Concepts for Review
	Quantitative Research Criteria	Qualitative Research Criteria		
Specific problem or research question (continued)	2. Relates problem statement or question directly to general problem area 3. Identifies independent (causal) and dependent (outcome) variables 4. Shows clear relationships or differences between variables 5. Describes population and setting used		identify the basic/applied nature of research? Do problems that are tested in laboratory settings using populations very different from your setting need more testing before application? Are the variables in the study similar to those operating in clinical setting?	(b) dependent (c) extraneous (Chapters 2 & 3) Basic/applied continuum (Chapters 1 & 4) Levels of Inquiry for research questions (Chapter 6) Specific problem statement (Chapter 4) Population and setting (Chapter 8)
		5. Criterion presented in detail		
Hypothesis or question	1. Has appropriate hypotheses or questions for study design 2. Has a specific prediction as to relationship between independent and dependent variable(s), or states the expected end result of study	1. Uses a question; never a hypothesis Criteria 2 & 3 not applicable	Will an answer to the research problem provide a possible answer to a clinical one? If predictions are made, are they logical from a clinical viewpoint? Has the researcher based prediction on theory or concepts relevant to nursing? Will further understanding	Hypotheses; research question Conceptual and theoretical frameworks and rationale (Chapter 4) Qualitative approaches to research

Component	Criteria		Questions	Where Discussed
	3. Answers research question with prediction	4. Has explicit philosophic perspective and related design methods	of the phenomena be helpful in practice?	Purpose of research (Chapter 4)
Purpose	1. States specifically why the researcher is carrying out the research study	Criterion 1, same	Does the purpose of the research provide further insight into the basic/applied nature of the research? Problems that primarily aim to build knowledge have possible cognitive applications; studies that clinically test knowledge in relation to interventions have possible direct applications to practice.	Clinical applicability, direct and cognitive applicaton—Stetler/Marram (1976) Model (Chapter 3) Basic/applied continuum (Chapters 1 & 3) Levels of inquiry for research question (Chapter 6)
Definition of key concepts	1. Defines all important concepts associated with the research problem operationally as variables	1. May be a finding and appear at the end of the study	Are clinically usable concepts defined to permit clinical measurement or observation of variables in the study? This is	Operational definitions Theoretical definitions (Chapter 4)

(continues)

Elements of Research	Scientific Adequacy		Implications for Clinical Applicability	Concepts for Review
	Quantitative Research Criteria	Qualitative Research Criteria		
Definition of key concepts (continued)	2. Establishes how the researcher is measuring and using the variables in the study	2. Detailed in the analysis section	vital as studies are tested or replicated in your setting.	
Philosophical, theoretical, or conceptual rationale and framework	1. Presents a well developed explanation of how the key variables in the research problem are connected or related 2. Explains the stated hypothesis(es) or question 3. Presents evidence that the conceptual or theoretical framework is applied to all aspects of the study	Criteria 1–3 may be the findings of the study and appear at the end	Does researcher show the relevance of the theory to nursing practice as well as to the problem if the theory used is not a nursing one? Quantitative studies that are based upon well-tested theory, when applied to clinical problems, are more likely to be directly applicable to practice.	Theoretical framework Conceptual framework Assumption Rationale Concept Theory (Chapter 4)

Literature review			
4. States the researcher's underlying assumptions and reasonableness	Criterion 4, same	Quantitative studies initiated with loose conceptual frameworks, or that primarily aim to develop theory, provide cognitive insights, but usually require more research before direct application is indicated.	Literature review (Chapter 4)
	5. Clearly states philosophical perspective		Comparative evaluation for applying findings to practice (Chapter 3)
1. Presents evidence of a clear, comprehensive, critical, and relevant literature review	Criterion 1 same, except it might appear at the end of the report to put findings into context; literature used as data; or no use of the literature if no relevant work exists or if the researcher decides it would bias and cloud the research process	Is the review of related literature a useful source of similar or replicated studies in making a comparative evaluation of the study's findings to other research?	
2. Presents sufficient information to show the relationship between the stated research problem and prior research and theoretical work			
3. Includes important recent studies and theoretical work			
4. Documents sources of reviewed studies to permit further review by reader			

(continues)

Elements of Research	Scientific Adequacy		Implications for Clinical Applicability	Concepts for Review
	Quantitative Research Criteria	Qualitative Research Criteria		
Literature review (continued)	5. Cites studies and theory which both support and conflict with researchers' predictions 6. Relates the review to this study			
Protection of human rights	1. Has scientifically significant research design, from problem or phenomenon to analysis methods 2. Has designed research to minimize risk and maximize benefit to human subjects 3. Has ethically appropriate selection of subjects to study the problem or phenomenon	Criteria 1–3, same	Will an answer to the problem or an explanation of the phenomena benefit clients or contribute to nursing knowledge? Are findings appropriate for clinical application? Are the research subjects subjected to undue risk, and is benefit to subjects and knowledge generated low? (Risk to clients is a primary considera-	Responsibility of research problems (Chapter 4) Ethical guidelines for nursing research (Chapter 7) Research design (Chapter 6) Clinical application, comparative evaluation (Chapter 3) Informed consent Human rights guidelines (Chapter 7)

(continues)

4. Indicates that subjects gave voluntary, informed consent	4. Allows informal informed consent which may be reiterated over the course of the study Criterion 5, same	tion before deciding to adopt findings into practice.) Failure to follow ethical guidelines for subject selection would prohibit application of findings to practice. Failure to obtain voluntary informed consent from subjects or appropriate representatives violates human rights; findings cannot be applied ethically to practice. Lack of promised protection of anonymity and confidentiality violates human rights; findings should not be applied to practice. (This may not always be mentioned in published nursing research reports. Research appearing in refereed journals and funded
5. Did not invite consent under highly stressful circumstances without reiteration later		
6. Does not identify individual subjects in the report	6. Makes ramifications clear if anonymity not desirable or feasible	
7. Shows evidence of ethics review by an institutional review board or committee	7. Requires informal approval by the group under study	

Elements of Research	Scientific Adequacy		Implications for Clinical Applicability	Concepts for Review
	Quantitative Research Criteria	Qualitative Research Criteria		
Protection of human rights (continued)			research is usually required to be subjected to independent ethics review. If no evidence is given and you are concerned about this before using findings in practice, a request for evidence of ethics review can be directed to the journal or author.)	
Sampling and setting population	1. Describes carefully the target population to which the study applies 2. Describes research setting carefully	1. Has subjects who are members of the population that exhibits the phenomena of interest 2. Describes in detail relation to the phenomena under study	The degree of similarity of study's population sample and setting to client populations in the clinical setting is an important consideration in doing a comparative evaluation. Certain biases	Population Sample (Chapter 8) Clinical application (Chapter 3) Extraneous variables operating in setting and population (Chapter 8)

3. Discusses bias in selecting and assessing population and setting	3. Expects bias within subjects for effect on meanings	operating in the selection and assessment of population and setting may limit applicability to your practice. The sample should yield knowledge about clinically significant variables for direct application of findings to practice. Generally a larger random sample yields more generalizable findings. If the sample size is small and chosen nonrandomly, the findings may not be scientifically valid for immediate application. (In making the decision about the appropriateness of sample size, you will need to consider this in relation to your experience with clients and problems similar to those under study.) Sampling bias	Fit of sampling strategy to research question and design (Chapter 8)
4. Uses appropriate method of sampling to fit research design and level of inquiry of study	Criteria 4 & 5, same		Sampling methods Random Nonrandom
5. Uses a sampling strategy with the potential to enhance knowledge and/or meaning			Sample size (Chapter 8)
6. Describes the method for determining sample size	6. Eventual size determined during the data collection/analysis phase		Sampling bias (Chapter 8)
7. Has adequate sample size given study question, design, variables, and phenomena under study	Criterion 7, same		Sampling error (Chapter 8)
8. Discusses known and probable sources of bias in sampling	Criteria 8 & 9 Describes rationale and approach used for selection of representative key informants		Threats to external validity (Chapters 6 & 12)

(continues)

Elements of Research	Scientific Adequacy		Implications for Clinical Applicability	Concepts for Review
	Quantitative Research Criteria	Qualitative Research Criteria		
Sampling and setting population (continued)	9. Controls or minimizes sources of sampling error		should be evaluated in terms of how critical this is to application in your clinical situation. Also you may identify other sources of bias which may be operating in the study based upon your clinical experience. If the sample does not adequately represent the clinical group the study purports to examine, the findings cannot be generalized beyond the sample.	
Design of the study	1. Has appropriate research design for the level of inquiry of research question and purpose of research 2. Shows that research design could yield meaningful results	Criteria 1 & 2, same	If the methods used by the researcher do not fit the research question, then the findings are not valid for applications. If application is to be feasible, a design must yield results that are shown to	Research design (Chapter 6) Levels of inquiry of research questions and research design (Chapter 6) Causality and research designs (Chapter 6)

3. Indicates consideration of potential effect of unwanted variables and use of the best possible measures to control for effect of extraneous variables on results	3. Control not used	be meaningful to your practice situation. Uncontrolled extraneous variables can seriously affect the validity of study results. Clinical experience and knowledge should assist you to identify some of the extraneous variables that may be operating in a study. The type of design used will also affect the way in which you can apply findings. Experimental designs that allow testing interventions in clinical situations have more potential for direct application to practice than designs that aim to examine phenomena and relationships. The latter may have some potential for cognitive application. In most cases research studies require formal or informal testing in your	Risks to internal and external validity (Chapter 6) Application of research findings to practice (Chapters 1 & 3)
4. Discusses limitations of design used to investigate research question	Criterion 4, same		
5. Has enough information about methods used to permit replication	5. Replication not usually possible, for meanings are expected to change		

(continues)

Elements of Research	Scientific Adequacy		Implications for Clinical Applicability	Concepts for Review
	Quantitative Research Criteria	Qualitative Research Criteria		
Design of the study (continued)			own clinical setting before direct application of findings. The researcher must provide enough detail about the methods used to allow replication if needed.	Methods of data collection Reliability Validity (Chapter 9)
Instruments or methods for data collection	1. Describes instruments for data collection 2. Gives rationale for development or selection of instruments 3. Fits instruments to research question 4. Has clear and convincing procedures for testing reliability and validity of instruments	Criteria 1–3 Focus on researcher's method for data collection; instruments seldom used 4. Rarely discusses reliability and validity of concepts; takes precautions to ensure representative data collection are described and strategies employed to enhance reliability and validity of data for analysis	In order to apply findings into practice, you must be convinced that the researcher has actually measured or observed the variables intended to be studied, and that these methods are reliable and valid for use with the study sample. Usually entire questionnaires or other self-report measures are not presented in detail in the report. However, these measures should be described well enough to allow you to decide on the potential for using them to replicate data	

	5. Has instruments that appear suitable for use with study sample	5. Has method suitable for the subjects	collection in your setting. If you decide to test or replicate the data collection procedure in your setting, information should be provided in the report on where the complete instruments can be located. In some cases, the findings of a study may not be directly applicable to practice, but reliable and valid instruments used in the study may have more direct implications for your assessment of clients in performing nursing process.	

Data analysis	1. Presents data analysis summary in a clear, well organized manner
	2. Labels and describes descriptive tables and graphs clearly and carefully
	3. Selects and uses statistical tests appropriately
		Criterion 1, same
		
		Criteria 2 & 3
		Seldom used
			Many factors determine the selection of statistical procedures to examine and summarize the data in light of the researcher's stated predictions. You will need to understand these factors if replication of the study is to be carried out in	Data analysis
				Levels of measurement
				Descriptive statistics
				Inferential statistics
				  (Chapter 10)
				Analysis of qualitative
				  data
				  (Chapter 10)
				Reliability and validity
				  of qualitative data
				  (Chapter 9)

(continues)

Elements of Research	Scientific Adequacy		Implications for Clinical Applicability	Concepts for Review
	Quantitative Research Criteria	Qualitative Research Criteria		
Data analysis (continued)	4. Has clear steps in analysis so that procedures could be replicated 5. Fits analysis to question and design	4. Describes qualitative methods for analysis in detail, describes steps taken (e.g., triangulation) to enhance validity of analysis procedures Criterion 5, same	your setting. Inappropriate data analysis will invalidate the findings of the study for application.	External and internal validity (Chapter 6) Findings (Chapter 12)
Conclusions and recommendations	1. Explains results of data analysis in specific reference to study questions, hypothesis(es), conceptual framework, and/or phenomena. 2. Bases conclusions upon data analysis 3. Has appropriate generalization of significant findings beyond the research study to the study population 4. Makes recommendations for nursing practice and/or further research relevant to the findings	Criteria 1 & 2, same 3. Provides sufficient evidence to support researcher's interpretation	Overgeneralization of results by the researcher can present a serious problem when incorporating the findings into practice. The reader must critique the scientific merit of the study to determine if generalization is warranted. A study which is seriously lacking in conceptualization will require further research before application of findings into practice.	

EXERCISES ▬▬▬▬▬▬▬▬▬▬▬▬▬▬▬▬▬▬▬▬▬▬

From the following brief descriptions of three research studies, decide which ones, if any, you would select to evaluate in entirety for *direct application* or *cognitive application* to clinical practice. State why.

Relationship Between Client Diagnosis and Quality of Care*

Chouinard, Galvin, and Quigley (1987) assessed the relationship between client diagnosis (acute or chronic) and the quality of care that clients perceive they are receiving. Fifty clients with medical diagnoses of acute illnesses and fifty clients with chronic medical diagnoses were administered questionnaires regarding the quality of nursing care received. The results of both client groups were statistically compared showing higher scores for quality of care perceived by acutely ill clients than for chronically ill clients.

A Qualitative Research Method to Study the Elderly in Two Residences[†]

Bailey (1985) investigated the nature of life patterns and health and well-being among two groups of elderly clients residing in one private and one government-subsidized housing facility. Through use of a diary and interviews, the researcher made observations and documented conversations and events occurring among the clients in both settings on a weekly basis over a three-year period. As a result of the study the researcher noted considerable differences between the residents in both settings. The government-subsidized residents were more involved in community activity than the private residents. The researcher inferred that activity level affects ability to be active and as such has nursing significance for care of the elderly.

Comparison of Intramuscular Injection Techniques to Reduce Site Discomfort and Lesions[††]

Keen (1986) compared the Z-track injection technique with standard intramuscular injection techniques for the amount of

---

* Adapted from a research proposal by N. Chouinard, M. Galvin, and A. Quigley (1987). Year IV students, Queen's University School of Nursing, Kingston, Ontario.

[†] Adapted from M. Bailey (1985). A qualitative research method to study elderly in two residences. In M. M. Leininger (Ed.), *Qualitative research methods in nursing.* New York: Grune & Stratton.

[††] Adapted from M. F. Keen (1986). Comparison of intramuscular injection techniques to reduce site discomfort and lesions. *Nursing Research, 35*(4), 207–210.

discomfort and lesions noted at the injection site. Fifty subjects who were receiving repeated injections of a narcotic for pain received injections using both methods. Subjects were asked to report level of discomfort from both injection techniques, and the skin surface was examined for lesions. The researcher concluded that the Z-track method can decrease the incidence of lesions and possible secondary discomfort from leakage of medication into the tissue more than can the standard technique.

REFERENCES

American Nurses' Association, Commission on Nursing Research. (1981). *Guidelines for the investigative function of nurses*. Kansas City, Mo.: American Nurses' Association.

Baily, M. (1985). A qualitative research method to study elderly in two residences. In M. M. Leininger (Ed.) *Qualitative research methods in nursing*. New York: Grune & Stratton Inc.

Chouinard, N.; Galvin, M.; & Quigley, A. (1987). *Relationships between client diagnosis and quality of care*. Unpublished research proposal. Queen's University, School of Nursing, Kingston, Ontario.

Downs, F. S. (1979). Clinical and theoretical research. In F. S. Downs & J. W. Fleming (Eds.), *Issues in nursing research* (pp. 67–87). New York: Appleton-Century-Crofts.

Fawcett, J. (1984). Another look at utilization of nursing research. *Image, 16*(2), 59–62.

Gerber, R., & Van Ort, S. (1981). Topical application of insulin to pressure sores: A questionable therapy. *American Journal of Nursing, 81*(6), 1159.

Hefferin, E. A., Horsley, J. A., & Ventura, M. R. (1982, May). Promoting research-based nursing: The administrator's role. *The Journal of Nursing Administration*, 34–41.

Horsley, J. (1985). Using research in practice: The current context. *Western Journal of Nursing Research, 7*(1), 135–139.

Horsley, J. A.; Crane, J.; & Bingle, J. D. (1978). Research utilization as an organizational process. *Journal of Nursing Administration, 8*, 4–6.

Horsley, J. A.; Crane, J.; Crabtree, M. K.; & Wood, D. J. (1983). *Using research to improve nursing practice: A guide (CURN project)*. New York: Grune & Stratton.

Keen, M. F. (1986). Comparison of intramuscular injection techniques to reduce site discomfort and lesions. *Nursing Research, 35*(4), 207–210.

Kirchhoff, K. T. (1983). Using research in practice: Should nurses be expected to use research? *Western Journal of Nursing Research, 5*, 245–247.

Roberts, C., & Burke, S. O. (1986, May). Applying nursing research: Getting started. *Canadian Nurse,* 20–22.

Stetler, C. B. (1983). Nurses and research: Responsibility and involvement. *NITA: The Official Journal of the National Intravenous Therapy Association, 6,* 207–212.

———— (1984). Nurses and research: Responsibility and involvement. In *Nursing research in a service setting,* Massachusetts General Hospital (pp. 5-18–5-23). Reston, Va.: Reston Publishing.

Stetler, C. B., & Marram, G. (1976). Evaluating research findings for applicability in practice. *Nursing Outlook, 24*(9), 559–563.

Van Ort, S. R., & Gerber, R. M. (1976). Topical application of insulin in the treatment of decubitus ulcers: A pilot study. *Nursing Research, 25,* 9–12.

4

The Research Problem: Formation and Critique

All research begins with a problem that provides direction for a research-based study. The problem may evolve from day-to-day practice. The problem is also the primary focus in reading a research report. Once the problem has been established, the best method for studying it must be determined. The feasibility of the study is also an important consideration.

In this chapter we will discuss the activities required of the researcher in selecting and defining a problem for research; we will then examine the steps taken by the consumer to evaluate this process as it is presented in a research report.

OUTLINE

Where Do Nurse Researchers Find Problems?

What Problems Are Suitable for Nursing Research?

How Do Nurse Researchers Define a Specific Problem?

What Are the Theoretical Underpinnings of the Research Problem?

Stating a Research Hypothesis

Determining the Feasibility of Research Problems

Beginning the Review of the Research Report

OBJECTIVES

After reading this chapter, you will be able to

1. Describe how nurse researchers formulate problems for study.
2. Determine what problems are researchable using the scientific method and what problems are more appropriately studied using qualitative methods.
3. Discuss the feasibility of research problems.
4. Write a research hypothesis.
5. Gain a beginning skill in performing a research critique of the problem, theoretical background, and literature review.

NEW TERMS

Theory

Variable

Operational definitions

Research question

Causal variable

Independent variable(s)

Outcome variable

Dependent variable(s)

Phenomenon

Theoretical framework

Assumptions

Conceptual framework

Research hypothesis

Scientific adequacy

Critique

WHERE DO NURSE RESEARCHERS FIND PROBLEMS?

Nursing Practice

Where do problems come from in nursing research? The richest and most basic source of clinical research problems comes directly from our day-to-day experience with clients. As nurses, we are constantly challenged to determine the best approaches to assess, plan, implement, and evaluate our care. For example, an evaluation of the client's status might require us to reassess and try another approach. As was discussed in Chapter 2, nursing approaches traditionally have been based upon experience and trial and error, rather than systematically derived from research findings.

Consider how a staff nurse's experience can generate a research problem. Suppose a staff nurse is to teach a group of newly diagnosed, adolescent diabetic clients about self-care using the hospital's teaching guidelines and audiotapes. The nurse discovers, however, that the clients are uninterested and uncooperative. In reassessing the situation, the nurse may suspect something is wrong with the teaching approach. Here is a clinical problem that can lead to more specific questions based upon the nurse's knowledge and experience. He or she may ask, Do these young clients have special learning needs that are not addressed by my approach? What are these learning needs? What is a more effective teaching approach? Questions such as these can be the beginnings of a research endeavor.

The next step should lead the nurse to the library to find out more about teaching young diabetic clients. The *Index Medicus* and the *International Nursing Index* are two good sources for identifying research studies conducted in nursing, medicine, and other health care disciplines. Alternatively, the nurse may use a computer-assisted search. (Resources and how to use them are discussed in Chapter 5.) Some research articles related to the problem will assist the nurse in focusing further on ideas and questions. In addition, many research studies actually suggest questions that may serve as greater motivaters for future investigation.

At this point, the staff nurse may wish to consult an experienced nurse researcher to discuss the possibility of investigating the problem through research. If the hospital does not employ a professional nurse researcher, a university nursing faculty is usually a good source of such help.

Nursing Literature

Often the literature itself serves as a starting point for the development of a research problem. In this case, the nurse researcher begins to question suggested approaches and findings presented in the literature about a particular topic and to consider alternate approaches and explanations. This thinking process can be generated by a variety of types of literature. As we already noted, published research reports always encourage further questioning. However, many unsubstantiated textbook approaches to client care can, and indeed should, be challenged. For example, many common clinical skills presented in basic nursing texts have recently been examined through research, and the research findings will eventually lead to changes in nursing practice. One good example of this research includes several recent studies that have tested different body positions to reduce client discomfort when giving intramuscular injections (Kruszewski, Lang, & Johnson, 1979; Rettig & Southby, 1982).

Theoretical Literature and Models

The theoretical literature of nursing and other disciplines offers another logical base for studying research problems. A **theory** provides an explanation of how certain concepts or abstract ideas are related to each other and serves as a basis for predicting future events. Over the past thirty years or so, as an outgrowth of the movement toward expanding the scientific base for professional nursing, a number of nursing theories and models have been proposed. (A model is a descriptive representation that often precedes the development of theory.) Among the major themes in nursing theory are stress, adaptation, systems, and development (Roy, 1980; Neuman, 1980; Johnson, 1980; King, 1981; Levine, 1967; Peplau, 1952). Several nurse theorists have devoted entire texts to the description of their theories; they often propose specific research questions to test a theory empirically in clinical practice situations. It would be impossible in this text to discuss in depth all of the nursing models and theories, which require further testing through clinical research. It is very important, however, that the research consumer understand the underlying concepts and predictions proposed by a nurse theorist before attempting to critique the use of a particular theory in a study. The best approach to learning about an unfamiliar theory is to read about it in the original published works of the theorist.

As an example, Table 4.1 summarizes how the nurse and client are viewed in nursing models proposed by King (1981), Roy (1980), and

_____ Table 4.1 _____

EXAMPLES OF CONCEPTS FROM THEORETICAL NURSING MODELS

	King	Roy	Orem
Basic underlying assumptions	Perceptions important to all therapeutic relationships	Individual adaptation related to residual, focal, contextual stimuli	Individuals responsible for self-care
Client	An active participant in care	An individual who is having difficulty adjusting to stimuli	An individual with a self-care demand that goes beyond the individual's self-care agency
Nurse	A partner in attaining therapeutic goals	Supporting adaptation through the nursing process	Promoting and supporting self-care

Orem (1985). The predictions that emerge from such models can provide numerous challenges for research.

One nursing theory that has generated proposed nursing research problems is the Neuman Systems Model (Neuman, 1982). In an analysis of this model, Hoffman (1982) outlines a number of relationships requiring validation through research. Let us consider the following prediction derived from the Neuman Model: "In the nurse-patient interaction, nursing action based on the identification of stressors in the patient situation will affect the reduction of stress in the patient system" (p. 47). This idea can sow the seed for a variety of research projects in almost any clinical setting. In fact, it did for the present authors. Based upon results obtained from client satisfaction questionnaires and predictions drawn from the model, we conceived a research project in an outpatient surgery setting. First, we considered the following question: What are the common stressors, as defined by Neuman, that affect outpatient surgery clients (Roberts, C.; Darbyshire, J.; & Dubenofsky, N., 1984)? Next, we plan to develop and pilot test a preoperative teaching and support program that is predicted to reduce the identified stressors.

In addition to nursing theory, theories from many other disciplines can be, and have been, the basis for many nursing research problems. The nursing research literature is rich with problems that have emerged from a variety of theories coming from the physical, social,

---

Example 4.1 ———————————

PSYCHOLOGICAL THEORY AS THE BASIS FOR A RESEARCH STUDY

McNett (1987) developed a research study based upon Lazarus' psychological theory of stress and coping. The researcher tested her predictions with 50 disabled wheelchair-bound clients. She investigated subjects' perceived availability of social support, the effectiveness of social support, and personal constraints as directly and indirectly affecting coping.

———

See McNett, S. C. (1987). Social support, threat and coping responses and effectiveness in the functioning disabled. *Nursing Research, 36*(2), 98–103.

---

and behavioral sciences. Example 4.1 depicts how a psychological theory frequently used in nursing serves as a basis for developing a nursing research problem.

——————— WHAT PROBLEMS ARE SUITABLE FOR ———————— NURSING RESEARCH?

We have already described the use of the scientific method as one of the basic underlying approaches for studying problems in nursing research. In formulating a specific problem for study, the researcher must be certain that the problem to be studied is suitable for this method. Not all problems that we encounter in nursing can, nor indeed should, be examined using the systematic steps of the scientific method, which aims to uncover measurable data for analysis to produce causal answers. For example, the following questions have definite moral and legal implications.

- Should therapeutic abortions be legalized?
- Do nurses have the right to strike?

These questions would elicit a wide range of reasoned opinions and are dependent upon individual values. There are no precisely right or wrong answers to them, and it is only through logical debate that further knowledge can be gained. There are, however, aspects of these questions that can be examined through the scientific method. For example, it is possible to conduct a research project to answer the following questions:

- What are the age characteristics of women who seek therapeutic abortions?
- Is group counseling more effective than individualized counseling in reducing clients' stress following a therapeutic abortion?
- In a labor dispute, will baccalaureate-prepared nurses support a strike action more than will diploma-prepared nurses?

An investigation of these questions certainly can provide some information surrounding the initial questions but can never provide the full answers.

The researcher must consider the key concepts in the problem to determine the extent to which they can be measured. In Chapter 2 we discussed the idea that through the scientific method the researcher attempts to make meaningful conclusions based upon quantifiable data or on information that surrounds the key concepts in the research problem. In order to collect these data, the key concepts must be made operational and measurable in the form of variables. A **variable** is simply a concept that has measurable changing attributes, and the **operational definition** describes how these attributes will be measured or observed in the study by the researcher. Often this definition is very challenging for the researcher, but it is extremely important if quantitative research is to be meaningful.

Some concepts in health care lend themselves easily to operational definitions and variability. Birth weight, for example, can be operationally defined with ease as a child's weight recorded in grams on a particular type of scale, in the delivery room, by trained personnel immediately following birth. Variations in weight can be easily measured and categorized as high, average, or low according to specified percentiles on a growth chart that summarizes norms for the population.

However, suppose one wished to examine the concept "maternal happiness." This concept is much more abstract and difficult to measure. In attempting to render this concept operational, one could start by examining the physical evidence for the existence or nonexistence of maternal happiness. For example, it is possible to observe what mothers report about their inner feelings and how they interact with their children, but can one be certain these parameters are adequate measurements of this concept? Unless the researcher can find observable and measurable dimensions that are valid reflections of the concept of maternal happiness, the problem cannot be subjected easily to quantitative study.

If little is reported in the research literature about the study concepts and how to quantify them meaningfully, the nurse researcher may first take a more inductive approach to studying the problem using qualitative methods. In this way, the researcher can collect a great deal of circumstantial information through interviews or other unstructured techniques to develop meaningful definitions that can be used in the development of more quantitative measures for later empirical testing.

In nursing practice we are constantly concerned about many abstract and complex concepts that are not easily quantified. Grief, pain, stress, coping, and chronicity are a few such complex phenomena. Many nurse researchers agree that the essential contextual meaning of these concepts needs further study using qualitative approaches in everyday environments.

The significance of finding an answer to a problem in nursing is the key issue in determining it suitable for study. The nursing research process is broad enough to include inductive, deductive, and combined approaches to study problems. However, this process must be used appropriately in order to find answers that can be meaningfully applied to practice. Many problems can be studied using a combination of both qualitative and quantitative methods. In Chapter 6 we will discuss further the issue of how researchers choose an appropriate design to fit the research problem.

HOW DO NURSE RESEARCHERS DEFINE ~~2 forms~~ A SPECIFIC PROBLEM?

Once the nurse researcher has identified the general problem or possible problem for research, as represented in Figure 4.1, the next step involves a great deal of thinking to narrow this down to a specific written statement, the **research question.** This statement provides guidance for the application of each successive step of the research process throughout the entire study. There are two generally accepted

Figure 4.1

RESEARCH PROCESS FLOWCHART

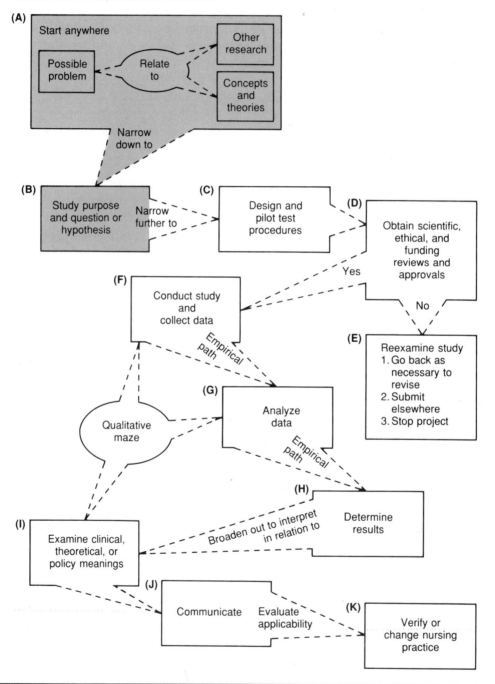

forms for stating the specific problem: declarative and interrogative. The declarative format simply states what will be investigated in the study and is often referred to as the purpose of the study. An example of this format is

> The purpose of this study is to determine if different levels of anxiety are reported during the third stage of labor by first-time mothers who have attended prenatal class and first-time mothers who have not attended classes.

The interrogative format simply asks a question and is often more direct. The declarative statement above can be rephrased in the interrogative form as

> Do first-time mothers who have attended prenatal classes report different levels of anxiety during the third stage of labor than first-time mothers who have not attended classes?

Many researchers favor the interrogative format over the declarative because of its simplicity and the clear distinction made between the specific problem statement and the purpose of the study. Ideally, the purpose of the study should outline why the problem is being investigated, while the problem statement defines what is being studied.

A good specific problem statement not only guides every aspect of the study but also indicates exactly what is being studied. It also identifies the key concepts under study and the kind of population in which these concepts will be studied. In quantitative causal studies, usually two or more concepts should be identifiable as variables. The causal variable is known as the **independent variable(s),** which is expected to have a measurable effect on the **outcome variable,** referred to as the **dependent variable.** In the above example it is clear that "attendance at prenatal classes" is the causal or independent variable and "levels of anxiety" is the outcome or dependent variable being measured. The population being studied is first-time mothers undergoing the labor experience.

In qualitative studies a clear description of the **phenomenon** (circumstance to be investigated) should accompany the problem statement. The following statements from Parse, Coyne, and Smith (1985, p. 28) show the difference between the research question and the description of the phenomenon.

Research Question: The investigation sought to answer the
question: What are the common elements in experiencing a feeling
of health among several different age groups?

Phenomenon: The phenomenon central to the study is the feeling
of health. Health has been defined in a number of ways....

The authors continue to present a variety of definitions of health
reported in the literature.

The specific problem statement appears simple enough when expressed on paper, but it requires much conceptual thinking and work
on behalf of the researcher. Again, by observing the researcher's
activities outlined in the left-hand box in Figure 4.1, you will see a
constant two-way path between possible problem, other research, and
concepts and theories.

We have already discussed how a researcher can form a possible
problem through reading other research and published theory. To define the problem, a further review of this literature is necessary. Other
published research presents the available evidence for the researcher
to make important decisions about selecting specific study concepts,
study population, and procedures for data collection. Other research
reports often discuss the feasibility of measuring key concepts.

WHAT ARE THE THEORETICAL UNDERPINNINGS OF THE RESEARCH PROBLEM?

All research begins with conceptual thinking about the problem.
Earlier we discussed how the researcher develops this reasoned thinking
or rationale through reviewing the related literature concerning the
problem and making mental predictions about the relationships of
concepts in the problem. If the researcher concludes that enough data
exist to explain the formulated mental predictions, then he or she may
proceed deductively to test these predictions empirically in light of the
explanations found in the literature. This situation relates back to the
earlier example in this chapter, where predictions about client behavior
resulted from the Neuman Systems Model (1982).

If the researcher can make predictions about how and why the
research concepts can be related to each other, or causally affect each
other, based upon an established theory, then that theory becomes the
theoretical framework or theory structure that guides the study. In

other cases the researcher may not find a strong formulated theory in the literature to guide the study of the problem. There may be enough evidence, however, to develop a well-reasoned explanation based upon generally accepted beliefs or **assumptions** about the problem, in combination with some fragmented conceptual or theoretical evidence derived from the literature. In this situation the framework developed by the researcher is referred to as a **conceptual framework.**

Silva (1986) completed an analysis of 62 nursing studies that used one of five nursing theories as a theoretical framework for research. The author discovered that in reality twenty-four of these studies used nursing models as frameworks in a very minimal way by simply summarizing the model without integrating it into the entire study. A second major use of nursing models in research involved employing the models to organize a particular part of the study such as data collection. The author identified only nine studies that actually tested nursing theory. Silva has developed criteria for evaluating adequate use of nursing theory as a framework for research. Her most important points include

—Testing the underlying assumptions of the theory in the study
—Deriving the study problem directly from the theory
—Empirically testing the study problem in an appropriate manner

Problems that are tested in light of a theoretical or conceptual framework are usually studied by using the scientific method of inquiry, depending heavily upon both deductive and inductive thinking. Conversely, when deciding to investigate a problem using primarily inductive thinking, as in many qualitative studies, the researcher usually finds little theoretical or conceptual evidence in the literature to guide the study. In these studies, the research problem is often derived from life experience and is investigated from the perspective of those involved in that experience. In purely qualitative studies, therefore, the research problem may not be explained in terms of a theoretical or conceptual framework at the beginning of the study. Instead, the researcher may present a philosophical rationale for studying the problem. Upon completion of analysis, however, the data obtained from research may be interpreted in light of theory. Examples 4.2 and 4.3 from the research literature demonstrate the conceptualization of a research problem using inductive and deductive approaches.

Example 4.2

INDUCTIVE APPROACH IN QUALITATIVE STUDIES

Kroska (1985) used qualitative research to explore the role of granny midwives in health care in the southern United States. The author provided rationale for selecting the ethnonursing approach (Leininger, 1978) in that she felt it was the most appropriate one to use in securing trust from informants and to gain a broad view of the contextual factors affecting the group. The author reviewed the literature and uncovered a number of specific historical and current facts which led her to develop the research problem. Through interviewing subjects a large amount of data was obtained. The data were qualitatively analyzed, and predicted relationships were stated at the conclusion of the report.

See Kroska, R. A. (1985). Ethnographic research method: A qualitative example to discover the role of "Granny" midwives in health services. In M. M. Leininger (Ed.), _Qualitative research methods in nursing_ (pp. 251–265). New York: Grune & Stratton.

Example 4.3

DEDUCTIVE APPROACH IN QUANTITATIVE STUDIES

Ziemer (1984) used the scientific method to investigate the effect of giving different types of information preoperatively on coping behaviors of post-surgical clients. The author reviewed the literature of past similar studies to demonstrate a need for the research. She used the Betty Neuman Health Care Systems Model (1980) to explain the expected relationships between surgical stress, giving various types of information, and use of coping strategies. Based upon this framework, a number of hypotheses were stated and tested in the study.

See Ziemer, M. M. (1984). Effect of information on post-surgical coping. In F. S. Downs (Ed.), _A source book of nursing research,_ 3rd ed. (pp. 117–131). New York: F. A. Davis.

STATING A RESEARCH HYPOTHESIS

Once the research problem has been carefully thought through, the researcher may write a formal research hypothesis in addition to the specific problem statement. The **research hypothesis** is essentially the researcher's prediction of how two or more variables are related. Usually the hypothesis is derived directly from the underlying theory that supports the research problem. In fact, in quantitative studies, the hypothesis becomes the working statement for the abstract theory that guides the study. Let us consider the following hypothesis:

> Day surgery clients who receive a preoperative teaching program to reduce identified stressors will report less anxiety in the early postoperative period than day surgery clients who received the usual preoperative teaching program.

This statement contains two variables. The independent variable, type of preoperative teaching program, is predicted to have an effect on the outcome or dependent variable, degree of reported anxiety. This prediction alone would have little meaning, but coupled with a clear explanation of how and why a teaching program can reduce stressors using the Neuman Systems Model (1982), it represents a working hypothesis for this theory.

The researcher must remember two important points in stating a workable hypothesis

1. That the prediction clearly depicts a relationship
2. That this relationship is predicted between at least one independent and one dependent variable

Consider whether the researcher who makes the following statement is formulating a workable research hypothesis.

> Day surgery clients who receive a preoperative teaching program to reduce identified stressors will report less anxiety in the early postoperative period. ← not a hypoth

This statement clearly fails to depict a relationship and only one concept is shown to vary, that is, degree of reported anxiety.

It should be noted that research hypotheses are not limited to predicted relationships between only one independent and one dependent variable. Often, researchers will make predictions about two or more independent and two or more dependent variables in the same hypothesis statement. Referring to the above example, the researcher may predict the following:

> Day surgery clients who receive a preoperative teaching program to reduce identified stressors will report less anxiety and less physical symptoms in the early postoperative period than day surgery clients who received the usual preoperative teaching program.

Provided that the underlying theory supports the predicted relationship between the type of preoperative teaching program and number of reported symptoms, this format can be considered as an acceptable hypothesis. However, a hypothesis that contains several variables often becomes lengthy and confusing for both the researcher and the reader of the final report. In this situation, the researcher might consider making two or more separate hypothesis statements.

Researchers who are engaged in qualitative research may not formally state a specific hypothesis at the beginning of the study. However, the researcher may have an hypothesis in mind, and as data are collected and analyzed, more specific predictions emerge, often resulting in an hypothesis that is stated upon completion of the study.

In most quantitative studies of a causal nature, the hypothesis is vital in selecting the methods for testing theory. Results obtained from the data collection should always be interpreted in light of the hypothesized relationship(s) stated at the onset of the study. Chapter 6, which discusses research design, presents a more detailed discussion on the types of research that are formal hypothesis-testing studies.

DETERMINING THE FEASIBILITY OF RESEARCH PROBLEMS

Once the researcher has decided that the problem at hand is suitable for research, there are a variety of other factors that determine the feasibility of actually performing the study of the problem. One of the earliest considerations to be made by the researcher is the ethical feasibility of pursuing the research problem. Although all nursing research is usually subject to rigorous ethics review procedures by a university or health care agency which employs or sponsors a nurse researcher, it is the responsibility of the researcher to consider all the ethical implications of studying a problem involving human subjects. Some problems, which cannot be studied without exposing subjects to undue stress, or which pose safety hazards to the emotional or physical well-being of subjects, must be terminated at the problem stage. (See Chapter 7 for a complete discussion of ethics review procedures.) If the problem appears to be ethically feasible, then the researcher must consider the number of personal and external resources necessary if the study is to be successful.

Financial considerations are always a prime concern when planning is done. Research is expensive: even very small projects require some source of funding, and usually all stages of the research process require money. Extensive library searches are very time consuming at the start of the study when the researcher is attempting to formulate the problem in the light of past and current investigations. Nurse researchers who conduct research as only one aspect of their professional role, or who conduct research on a full-time basis and have several studies operating concurrently, often require assistance with the task of reviewing the literature. This requirement involves paying a research assistant to do some of the "leg work." Computer searches of the literature can be helpful in conserving time but are costly. The money necessary simply to reproduce materials and buy paper can quickly add up to hundreds of dollars. In some situations the researcher may need to rent additional office space, and rent or buy office equipment if the study is an extensive one and extra personnel are hired.

Data collection is usually the most expensive part of a project. Many studies in nursing research require client interviews or surveys with face-to-face contact with an interviewer. This often necessitates the hiring of one or more paid research assistant(s). Perhaps funds are necessary to cover the cost of travel for these personnel, if data are collected in the client's home or other facility that is some distance from the office where the research activity is coordinated. Sometimes research questions require the use of expensive equipment for the collection of data. If this equipment is not available to the researcher, it may need to be purchased or rented.

Many research studies require the use of a computer for data analysis. If the researcher is unable to secure these services free of charge from the employing agency, computer use can be expensive. In addition, many nurse researchers who are not experts in the area of statistics find it necessary to consult an expert for advice on analyzing the data. This usually involves a fee.

These are only a few of the likely costs involved in the conduct of a research project. From the very inception of the problem, the researcher must plan for these expenditures if the research project is to be a feasible endeavor. For small research projects, researchers may approach the employing agency for assistance with funding. This is particularly important if the research findings will likely benefit the agency directly. Most large projects costing more than one or two thousand dollars require proposals for external funding from private or government agencies. In applying for external funds the nurse researcher must prepare an extensive, detailed proposal outlining the scientific merit and cost of the project in light of the specific goals of the prospective funding agency. This is nearly always an extremely difficult, time-consuming, and competitive task. Often, nurse researchers must compete with other professional groups for limited funds. A nurse researcher who is applying for a large sum of money must be extremely skillful in selling a significant, well-thought-out and designed project to the scientific experts and bureaucrats who will be assessing its merit and deciding whether or not to provide funding.

(3) Time is closely tied to money in conducting nursing research. Grant-issuing agencies that support nursing research often expect precise timelines for a project and its budget. Therefore, it is extremely important that the scope of the research problem to be studied is narrow enough to fit into an acceptable time period. For example, the authors proposed to examine the relationship between child-rearing practices and the accomplishment of developmental tasks by AmerIndian children from birth to three years. We wanted to study the same group of children for a three year period, and this would have required funding for a relatively prolonged period. However, since little information was available about child-rearing practices in this population, considerable time would be needed to explore such practices before examining the main issue. In this instance, a shorter study was planned and submitted for funding to collect data regarding child-rearing practices. The short project was challenging and time-consuming, but it was necessary in order to lay the foundation for a more time-feasible study of relationships at a later date.

Many inexperienced researchers fail to assess accurately the time needed to accomplish the basic steps of the research process as outlined in Chapter 6. Even if beginning with a seemingly feasible and carefully defined problem, it is advisable for the researcher to consider all the possible problems that might occur at each step of the process, and to schedule ample time to deal with the unforeseen complications that inevitably occur with even the simplest of projects.

(4) The researcher's interest in, and commitment to, the problem area are critical to feasibility. Research projects require a great deal of

time and effort; however, most nurse researchers pursue this interest in addition to many other professional roles such as clinician or teacher. It would be extremely difficult to spend long hours, often outside of working time, reviewing the literature or collecting data concerning a problem of little personal interest.

⑤ The experience of the researcher is another factor important to feasibility. Not only do beginning researchers usually need more time to negotiate the basic steps of the process, but they often lack the experience and skills needed to design complex projects and carry out elaborate data analysis. Problems which require sophisticated skill and knowledge of research methodology may only be feasible for study by the experienced investigator.

Two other related considerations which can influence the feasibility of studying a research problem involve the ability to secure an appropriate group of individuals to study and to gain the cooperation of key persons who can facilitate this process. Since the majority of nursing research involves human subjects, getting an appropriate and representative sample for the study of a proposed research problem is always a major concern. Sometimes individuals who may be stressed by an illness and hospitalization will not consent to participate in a research project. Others may simply refuse because they feel they do not have the time. In other situations the researcher may have difficulty accessing the desired population. Consider the nurse researcher in a small urban hospital who is interested in studying the effect of preoperative teaching on the postoperative anxiety of open-heart surgical clients. If only one or two open-heart surgeries are performed monthly in the immediate geographical area, it may be very difficult to obtain a reasonable sample to study the proposed problem in this setting.

Often there may be sufficient prospective subjects available, but access to this desired population requires the cooperation of key individuals or groups. For example, a nurse researcher who is seeking prospective subjects in a hospital environment or other health care facility usually requires the permission of the administration of that facility before proceeding. Generally, prior to permission being granted, the proposed project must be submitted to a rigorous ethics review process (see Chapter 7). Without this administrative approval and cooperation, the project cannot begin.

Securing the stamp of approval from administrative bodies, however, does not ensure easy access to prospective subjects in many research settings. The nurse researcher who plans to study a problem in a hospital or clinic environment must also consider the philosophies, roles, tasks, and objectives of health care providers in these environments. Usually a formal consent is not required from these individuals. It is politically very wise, however, to ensure that their cooperation and support will be sustained throughout the study. Nurses, physicians, and other health care professionals who maintain daily contact with subjects and are sold on the proposed study can do much to facilitate the nurse researcher's tasks of subject selection and data collection. If these professionals are not supportive of the project, the nurse researcher may have difficulty gaining access to subjects to request their consent to participate or collect the necessary data. Unfortunately, many nurse researchers still must face the reality that a large number of physicians and professional nurses have not yet grasped the significance of nursing research in promoting better client care. If the nurse researcher is unable to sell the proposed idea to supporting bodies in the research setting, another location must be found or the project may have to be aborted at the proposal stage.

_____ BEGINNING THE REVIEW OF THE _____
RESEARCH REPORT

So far in this chapter we have discussed the important tasks of the nurse researcher in planning a research project: the selection and conceptualization of a feasible and researchable studying problem. The evidence for this activity should be clearly presented in the beginning sections of the researcher's report. How well the researcher has accomplished this task is vital to the overall scientific validity of the project and the applicability of the research findings to nursing practice.

The process of establishing the **scientific adequacy** of a piece of research requires that the reader carry out a careful **critique** or evaluation of the research activities involved in each step of the research process as they are described in the research report. This can be difficult if you are a beginning reader of published research. The best way to start learning this skill is to select a short research report that is relatively easy to read, is of interest to you, and is not filled with statistics or jargon. Second, you will need a set of criteria to guide your evaluation. The guidelines in Table 4.2 should help you critique the introductory section of a research report. The exercise section at the end of this chapter provides direct practice in evaluating the researcher's conceptualization and statement of the problem in the introductory section of a research report.

_____ *Table 4.2* _____

EVALUATING THE CONCEPTUALIZATION AND STATEMENT OF THE PROBLEM

| Elements of Research | Scientific Adequacy | | Clinical Applicability |
	Quantitative Research Criteria	Qualitative Research Criteria	
Problem area or phenomenon *Jen*	1. Begins with a discussion of the general problem area or phenomenon 2. Presents sufficient background information 3. Discusses problem or phenomenon relation to nursing	Criteria 1–3, with more emphasis on a phenomenon	Is enough information given to convince reader of clinical significance of the problem or phenomenon and the feasibility of researching the problem in a clinical setting?
Specific problem or research question	1. Identifies specific problem(s) by end of introduction 2. Relates problem statement or question directly to general problem area 3. Identifies independent (causal) and dependent (outcome) variables 4. Shows clear expected relationships or differences between variables 5. Describes population and setting used	Criteria 1–4 usually not applicable at onset of study Criterion 5 presented in detail	Does the specific problem statement help reader begin to identify the basic/applied nature of research? Do problems that are tested in laboratory settings using populations very different from your setting need more testing before application? Are the variables in the study similar to those operating in the clinical setting?
Hypothesis or question Hypothesis or question (continued)	1. Has appropriate hypotheses or questions for study design 2. Has a specific prediction as to relationship between independent and dependent variable(s), or states the expected end result of study	1. Uses a question; never a hypothesis. Criteria 2–3 not applicable.	Will an answer to the research problem provide a possible answer to a clinical one? If predictions are made, are they logical from a clinical viewpoint? Has the researcher based prediction on theory or concepts relevant to nursing? Will further

(continues)

_____ Table 4.2 _____

(CONTINUED)

Elements of Research	Scientific Adequacy		Clinical Applicability
	Quantitative Research Criteria	Qualitative Research Criteria	
	3. Answers research question with prediction		understanding of the phenomena be helpful in practice?
		4. Has explicit philosophic perspective, and related design methods	
Purpose	1. States specifically why researcher is carrying out the research study	Criterion 1, same	The purpose should provide further insight into the basic/applied nature of the research. Problems which primarily aim to build knowledge have possible cognitive applications; studies that clinically test knowledge in relation to interventions have possible direct applications to practice.
Definition of key concepts	1. Defines as variables all important concepts associated with research problem 2. Makes clear how researcher is measuring and using variables	1. Concept definition can be a finding and appear at the end of the study 2. May be detailed in the analysis section	To be clinically usable, concepts must be defined to permit clinical measurement or observation of variables in the study. This is vital as studies are tested or replicated in your setting.
Philosophical, theoretical, or conceptual rationale and framework	1. Presents well developed explanation of how key variables are connected or related 2. Has an adequate explanation for a stated hypothesis(es) or question	Criteria 1–3 may be the findings of the study and appear at the end	Quantitative studies based upon well-tested theory, when applied to clinical problems, are more likely to be directly applicable to practice. The researcher must show the relevance of the theory

_____ Table 4.2 _____
(CONTINUED)

| Elements of Research | Scientific Adequacy | | Clinical Applicability |
	Quantitative Research Criteria	Qualitative Research Criteria	
Philosophical, theoretical, or conceptual rationale and framework (continued)	3. Shows that conceptual or theoretical framework is applied to all aspects of the study 4. States researcher's underlying assumptions	4. Same 5. Philosophical perspective must be clearly stated.	to nursing practice as well as to the problem if the theory used is not a nursing one. Quantitative studies initiated with loose conceptual frameworks or primarily aiming to develop theory provide cognitive insights, but usually require more research before direct application is indicated.

Hints on Reading

The first step in examining a research report is to read it over carefully to get a general idea of what has been studied. Frequently, researchers will preface a report by presenting a brief overview of the study and its findings. This abstract can be enormously helpful in assisting the reader to focus on the content of the report, particularly when reports are lengthy. A more complete discussion of how to evaluate an abstract is presented in Chapter 5.

Finding the Problem

Step two involves another reading of the report to identify the research problem and the sections of the report that describe how the researcher has attempted to examine the problem using the research process. This may sound easy, but that is not always the case. The researcher may proceed with introductory comments for a couple of pages or more before a clear statement of the general problem is presented. This is obviously confusing for any reader. The general problem should be introduced very early in the report, within the first

[handwritten: good intro should have ① gen prob ② background info ③ purpose of study ④ specific prob]

paragraph if possible (Downs, 1984). Likewise, a specific problem statement should appear at the end of the report's introduction. A good introduction would include (a) general problem area; (b) background (need for the study briefly summarized); (c) purpose of the study (why the study is being done); and, (d) specific problem statement or description of phenomenon being studied in qualitative research.

Identifying Key Variables

Once you have identified the specific problem in a quantitative study, it is usually easy to find the key variables that were studied. It should be evident from the problem statement which variables are independent and which are dependent. Earlier in this chapter we discussed how concepts are operationalized in research. Early in the report, following the specific problem statement, the researcher should define how key concepts are being measured or observed and used in the study. Often the researcher will discuss this process under the heading operational definitions. *[handwritten: (defines variables & makes them meas &/or observable in a partic study)]*

Examining the Conceptual Background for the Problem

The researcher's rationale, theoretical or conceptual framework, the hypothesis(es), and the literature review all provide evidence of how the researcher has thought through and developed the problem. Unfortunately, in many early nursing research reports on quantitative research, the theoretical or conceptual frameworks may not be clearly evident but are merely hinted at in the literature review. This situation has gradually changed in more recent studies, as nurse researchers become more cognizant of theory and theory development. A well written research report should provide an explanation of the theoretical or conceptual rationale and framework for the study problem in a section of the report that is apart from the literature review. It is confusing for the beginning research reader to identify and examine a conceptual or theoretical framework that is embedded in the literature review. You may find it helpful in this situation to write a short summary (in your own words) of the researcher's explanation of how and why the key variables in the problem are presented along with the literature that supports those ideas. This may help you identify the theoretical or conceptual framework in the report before proceeding to the critique.

In qualitative studies the philosophic perspective used by the researcher should be stated and related to methods selected for data collection in the study. The problem is usually discussed in relation to theoretical background following data analysis at the end of the report.

Examining the Literature Review

The literature review should place the problem in terms of other previous research concerning the problem or other similar problems. The best way to begin learning the skill of critiquing the literature review is to select a study that deals with a topic that interests you and of which you have some knowledge and experience. If you are reading a study that concerns a subject area with which you are not thoroughly familiar, you may have difficulty determining whether or not the researcher has adequately reviewed all important reported studies to present an unbiased viewpoint. The only way you can be certain that your critique will be reasonably accurate is to conduct a brief review on your own. The following chapter will provide you with more specific guidelines for doing this review. A quick check of the library indices, which report research studies conducted in the subject area over the five-year period preceding the study, should reveal most publications cited in the literature review. If additional works are found that appear related to the study question, you should secure and review these articles before making a decision. Occasionally you will find studies discussed in the review that may seem outdated. These studies must be evaluated according to the importance of the findings to the present study. A piece of research conducted twenty or thirty years prior to the study may be a crucial link to investigating the problem.

Inexperienced research consumers are often highly critical when evaluating the scope and number of citations in published reports. In reality, researchers who submit their works to learned journals are usually limited in space for presentation of their report. If the study problem is one that has been extensively investigated in the past, the literature review can be very lengthy. Many times the researcher must select only the most important current and relevant findings for publication.

SUMMARY

Chapter 4 provides the reader with considerable detail concerning how researchers find and conceptualize problems for study. Through the use of examples and discussion, the reader is guided toward understanding how research problems originate from nursing practice, research, and theory. Nursing research problems are discussed in light of the basis for selection of approaches used by researchers to study problems effectively. For example, certain research problems can be studied more effectively using qualitative rather than quantitative methods, while other problems are best studied through logical debate.

This chapter also describes how researchers narrow and define problems in order to state a specific research problem to guide the study. This discussion applies to both quantitative and qualitative research. Considerable attention is given to the theoretical underpinnings of research problems. The purpose, meaning, and use of theoretical and conceptual frameworks are explained in relation to quantitative and qualitative studies. Research examples illustrate these points. The definition, use, and statement of the research hypothesis is discussed in relation to the theoretical background of the study and its use in quantitative and qualitative investigations.

Several factors may affect the feasibility of undertaking a research project. For example, ethical implications, financial considerations, time available to conduct the study, the reseacher's experience, and the co-operation of others are all factors that must be considered before carrying out a research study. The last section of the chapter describes how to begin critiquing the researcher's conceptualization and statement of the research problem.

EXERCISES

1. The following research example is taken from a research proposal formulated by a group of fourth-year baccalaureate nursing students. Read it carefully and, using the guidelines in Table 4.2, write a brief evaluation of the problem, the conceptual or theoretical framework, and the rationale. If you have not read a great deal on the topic area of this study, you should go to the library and review some of the following references before beginning your critique.

   Foster, S. B. (1974, March-April). An adrenal measure for evaluating nursing effectiveness. *Nursing Research, 23,* 118–124.

   Frank, K. A.; Heller, S. S.; & Kornfeld, D. S. (1972). A survey of adjustment to cardiac surgery. *Archives of Internal Medicine, 130,* 735–738.

   Hackett, T. P., et al. (1968, December 19). The coronary care unit: An appraisal of its psychologic hazards. *New England Journal of Medicine, 279,* 1365–1370.

Klein, R. F., et al. (1968, August). Transfer from a coronary care unit: Some adverse responses. *Archives of Internal Medicine, 122,* 104–108.

Lethbridge, B.; Somboon, O.; & Shea, H. (1976). The transfer process. *Canadian Nurse,* 10.

Minckley, B. B., et al. (1979). Myocardial infarct stress of transfer inventory: Development of a research tool. *Nursing Research, 28*(1), 4–10.

Pride, F. L. (1968). An adrenal stress index as a criterion measure for nursing. *Nursing Research, 17,* 292–303.

Roy, C. (1976). Adaptation as a model of nursing practice. In C. Roy (Ed.), *Introduction to nursing: An adaptation model.* Englewood Cliffs, N.J.: Prentice Hall.

Schwartz, L., & Brenner, Z. (1979). Critical care unit transfer: Reducing patient stress through nursing interventions. *Heart & Lung, 8*(3), 540–546.

Toth, J. (1980). Effect of structured preparation for transfer on patient anxiety on leaving coronary care unit. *Nursing Research, 29*(1), 28–34.

Volicer, B. (1973). Perceived stress levels of events associated with the experience of hospitalization: Development and testing of a measurement tool. *Nursing Research, 22*(6), 491–497.

Introduction

In the last few decades, technology has been playing an increasingly greater role in methods of health care delivery. This is evidenced by the development of large numbers of "high tech" care areas such as Intensive Care Units (ICU) and Cardiac Care Units (CCU). Prior to discharge from hospital, patients are almost always transferred from these areas to a less acute care area such as a general medical or surgical unit. Transfer can cause a break in the continuity of care as well as a change in the consistency of care, and thus represents a period which can be emotionally traumatic to patients recovering from an episode of acute illness (Lethbridge et al., 1976).

The period immediately following cardiac surgery has been reported by patients to be very stressful. Feelings of anxiety, depression, confusion, and unreality are experienced by cardiac surgery patients as a result of the patient's encounter with the unfamiliar environment of the ICU and the ever present threat to the patient's physical integrity (Frank et al., 1972).

Coronary artery bypass graft (CABG) patients may feel anxious about transfer from the intensive care unit to a general hospital ward. Little research has been done to examine transfer anxiety of these specific patients. However, many studies have examined the anxiety experienced by coronary (MI) patients upon transfer from the CCU. Several recommendations have been generated on patient preparation in order to decrease transfer anxiety. This research endeavour investigates the effect of structured preparatory teaching, completed prior to transfer from ICU, upon CABG patients' anxiety level.

Literature Review

There has been evidence to both support and refute the idea that anxiety is associated with transfer. Volicer (1973) and Hackett et al. (1968) found in their research studies that patients did not find transfer stressful. In fact, in Hackett's study, the sample of MI patients viewed their transfer as evidence of progress. However, there have been other studies whose results indicate that transfer from ICU's and CCU's to a general floor is a negative and anxious experience (Lethbridge et al., 1976; Klein et al., 1968). Not only do anxiety levels increase but it has been noted that for MI patients their cardiovascular status was unstable and that arrhythmias were likely to occur within two hours after transfer (Minckley, 1979; Klein et al., 1968). Toth (1980) found that patient anxiety upon transfer was indicated by physiological parameters without corresponding expression in psychological parameters. Increased communication between nurse and patient, continuity of care after transfer, and patient preparation for transfer have been methods shown to be effective in reducing patient transfer anxiety (Klein, 1968; Schwartz & Brenner, 1979; Foster, 1974; Pride, 1968).

More specific to transfer patients, Toth (1980) researched the effect of structured preparation for transfer from CCU, on patient anxiety. Physiological data supported the notion that structured pretransfer teaching significantly lowered the anxiety of the experimental group. Psychological parameters of anxiety, however, were not influenced.

Theoretical Framework

Sister Callista Roy (1976) views man as a biopsychosocial being in constant interaction with a changing environment. Man's biopsychosocial integrity constitutes a basic human need which must be maintained during these environmental changes. A positive response to change is known as the process of adaptation. According to Roy, man's ability to adapt depends on (1) the degree of environmental change and (2) the state of the person coping with the change (also known as the adaptation level) which is determined by focal, contextual, and residual stimuli. Maladaptive responses to change are disruptive to the individual.

Two main types of mechanisms aid the individual in coping with change (Roy). The regulator mechanism works via the autonomic nervous system; as it increases heart rate and blood pressure, it causes tension and excitement. The individual is prepared for "fight or flight." The cognator mechanism identifies, stores, and relates stimuli. It involves man's thought processes and decision making abilities. Roy believes that these two mechanisms should be analyzed when assessing a person's adaptive responses to change, and when planning further nursing care.

CABG patients are faced with environmental and psychological change when transferred from an ICU to a general floor. Gone is the intensive surveillance by personnel and machines. The patient is asked to increase his independence even though he still may think of himself as critically ill. Therefore, nursing interventions designed to reduce anxiety-producing stimuli and strengthen patients' adaptive responses as defined by the Roy model (1976) should reduce transfer anxiety.

2. Write an appropriate hypothesis for the study described in Exercise 1.

REFERENCES

Downs, F. (1984). *A source book of nursing research,* 3rd ed. Philadelphia: F. A. Davis.

Hoffman, M. K. (1982). From model to theory construction: An analysis of the Neuman health care systems model. In B. Neuman (Ed.), *The Neuman Systems Model—Application to nursing education and practice* (pp. 44–52). Norwalk, Conn.: Appleton-Century-Crofts.

Johnson, D. (1980). The behavioral system model for nursing. In J. Riehl & C. Roy (Eds.), *Conceptual models for nursing practice* (pp. 207–216). New York: Appleton-Century-Crofts.

King, I. M. (1981). *A theory for nursing systems, concepts, process.* New York: Wiley.

Kroska, R. A. (1985). Ethnographic research method: A qualitative example to discover the role of "Granny" midwives in health services. In M. M. Leininger (Ed.), *Qualitative research methods in nursing* (pp. 251–265). New York: Grune & Stratton.

Kruszewski, A.; Lange, S. H.; & Johnson, J. (1979). Effect of positioning on discomfort from intramuscular injections in the dorsogluteal site. *Nursing Research, 28*(2), 103–105.

Levine, M. (1967). The four conservation principles of nursing. *Nursing Forum, 47,* 45.

McNett, S. C. (1987). Social support, threat and coping responses and effectiveness in the functioning disabled. *Nursing Research, 36*(2), 98–103.

Neuman, B. (1980). The Betty Neuman health-care systems model: A total person approach to patient problems. In J. Riehl & C. Roy (Eds.), *Conceptual models for nursing practice,* 2nd ed. (pp. 119–134). New York: Appleton-Century-Crofts.

———— (1982). *The Neuman Systems Model—Application to nursing education and practice.* Norwalk, Conn.: Appleton-Century-Crofts.

Orem, D. E. (1985). *Nursing concepts of practice,* 3rd ed. New York: McGraw-Hill.

Parse, R. R.; Coyne, A. B.; & Smith, M. J. (1985). *Nursing research: Qualitative methods.* Bowie, Md.: Brady Communications.

Peplau, H. (1952). *Interpersonal relations in nursing.* New York: Putnam.

Queen's University School of Nursing Year IV Students. (1983). *The effect of structured pretransfer teaching on patient anxiety.* Unpublished research proposal. Queen's University, School of Nursing. Kingston, Ontario.

Rettig, F. M., & Southby, J. R. (1982). Using different body positions to reduce discomfort from dorsogluteal injection. *Nursing Research, 31*(4), 219–221.

Roberts, C.; Darbyshire, S.; & Dubenofsky, N. (1984). Client and caregiver satisfaction and welfare after day surgery: A pilot project. *Proceedings: Nursing Research and the Clinical Staff Nurse,* November 1984. Montreal: Sir Mortimer B. Davis Jewish General Hospital.

Roy, C. (1980). The Roy adaptation model. In J. Riehl & C. Roy (Eds.), *Conceptual models for nursing practice,* 2nd ed. New York: Appleton-Century-Crofts.

Silva, M. C. (1986). Research testing nursing theory: State of the art. *Advances in Nursing Science, 9*(1), 1–11.

Ziemer, M. M. (1984). Effect of information on post-surgical coping. In F. S. Downs (Ed.), *A source book of nursing research,* 3rd ed. (pp. 117–131). New York: F. A. Davis Co.

5

Reviewing the Literature: An Essential Skill

INTRODUCTION

Literature review is an essential aspect of the research process and the research consumer's process. The ability to review critically individual reports of clinical nursing research is at the heart of this process and as such is the focus of this chapter.

The knowledge base of professions, however, is not built on individual studies, but is an accumulation of research findings along with theoretical development. To access this body of literature, understand it, and finally come to some scientifically logical and clinically meaningful conclusions is a lengthy and complex process. This chapter will explain the steps involved and illustrate some of the tools you can use in a literature review.

OUTLINE

OBJECTIVES

After reading this chapter, you will be able to

1. Understand the steps in the process used by research consumers and researchers to do a critical review of the literature on a specific topic.
2. Appreciate the need to do thorough and repeated literature reviews at several steps within the consumer's process.
3. Recognize the essential elements of a good research literature review.

NEW TERMS

Abstract
International Nursing Index
Index Medicus

Data base
Secondary source
Primary source

THE LITERATURE REVIEW AND THE _____ RESEARCH PROCESS

Literature review is a process that involves finding, reading, understanding and forming conclusions about the published research and theory on a particular topic. In most research studies, a literature review is done at the onset of a study and is updated or extended during the final phases of the project. In Figure 5.1 the steps in cells A and I almost always require a literature review. When the possible research problem is being identified or narrowed, and when interrelationships between previous studies, theories, or concepts are being explored, a critical literature review is essential. Perhaps less obvious is the value of the review when making decisions on the best design for the study (cell C), including the data collection strategy (cell F), and data analysis procedures (cell G).

Reporting on the Literature Review

In most research articles, there will be a synopsis of the conclusions of the literature review near the beginning of the report along with a few details on the studies or theoretical works critical to interpreting the study's findings. At the end of the report the researcher will contrast and compare the study findings and conclusions with those of the updated literature review. This is the standard pattern for most studies. It is consistent with the scientific method as introduced in Chapter 2: that is, collect and organize all currently available related facts (step 2 of the scientific process), then check the conclusions against other related facts (step 6).

The report of the literature review is only the tip of the iceberg. In this chapter you will learn to do the entire process, although you will rarely give all these details in your reports. (An exception to this rule is when a separate article is published with the full literature review, for example, the Moore, Guenter, Bender, and Hogan [1986] review of nutrition-related nursing research. A section below discusses review articles as a special case.) As a research consumer you will critique the brief review of the literature section along with the rest of the report. Guidelines for this portion of the critique of a research report are detailed at the end of this chapter.

Variations in Qualitative Research

Qualitative researchers approach the literature in different ways and often at different points in the research process. A researcher with a

Figure 5.1

RESEARCH PROCESS FLOWCHART

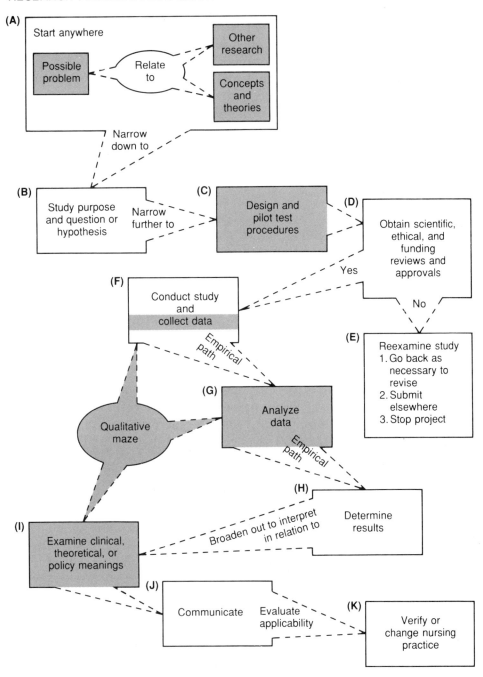

qualitative as opposed to a quantitative perspective will tend to view the literature with more skepticism, or will see it as merely an additional source of data. Thus, the literature review will be placed in different sections of the report than is the case with quantitative study reports.

Opinions differ among qualitative researchers on the value and place of the literature review prior to data collection, which a qualitative researcher often calls fieldwork. Field and Morse (1985) have grouped these opinions into three main viewpoints. Those who ascribe to the first view do not consult other studies or theories before or during data collection to avoid clouding or misleading the researcher's understanding of the phenomena under study. Phenomenologists (see Table 6.2 for a description of this type of research) commonly use this approach.

A second point of view is held by researchers who use a method called grounded theory (Glaser, 1978; Chenitz & Swanson, 1986, p. 45; see Chapter 10 of this book for an explanation of grounded theory). Grounded theorists advocate simultaneous data collection and analysis with the literature as a source of data and an aid to analysis. Although the openness of the researcher to new perspectives is desirable, ignoring the literature can be inefficient, since the researcher can rediscover time and time again what is already known and well documented in the literature.

A third point of view is that all available literature on the research topic should be read and findings should guide the study. This approach is not usually consistent with the purpose of a qualitative study because it can prematurely and severely narrow the range of observation, and thus yield results that do not fully describe the phenomena. This problem is compounded if the previous work is not critically examined for assumptions and biases that could influence the current study. Such an approach is best left to the quantitative researchers who are operating from the perspective of a logical, positivist scientific method rather than from the phenomenological, qualitative perspective.

Thus, Field and Morse advocate a middle ground, which is to review critically all relevant literature for biases, assumptions, and unfounded conclusions. Those who ascribe to this view conduct a detailed content analysis (see Chapter 10 for a description of this procedure) of the relevant literature. They use the results of their content analysis to derive meanings from previous studies and prevailing theories only. Thus, they consider themselves to be both open and informed as they move to the data-collection phase. They proceed to collect data by using the literature review as an additional source of data, and then they contrast their findings with findings from the literature. This approach is efficient in the use of the literature but, from the qualitative perspective, is efficient only to the extent that the researcher can "forget" the previous findings and theories during the data-collection and analysis phases.

THE RESEARCH CONSUMER'S LITERATURE REVIEW

As a research consumer, you will sometimes conduct a literature review with as much rigor as that of a researcher. The purpose of your reviews might differ from that of the researcher, whose purposes are linked to the conceptualizations and interpretations of findings for a study. Your focus is likely to be the clinical applicability of a single study or a group of studies.

There are specific steps that both a researcher and a research consumer take in conducting a literature review. You will find that the process is more systematic, complex, and thus more lengthy than the less formal literature reviews that you may have conducted either to prepare term papers or to explore a clinical question. The steps are

STEP 1 Define the topic and purpose.

STEP 2 Search for relevant articles, books, or reports.

STEP 3 Select and critically read the pieces.

STEP 4 Synthesize and critique the body of literature.

STEP 5 Form conclusions linked to the purpose of the review.

Defining the Topic and Purpose

In this step you will write out the topic and the specific purpose of the literature review. The topic is often written as a question.

- What is the best approach to . . . ?
- Is it safe to use . . . ?
- What is the scientific evidence for our current practice of . . . ?

This initial question will probably be fine tuned as you proceed. For the researcher it is often the first draft of what will become the research question.

The purpose of the literature search is also explicitly stated. This is the reason why you are asking the question. If the reasons are primarily clinical you might want to pay particular attention in the topic question to articles that document the use of the technique or approach. If the reasons are primarily scientific, as they are for most research, you will want to pay particular attention to research reports. These two general types of purposes, however, are not mutually exclusive. Most articles or books in the nursing literature contain suggestions both for practice and some scientific evidence. An example of a literature review that could have both clinical and research uses was done by Burke for a study she was about to begin with her colleagues on the reliability and validity of the use of the Denver Developmental Screening Test for Cree Indian children. This was an unpublished document that was used to guide various aspects of the study such as those highlighted in Figure 5.1. Portions of this review will be used as an example in this chapter.

The statements of the topic, question, and purpose will direct the review and help you broaden or narrow your search. For example, a community health nurse asked two nursing professors, "Is the Denver Developmental Screening Test (DDST) appropriate to use with the Cree Indian children in my caseload?" An initial look at the references and original studies from which the DDST was developed did not provide assurance that it would be clinically appropriate for this population. Indeed, the Cree children seemed substantially different from the population on which the DDST was standardized. The faculty member then approached Burke for her opinion as a maternal and child nurse and a researcher. The topic was broadened slightly to, "What is the clinical and scientific evidence for the use of the DDST for children of ethnic or cultural backgrounds very dissimilar to those of the standardization sample?" The purpose was thus to answer the clinical question and, if that were not possible, to provide information for the conceptual framework and study methods for a study to answer the initial question asked by the community health nurse. This eventually led to the study that is excerpted in Example 5.1.

At this stage of defining your question and the purpose of the literature review, you will usually consult and read a few reference works, and come to an initial understanding of the answer or lack thereof. In the example of the DDST, pediatric nursing texts, the DDST manual, and the developers of the DDST were consulted at this stage. However, a satisfactory answer was not found.

Occasionally, the question is completely answered at this step and there is no need to proceed further. Most often, however, the question

(text continues on p. 120)

___ *Example 5.1* ___

A LITERATURE REVIEW

Abstract

Reported cross-cultural uses of the Denver Developmental Screening Test (DDST) cast some doubt on its applicability with Canadian Indian children. We did a longitudinal study of the validity of the DDST with Cree Indian children from Moose Factory and Moosonee. We collected data in 1980 using the DDST, other developmental measures, and a maternal questionnaire. The hospital and outpatient record searches were repeated in 1983.

The DDST was slightly related to some developmental measures, but sensitivities were very low. There were no significant relationships with any of the concurrent measures of illness or risk of handicap. Results three years later were mixed, with some small relationships with measures of health or developmental status, but again the sensitivities were very low. Interpretative traps and cross-cultural pitfalls as well as the limited recommended use of the DDST with these children are presented.

Introduction

The Denver Developmental Screening Test (DDST) (Frankenburg & Dodds, 1967) is widely used for assessing developmental status of infants and children up to age 6, both in clinical practice and in research (Crane et al., 1981; Davidson et al., 1978; Kirkconnell & Hicks, 1980; Majeres & Timmer, 1981; Morrison & Newcomer, 1975; Morrison & Pothier, 1972; Rothenberg & Varga, 1981). It can be used without extensive training in psychological testing: only a simple scoring sheet, manual, and small kit of standard equipment are required.

Nonetheless, important questions about its reliability and validity remain unanswered (Cahoon, 1973; Coons et al., 1980; Lichenstein, 1981; Meier, 1975; Werner, 1972). One question is whether the DDST is appropriate with various ethnic or minority groups (Erickson, 1976; Mercer & Lewis, 1978; Nugent, 1976). While there are reports of successful use with Native Canadians (Bell & Gosselin, 1983; Newton, 1973), there have not been any validity studies with these groups.

(continues)

Example 5.1 (Continued)

In cross-cultural studies of the DDST with other groups, the results have been mixed (Barnes & Stark, 1975; Jaffe et al., 1980; Olade, 1984; Sandler et al., 1970; Shapira & Harel, 1983; Sturner et al., 1982; Ueda, 1978; Williams, 1984). Most studies recommend cautious, continued use of the DDST. Two exceptions which questioned the validity of the DDST were studies of Mexican Indian children and children referred for developmental delay (Applebaum, 1978; Solomons & Solomons, 1975).

We report on validity of DDST with Canadian Cree Indian children. We addressed three questions:

1. Does the DDST produce similar developmental results as other measures of developmental status?
2. Does the DDST identify children at risk or with current health problems?
3. Does the DDST provide early identification of children who will later be diagnosed as having health or developmental problems?

Discussion

As in most other cross-cultural studies (Barnes & Stark, 1975; Olade, 1984; Sturner et al., 1982), there was limited support for the DDST as a measure of current developmental status, but the relationships with other developmental measures were weak. The number of children whose mothers, other developmental tests, or the charts indicated had slow development, and whom the DDST completely missed and classified as normal is disturbingly high. The lack of sensitivity casts much doubt on its use to identify children with current developmental delays. This lack of sensitivity was also noted by Cadman et al. (1984).

The rate of children with abnormal or questionable DDSTs is within the range expected in the general population (Pless & Douglas, 1971; Whaley & Wong, 1983), but the relationship in this population between results and age is disturbing. Williams (1984) noted the same trend in Filipino children. With a good developmental assessment test, the results do not correlate with age, but in these Indian children only the 3 to 4 year olds had abnormal, questionable or untestable results.

Example 5.1 (Continued)

The findings do not support the use of the DDST to identify children with health problems which could be assumed to be reflected in altered developmental progress. None of the concurrent indicators of illness or health risk from the mothers, nurses, or hospital records were related to the DDST. It is our speculation that the DDST as a developmental test is too indirect a route for screening for health or risk of handicap.

As in another study of predictive validity (Coons et al., 1980), there was limited and mixed support for the DDST's ability to predict health and development problems three years later. Like the concurrent correlations there are some small, significant results, but an unacceptably high number of children with problems were classed as normal by the DDST. Thus, if it were the exclusive screening test, these children would have been missed.

Gaps and delays such as seen in these children are disturbing to the untrained tester. The widely available score sheets in the absence of manuals and equipment are hazardous because there is no indication on the sheet that further equipment and training is needed. Thus, the person who has only the score sheet is at great risk of not only administering the DDST incorrectly, but also of misinterpreting it after administration. The most common interpretive errors were either to conclude that a delayed individual item indicates an abnormal DDST result or the presence of an item in which the child has had no experience results in an untestable child. Neither are true. Our experience in the study and elsewhere is that with training, the interviewers rarely have an untestable child.

Recommendations

For this population of Cree Indian children it would be hazardous to use the DDST as an exclusive screening test for either developmental or health risk. However, the usefulness of the DDST to focus the health professionals' attention on child development and as a vehicle for facilitating discussion with parents around developmental issues has not been studied, so it would be premature to discontinue the DDST for these purposes at this time.

(continues)

Example 5.1 (Continued)

Based on our experience in conducting this study and reports on DDST studies in other ethnic groups, we have several further recommendations. To avoid the illusion of easy administration and interpretative traps, the DDST's one page score sheet should have a warning printed on it to the effect that (a) standard testing materials must be used, (b) the manual is required for accurate testing and interpretation, and (c) training is required to accurately administer and score the DDST. A translator or a bilingual tester is needed if the mother or child does not have the same first language as the tester (Miller et al., 1984).

Conclusions

Developmental tests, of which the DDST is only one, are a fundamental part of professional nursing and other health professionals' practice with children. What developmental assessment tools do best is provide an indication of current developmental status which is vital for working with children and families. However, screening for health or illness status or future developmental status probably goes beyond the capabilities of such simple tests.

Excerpts from S. O. Burke, et al. (1985). Pitfalls in the cross-cultural use of the Denver Developmental Screening Test: Cree Indian children. *Canadian Journal of Public Health, 76,* 303–307.

is still somewhat open, or additional aspects of the question become clearer and thus require additional information.

Searching for Relevant Literature

Once the topic of the literature review and the purpose are clear, the systematic search of the literature can begin. It is important to determine the range of the search at this point. Key considerations in the range of the search are

- How many years back should you go?
- What bodies of literature should you search?
- What client or subject characteristics are of interest?

- How many articles and books can you reasonably read in the time you have available to answer the question?
- Do you need to go beyond the library resources most easily available to you?

You should discuss these considerations with others involved in examining the question. In addition, it is important to discuss the search with your librarian at this point. Larger health sciences libraries have the specialized help that you will need. Smaller institution libraries and general libraries might not. After reading the sections below on the use of literature indexes and computer-assisted searches, you will be able to ask the correct questions of your local librarian to determine how to reach the resources that you will need.

At this point you will be able to determine how to identify the articles, books, and reports on the topic of interest within the range you need. There are four basic types of resources for your search.

—The catalogue of books and journals available in a particular library system
—The indexes covering various fields of study
—The indexes printed at the end of each year for most journals
—Computer-accessed indexes of journals and reports within various broad fields.

These resources all require some expert librarian help and learning on your part to use them most effectively. Searches using these resources can be done by hand or with the aid of a computer. Any search may use one or all of these resources, depending on the review of the literature question, the purpose, and the range of the search to be done as described above. How you actually use each resource is described in the following section on tools and strategies for use in reviewing the literature.

In the example of the community health nurse and the use of the DDST, there were not sufficient library resources at the isolated health unit or local library to answer the question. Thus the nursing professors took the problem to their large university health sciences library. The range of the search was as follows: Literature back five years was reviewed; the nursing, medical, and psychology bodies of literature, in English or French, and all studies using the DDST were examined; the research focused on children only; and the researchers determined up to fifty studies could reasonably be reviewed. The library catalogue search for titles related to the DDST and Cree Indians yielded nothing. We decided to take a broad look at the literature and therefore used indexes of fields rather than indexes of specific journals. Since we wanted breadth, we used computerized searches of health science, psychology, and mental health indexes for the references on articles or reports of studies within the range of our interest. (For details on exactly how we did this see the section on computer-assisted searches below.) Our first search of these indexes did not yield the fifty references we had hoped for, so we went back another five years for a total of ten years. We still did not have fifty studies, but decided that older work would either be dated or already be listed in those studies for which we now had references. Table 5.1 lists the articles located in chronological order. Note that the articles span fifteen years because the review was updated when a follow-up study was done several years after the initial work.

Once you have a reference list of potentially relevant articles, reports, and books, you can begin a library search. Articles and shorter reports or chapters are usually photocopied. Books and larger reports are checked out. Even in the largest libraries you will not find every piece for which you have a relevant reference. For these references you will need to use interlibrary loan, which is done with the assistance of the librarian. You will usually need to have as much of the bibliographical information as possible (authors, data, title, journal, volume number, pages) and where you obtained the reference information (computerized search, reference list from a book or article, etc.). The librarian usually takes it from there and will let you know when the reference arrives. This can take a few weeks.

It is very important to read the references within each article as you collect them so that you may search for other relevant work to add to your list. As demonstrated, you will not get all the relevant material in a specific area with only a computer-assisted search. However, using the search of the reference lists as well, you will eventually find the vast majority of them.

Critical Reading of the Article or Report

Critical reading involves a preliminary phase—reading the abstract and then scanning the body for suitability in the review. A critical review is then done if the piece seems suitable for the purposes of the review.

Reading the Abstract   The first part of most articles or reports is the **abstract.** This is a concise statement of the contents of the entire

Table 5.1

CROSS-CULTURAL DDST STANDARDIZATION AND VALIDITY STUDIES[1]

Author	Population[2]	Number of Subjects	Type of Data[3] Collection Tool	Researchers' Conclusions
Sandler, et al, 1970	Puerto Rican and Black (4–6 year olds)	104	Standardization	Language and fine motor items not applicable; therefore, use with caution
Sandler, et al, 1971 & 1972	Lower class, Philadelphian Black (55–66 months)	373	Standardization	Generally similar results to DDST norms; only language showed differences with norms; therefore, use recommended
Chevrefils, 1973	French Canadians	1,200	Standardization of French translation	Use standardized French version
Bryant & Davies, 1974	Wales (16–375 days)	668	Standardization	No differences with DDST norms and no differences by sex, social class, or parity; therefore, use DDST
Barnes & Stark, 1975	Rural Canadian	226	Standardization	Adequate for use
Solomons & Solomons, 1975 & 1982	Mexican and Mayan Indian (2–54 weeks)	288	Standardization; criterion validity, Bayley Motor Scales	No cultural differences between groups; later in gross motor locomotion and advanced in fine motor; DDST failed to identify 16 of 17 "questionable" babies; therefore, of limited use
Appelbaum, 1978	Lower social class Texan (2–30 months)	76	Criterion validity with Bayley Scales	Correlations generally low, with marked underselection insensitivity of DDST
Ueda, 1978	Okinawan and Tokyo	1,786	Standardization	Using a Japanese version, Okinawan children were slower in gross motor and advanced in language; therefore, administer with adjusted norms and use caution

(continues)

_____ Table 5.1 _____

CONTINUED

Author	Population[2]	Number of Subjects	Type of Data[3] Collection Tool	Researchers' Conclusions
Jaffe et al, 1980	Israeli (9 months)	914	Standardization	Later in motor, but use routinely with adjusted norms
Song et al, 1982	Shanghai	1,041	Standardization	Recommended for screening
Sturner, et al, 1982	Rural North Carolinians 52–64 months	1,738	Criterion validity with Stanford-Binet	Sensitivity = .68; specificity = .95; recommend two stage PDQ and DDST screening in routine pediatric practice
Harper & Wacker, 1983	Rural disadvantaged preschoolers	1,018	Criterion validity with Stanford-Binet or Wechsler Primary & Pre-School Intelligence Scale	Low sensitivity
Shapira & Harel, 1983	Israeli	2,248	Standardization with Hebrew translation	Israeli children had earlier development in personal-social and later in motor skills; therefore, the Hebrew re-standardized version is recommended
Olade, 1984	Nigerian	94	Face validity	Useful, but needs standardization
Williams, 1984	Filipino	6,006	Standardization	Generally later development in all areas of DDST; discriminate analysis showed maternal and home factors, as well as age of child, are related to DDST scores

[1] Excludes studies where the DDST is used to measure the dependent variable of developmental status, those with samples similar to the DDST standardization study, very small samples, or extreme design flaws.

[2] Unless otherwise specified, covers approximately birth to age 6 years.

[3] See Chapter 9 for a discussion of data collection tools, the concepts of criterion validity and standardization as used in studies that focus on data collection tools themselves.

report (see Example 5.1). You can see that the writer is limited to about one sentence per section of the entire study report—purpose, question, variables, measures, sample, methods, analysis, discussion, conclusions, and so on. Well-written abstracts are a great help in deciding whether or not to read the entire article. Poorly written abstracts can waste your time since they might guide you to read an irrelevant article or, more seriously, to decide not to read a relevant article. If in doubt about the relevance after reading only the abstract, you should take the time to scan the entire article.

The abstract restates the key elements of the study in a succinct format, so you might want to use the abstract to double check your understanding of the full article or report while scanning and while critically reading. Interpretations for your clinical practice, however, should always come from the more fully described body of the report and not the abstract.

Scanning for Suitability Once you locate a likely article for your review, you will scan it to see if it fits with your particular purposes. Possible purposes include

—Determining the clinical applicability of a particular nursing assessment or intervention

—Determining the state of the research-generated knowledge base for practice in a particular field

—Discovering likely conceptual or theoretical models for use in practice and research

—Determining gaps or inconsistencies in the literature in order to determine the need for a study

—Determining the best research design for a particular study

As Fox and Ventura (1984) have demonstrated, clear written criteria for inclusion in or exclusion from the review are very helpful. Indeed, for a large review, and when there is more than one person involved, these written criteria for inclusion, based on your purposes, are essential. This is how you thin out the wheat from the chaff for the next phase of the review. If you are not finding enough material or if it is not what you want, you might reexamine and revise your purpose for the review.

From the titles and abstracts we had printed with the references in the computerized search, it was determined which ones to locate. These were further thinned out by omitting those studies that either were not data-based or focused on samples not of interest to the review.

This left the first nine entries in Table 5.1. Some of those studies omitted were helpful for other purposes and were put aside for later use. The clinical report of the use of the DDST with another Canadian Indian group (Bell & Gosselin, 1983) and a critical review of the DDST as a research data collection tool (Fleming, 1981) are examples of this.

Reading for Scientific and/or Clinical Merit   This phase of step 3 is the heart of the literature review and occurs once you have chosen the suitable studies. The quality of the critical reading will to a large extent determine the usefulness of the review. The bulk of this textbook describes how content is critically reviewed. The review process is outlined in the Appendix to Chapter 3. Each of the component parts of the content to be critiqued for each article is discussed in more detail in later chapters, and these chapters are cross-referenced in that Appendix. For example, you will evaluate the tools used to collect data in the process of critiquing each article. However, if the tools themselves are part of the purpose of your review, then you will also refer to the chapter on data collection, which will give you more explicit detail on the critique of this particular aspect of a report.

This phase requires careful recording. The mechanisms you can use to do this are discussed in some detail below in the Tools and Stategies section. For the DDST review, Burke used index cards, notes on the reprints, and notes on themes and concepts as well as an expanded version of Table 5.1 to record the content and her critique of the content of the articles reviewed.

Synthesizing and Critiquing the Body of Literature

In this phase you move away from the individual article, chapter, or report that you have reviewed. You will now be something of an expert in the field, for very few people will know as much about the topic of your review as you do. You will focus on the body of literature as a whole, basing your conclusions on what you have found. Now is also the time to make decisions based on your own judgments. You should examine the body of the literature for the following:

— Strengths and weaknesses

— Gaps

— Replication and duplication

— Contradictions

— Inconsistencies

Usually it is solely this portion of a researcher's literature review that you will see in an article. For example, the synthesis and critique of the DDST review can be seen in the introductory section of Example 5.1.

Forming Conclusions Linked to the Purpose of the Review

If the critique of the individual pieces of literature is the heart of a review, then forming a conclusion is the brains. The conclusion step brings you back to the beginning of the literature review process and the research question that led to the review. Now you will be able to answer the question to the extent that it is possible given the overall trends in the literature. For example, you may find there is a consensus on the findings across studies or that there is little agreement or conflicting results reported. You may find your question is only partially addressed.

The process of drawing conclusions requires careful analysis and often rereading of articles so that your conclusions are accurate representations of the individual studies. If the purpose of the review was to identify researchable questions, then these are listed in the conclusion section. If the purpose was to answer a clinical question, then the answer is stated in the conclusion section. If the purpose was not met or only partially met, this is explicitly stated in the conclusion section.

TOOLS AND STRATEGIES

A number of tools and strategies can be used to make your literature review more comprehensive. Among the most important tools in locating the relevant literature are the computer-assisted search and the manual search of indexes. If you do not already know how to use a card catalogue, you should learn that skill as well. Once you have the references for the literature, there are some skills you can use to keep track of what you have found. In addition, there are ways to organize the findings of the literature review that will assist you in coming to a conclusion about the question you are asking. Finally, in some areas of nursing, published reviews of the literature already exist. These can be very helpful if used correctly.

Indexes

The most important index for nursing research is the ***International Nursing Index,*** which is published by the American Journal of

Nursing. *Index Medicus* contains many nursing references as well as medical research that can be useful to nurses. Depending on your specific clinical interests, indexes in sociology and psychology might contain relevant references. Each index contains many volumes. Developing skills in using the volumes of these indexes will enhance your ability to locate nursing research that may be applicable to your practice.

Reference indexes are compiled yearly. (Parts of the current year might be in the library as well as monthly or quarterly updates. These will be incorporated into the annual issue at the end of each year.) References to articles within many specified journals and/or on specific topics are listed in these indexes. They are sorted and listed in two ways, by author and by topic. In addition, there are lists of all the topic categories and lists of the abbreviations used for the names of the journals.

Start with the most recent year's index. First, look for the list of topic categories that is at the beginning or the end of the book, depending on the index. Next, decide which of these topics are relevant to your search. If there are several, it will help to write them down. Next, find the section or the volume that has the references listed alphabetically by topic. Locate your topic and scan for titles of likely articles. Figure 5.2 shows an excerpt from the *International Nursing Index*. Note that journal names are abbreviated. If you need the full title, check the index's list of indexed journals and their abbreviations. If the title appears in brackets it has been translated into English.

Computer-Assisted Literature Searches

A computer-assisted literature search uses a computer to search through the references, keywords, and in some cases the abstracts of all the articles, reports, and books in a particular **data base.** Any of the references that meet the criteria you have set will be printed for you immediately or mailed to you within a few days. The MEDLINE (medicine, nursing, and hospital articles), PSYCH ABSTRACTS (books, reports, and articles), and ERIC (education books and reports) data bases have been in use since the mid-60s. They require the assistance of a specially trained librarian using a terminal that is connected via telephone lines to a large computer that contains the particular data base. Personal microcomputer data bases might be useful for more limited searches if access to the larger systems is not feasible.

A computer-assisted search is best used when the topic is well defined, but the literature is apt to be located in many journals. If the

_____ Figure 5.2 _____

READING AN INDEX CITATION

THE INTERNATIONAL NURSING INDEX (1986)

FEVER **(1)**
  see related
    ANALGESICS, . . . **(2)**
    CHEMICALLY INDUCED **(3)**

    . . .
    DIAGNOSIS

    . . .

    . . .
    DRUG THERAPY

    . . .

    . . .
    ETIOLOGY

    . . .

    . . .

    . . .
    NURSING **(3)**

    . . .
    Relationship of routine assessment of temperature and febrile illness. **(4)**
    Nations L. E. **Rehabil Nurs** 1986 Sep–Oct; 11(5):18–20.

    (5)   **(6)**   **(7)**   **(8)**   **(9)**

    . . .

    . . .

    . . .
    PHYSIOPATHOLOGY

    _____
    . . . = a reference
    (1) Main heading
    (2) Related main headings to search if relevant
    (3) Subheadings
    (4) Title of article
    (5) Author
    (6) Journal
    (7) Year
    (8) Volume and issue
    (9) Pages

topic is too broad or ill defined you will receive many references that are not applicable. For example, a search for all articles that used the terms "stress" and/or "coping" would probably yield hundreds of references per year. You would therefore have to modify the search to specific groups, ages, years, and so on. On the other hand, if you are relatively certain that most references will appear in only a few journals, it is more efficient simply to review the annual indexes of those particular journals.

In the example of the cross-cultural uses of the DDST search, we worked with the librarian and searched the three data bases named above. Less extensive data bases are less expensive, and might suit your purposes just as well. Your librarian can advise you on this. The MEDLINE and PSYCH ABSTRACTS searches both yielded a few relevant articles. There was some duplication between these data bases, but there were unique references in each search. The ERIC data base was also searched, but no relevant references were found. One reference from each of these searches is shown in Figure 5.3.

Note that each has a slightly different style, but that the same information is given for each. ERIC and PSYCH ABSTRACTS both have document retrieval numbers so that you could order the reference directly if it looks relevant to you. Note also the typing error (last name of the author) in the PSYCH ABSTRACTS reference. This points out the fallibility of the system, which is only as good as the quality of the information put into it. If titles or abstracts are not inclusive or specific, then a relevant article can be missed. In this search we looked for the terms, "Denver Developmental Screening" and/or "DDST." If the spacing or spelling were incorrect in the abstract, or if the text *per se* was not mentioned, or if it was titled in another way, then the reference would not be pulled and printed.

Thus, computer-assisted searches are a powerful tool for identifying relevant articles when the topic is very specific. They do cost money, however. Your librarian can give you an estimate. The more specific the search is, the cheaper it will be. The DDST searches were $10.00 to $20.00 each. If you are going to base nursing care on the findings of a review, then that is a good investment.

Note Taking and Record Keeping

It is very easy to get lost while doing a review of the literature. You have to be meticulous in your attention to detail and still maintain the perspective needed to address the relatively broad purpose of the review. Fortunately there are some techniques, both time honored and based on new technology, that can help immensely with this task. These strategies fall into several loose groups—keeping track of references, note taking, and compiling results. The key to all of these techniques is to be as systematic and complete as possible.

_____ *Figure 5.3* _____

READING COMPUTER-ASSISTED LITERATURE SEARCHES FOR 1983 DDST SEARCH EXCERPTS

MEDLINE

7 **(1)**
AU —Fleming J **(2)**
TI   —An evaluation of the use of the Denver Developmental Screening Test. **(3)**
SO —Nurs Res 1981 Sep–Oct; 30(5) : 290–3
      ‿‿‿ ‿‿ ‿‿‿‿‿ ‿‿‿
      (5)   **(8)**   **(6)**   **(7)**

PSYCH ABSTRACTS

9 **(1)**
AN 07122 68–4. 8210. **(4)**
AU SOLOMOS–HOPE–C. **(2)**
TI   CROSS-CULTURAL NORMS FOR INFANT DEVELOPMENT SCREENING. **(3)**
SO INTERNATIONAL JOURNAL OF REHABILITATION RESEARCH.
     ‿‿‿‿‿‿‿‿‿‿‿‿‿‿‿‿‿‿‿‿‿‿‿‿‿‿‿‿‿‿‿‿
                          (5)

1981 DEC VOL 4(4) 531.
‿‿‿‿ ‿‿‿‿‿‿ ‿‿
(8)   **(6)**   **(7)**

ERIC (EDUCATION AND INFORMATION RESEARCH CENTER)

1 **(1)**
AN EJ274444. **(4)**
AU Fewell, Rebecca R.: and Others. **(2)**
TI   Informant versus Direct Screening: A Preliminary Comparative Study. **(3)**
SO Diagnostique; v7 n3 p 163–67 Spr 1982. 82.
     ‿‿‿‿‿‿‿‿ ‿‿‿‿ ‿‿‿‿‿‿ ‿‿‿‿
     (5)   **(6)**   **(7)**   **(8)**

_____

(1) Computer-generated reference number for this particular search
(2) Author
(3) Title of article
(4) Reference number for reprints or microfiche directly from this data base
(5) Journal
(6) Volume and issue number
(7) Page numbers
(8) Year

References   Several ways to record bibliographic information are to use index cards, reference lists, the printout from a computerized search, or a reprint on which you write notes. The purpose of all these methods is to be able to locate the reference and also to communicate to others where you obtained your information. If possible, you should stay with one system for the entire search.

The essential information needed for all references is

— Author

— Title of article, chapter and/or book, or report

— Date

— Publication details; that is, journal or publisher, volume and number of periodical

— Pages

You might decide to keep track of other things as well, such as the author's address and affiliation, or the general topic area covered in the piece. You will find it easier in the long run if you always write or enter this information using the style of the American Psychological Association (1984), the one most frequently used in nursing research journals and psychology. Medical journals usually use another style, but the same information is included. Whatever style you use, learn to do it well and you will seldom have the annoying problem of not being able to locate the same reference at a later date. Examples of an article and a book in APA style are

> Thomas, S. P. (1986). A descriptive profile of Type B personality. *Image: Journal of Nursing Scholarship, 18,* 4–7.
>
> Glaser, B. G. (1978). *Theoretical sensitivity.* Mill Valley, Calif.: Sociology Press.

If you want to report on your review in writing, it is worth the effort to do the references in letter-perfect APA style from the beginning, to save rewriting and corrections later.

Many people use cards for recording their references. They are easy to carry and sort for use in the library or by a typist. You can also put a few notes on a card. A problem with cards is that many of the articles you think might be good do not fit within your purpose once you scan them; you can therefore spend a great deal of time making out cards that are not useful later. Another problem with cards is their size. They do not hold many notes, so if the article does seem relevant, you will have to switch to another system of note taking or start using multiple cards for each reference.

Other people use the original reference list such as that from a computerized search or a personal photocopy of the references from a review article or index. This can be awkward if the list is long. For example, it is most convenient to find all *American Journal of Nursing* references at one time when you have located that section of the stacks. Leafing through pages of printout or reprinted indexes is slow. People who use this method usually scan the article as they locate it in the stacks and then photocopy it for later critical reading. If you use this method, be sure to note why likely articles are not used in the review. Keep the notes with the lists of references, and as soon as an article or chapter is photocopied, the reference in APA style can be written at the top of the first page. A few journals will have all the necessary information in the article, but many do not. It is easy, for example, to lose track of the exact page numbers in the process of photocopying.

Note Taking Before you start to read the articles, reports, or books, you should have a list of what to look for to guide you. You can add to this list as new critical elements emerge, and you can go back to check articles already reviewed to include the new criteria. You will find that the reference cards are not large enough in most cases. If you have photocopied each article, then you might want to make notations right on the photocopy. Some researchers prefer to make notes separately. As you read you will find that expected and unexpected themes and ideas come to mind. Write them all down. You might keep a log. Burke likes to highlight on the reprint and then to make comments with self-adhesive notes on the article. These can then be rearranged by topic or idea for the report. Whatever system you prefer, use it for each article.

Compiling Results The time-honored method of compiling results is the construction of a table such as Table 5.1. This lists all the critical aspects of each study and begins to allow you to view the body of literature as a whole. Burke has recently begun to use an integrated software system's data base to compile such tables for literature review. Fields for each of the relevant categories to be looked for in each article are developed—for example, author, date, sample size, type of design, nursing diagnosis of subjects, variables, data collection tools, statistics used—and the findings for each article are entered as the article is read. As trends and relationships begin to emerge, tables of the relevant categories can be screened or printed for analysis. Furthermore, anything that can be logically counted can be displayed in

_____ Figure 5.4 _____

RESEARCH STUDIES PER YEAR ON CHRONICALY ILL OR DISABLED
CHILDREN IN SIX NURSING JOURNALS

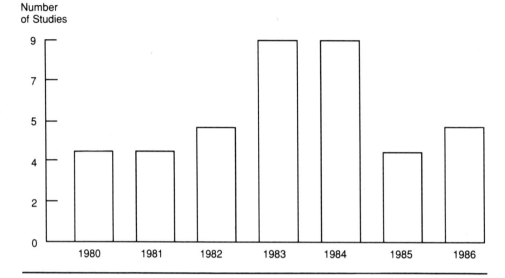

a graphic that is relatively simple to generate from such a data base. Figure 5.4 shows the number of research studies per year on a particular topic that was recently compiled by Burke (1987). It makes a clear point that the volume of studies in the particular area is not on the increase. This table was generated by using the computerized data base within the integrated software package Enable. Some other integrated software packages include DBaseIII, Lotus, and Symphony.

Secondary Sources

A **secondary source** is a report of the findings of one person by another person. In research literature reviews, this technically occurs whenever an author reports on the literature reviewed. However, usually the literature reviewed is available to you as well, and, if you check it yourself, it is no longer a secondary source. Literature that you have reviewed directly is a **primary source.** Occasionally, the author refers to unpublished material or to personal conversations or correspondence that you cannot easily confirm yourself.

The problem with secondary sources is the same one you probably encountered as a child when you played the game of whispering a secret from person to person around a circle. The content changes slightly with each telling and the final version can be completely different from the original. Thus, journal editors dislike the use of uncheckable secondary sources in articles and urge authors to avoid them.

As a research consumer, you will often rely on secondary sources. You should keep in mind, however, that the possibility of misinterpretation is greater with such information. Furthermore, if nursing care is to be based on such findings or conclusions, the primary source should always be located and checked.

Published Literature Reviews

Scholarly nursing journals regularly publish critical, state of the science reviews of the literature on topics of interest to their readers. These can be very helpful as they integrate a body of knowledge. Such reviews are often done by persons with expertise in the area, and thus, they can offer a sophisticated level of criticism. You cannot simply take such critiques at face value, however. Each one should be reviewed, using the same criteria you would for a research report (Ganong, 1987). (See the next section and Table 5.2.) Depending on your critique of the review, you might be able to rely on the conclusions and only update your own review. However, if you are in doubt about the thoroughness, rigor, or the quality of the logic in the conclusions, then you will have to use the review with some caution, or conduct your own independent review. If the published review is old, then you will need to update the review of the literature yourself. This should be done by going back a year or two before the publication date because it can take a year or so for a review to appear in print.

For example, a nurse administrator who is writing a job description for a new position might find a review of the McCloskey article (1981) on the effects of nursing education on job effectiveness very helpful. After a critical review of the article, the administrator might decide that it seems to be scientifically sound and applicable to the particular clinical setting. However, it is old and thus a review from a year or so prior to 1981 forward would be needed to round out the review or add new perspectives. Conversely, a nurse on a ward with many older clients might be concerned about their nutrition and review the article by Moore, Guenter, and Bender (1986). While it is up-to-date and seems scientifically sound, the content focuses on tube feedings, parenteral nutrition, and cancer patients. Since these were not the type of patients of concern to the particular nurse, it would be decided that the review was not clinically applicable.

An example of a review that was viewed with caution after a critique was that by Fleming (1981). This was one of the articles identified in the DDST computerized search described earlier. While the article had some helpful conclusions, it did not address at least two of our concerns in enough detail. These concerns were the cross-cultural uses of the DDST and the problems of quantification used as a research tool. Thus, we did not rely on this article, but conducted an independent search and critique.

CRITIQUING THE RESEARCHER'S REVIEW OF THE LITERATURE

The researcher will have reviewed the literature in some depth and detail, but the whole will rarely appear in the published report. You will read only the concise conclusions of the presumably relevant portions of that review. It takes several readings of an article or report and some careful thought to determine if the reported review is scientifically adequate or clinically applicable. The questions in Table 5.2 will guide you in this process.

A study should have a scientifically adequate review of the literature in order for it to build on the current state of knowledge in a particular area. A review should also be scientifically adequate for it to

Table 5.2

EVALUATING A LITERATURE REVIEW

Scientific Adequacy	Clinical Applicability
Purpose	
Is the purpose of the review clear and closely related to the study question?	Is the purpose of the review clinically relevant to you?
Thoroughness	
Does it cover the critical aspects of the study, i.e., the phenomena, concepts, variables, measures, design, or analysis issues relevant to the study?	Does it represent a thorough coverage of the pertinent clinical issues relevant to the study?
Do you know of relevent work that is not included?	Are there critical clinical issues that are not mentioned?
Is it concise with content that is apropos to the study?	Does it have the depth of understanding of the clinical concepts necessary to be convincing?

_____ Table 5.2 _____

CONTINUED

Scientific Adequacy	Clinical Applicability
Logical Rigor	
Does it critique the strengths and weaknesses of the existing work?	Would a nurse with experience with the types of clients in the study conclude that the review was consistent with the state of knowledge in the field?
Does it include the contradictions and inconsistencies in the body of literature?	
Does it point out the gaps in the literature relevant to the study?	
Review Conclusions	
Does the review weave the literature's findings together to form logical conclusions about the state of knowledge?	Are the conclusions meaningful for your type of clients and the nature of your practice?
Do the conclusions formed clearly flow in to the study question?	
Are the conclusions reached at the end of the review clear and concise?	
Study Discussion and Conclusions	
Are the findings of the literature review compared and contrasted with the findings of the study?	Is the literature used to enhance and/or question the applicability of the study results to practice?
Qualitative Studies Only	
• Is the strategy for the use of the literature clear, i.e., will it be used at the onset to direct the study, used as data or used at the end in the discussion only?	Does the approach to the use of the literature add to the clinical usefulness of the study or detract from it?
Is the approach to the use of the literature consistent with type of qualitative study?	
Quantitative Studies Only	
Is the literature reviewed at the onset of the study and used to guide the design?	Have the clinically relevant issues in the literature review been woven into the discussion and conclusions?
Are the data collection tools, design, and analysis methods substantiated with references to pertinent literature?	
Is there a return to the literature as the findings are discussed and study conclusions are made?	

be clinically applicable. However, it is possible to have a review (and indeed an entire study) that, while scientifically adequate, is not clinically relevant to you and your practice. Therefore, the two columns in Table 5.2 detail pertinent questions to ask for both scientific adequacy and clinical applicability. You will probably wish to address the question of scientific adequacy first because if a review is not creditable in this regard, it is highly unlikely to have clinical applicability.

SUMMARY

To evaluate the research findings and theories on a particular topic, the research consumer, as well as the researcher, must be able to review critically a group of reports or articles in order to make conclusions that are both scientifically logical and clinically relevant. The steps involved in this process involve defining the topic and purpose, searching for relevant reports, selecting and critically reading the material, synthesizing and critiquing the body of literature, and making conclusions that answer the purpose of the review. The researcher or consumer of research may consult published literature reviews, conduct a manual search of indexes, or do a computer-assisted literature search. This chapter outlines various strategies that will aid the reviewer in keeping track of information and in organizing and synthesizing it.

EXERCISES

1. Using the excerpt from the Burke et al. article in Example 5.1, critique the scientific adequacy of the literature review. Use the first column of Table 5.2. Assume that it is a quantitative study.

2. Assume that you are a pediatric nurse working with Cree Indian children such as those in the study. Answer the clinical applicability questions in the second column of Table 5.2.

3. Assume that you are a pediatric nurse working with a population of children very much like those with whom the original DDST was developed. Answer the clinical applicability questions in Table 5.2.

4. Now assume that you work in an adult intensive care unit and answer the same clinical applicability questions.

5. How are your answers to Exercises 2, 3, and 4 different? Why is this?

6. How could the literature review have been changed to make it more scientifically convincing or more clinically applicable?

REFERENCES

American Psychological Association. (1984). *Publication Manual of the American Psychological Association,* 3rd ed. Washington, D.C.: American Psychological Association.

Applebaum, A. S. (1978). Validity of the revised Denver Developmental Screening Test for referred and non-referred samples. *Psychological Reports, 43,* 227–233.

Barnes, K. E., & Stark, A. (1975). The Denver Developmental Screening Test: A normative study. *American Journal of Public Health, 65,* 363–369.

Bell, M., & Gosselin, C. (1983). Early intervention in the Eastern Arctic. *The Canadian Journal of Mental Retardation, 33*(4), 14–18.

Bryant, G. M., & Davies, K. J. (1974). The effect of sex, social class and parity on achievement of Denver Developmental Screening Test items in the first year of life. *Developmental Medicine and Child Neurology, 16,* 485–493.

Burke, S. O. (1987). Caring for handicapped children: Has nursing research helped? Keynote address at the International Symposium on Clinical Pediatric Nursing Research, Montreal Children's Hospital and McGill University School of Nursing.

Burke, S. O.; Sayers, L. A.; Baumgart, A. J.; & Wray, J. (1985) Pitfalls in the cross-cultrual use of the Denver Developmental Screening Test: Cree Indian children. *Canadian Journal of Public Health, 76,* 303–307.

Cadman, D.; Chambers, L. W.; Walter, S. D.; Feldman, W.; Smith, K.; & Ferguson, K. (1984). The usefulness of the Denver Developmental Screening Test to predict kindergarten problems in a general community population. *American Journal of Public Health, 74,* 1093–1106.

Cahoon, M. (1973). Discussion of standardization of the French adaptation of the Denver Developmental Screening Test for use among French-speaking Canadians, presented by Monique Chevrefils. *Proceedings of the Colloquium on Nursing Research,* Part 3. Montreal: McGill University.

Chenitz, W. C., & Swanson, J. M. (1986). *From practice to grounded theory: Qualitative research in nursing.* Menlo Park, Calif.: Addison-Wesley.

Chevrefils, M. (1973). Standardization of the French adaptation of the Denver Developmental Screening Test for use among the French-speaking

Canadians. National Health Grant, Project No. 605-22-33. *Proceedings of the Colloquium on Nursing Research.* Montreal: McGill University.

Coons, C. E.; Frankenburg, W. K.; Fay, E. C.; Fandal, A. W.; Lefly, D. L.; & Ker, C. (1980). Preliminary results of a combined developmental/environmental screening project. In N. J. Anastasliow, W. K. Frankenburg, & A. W. Fandal, *Identifying the Developmentally delayed child.* Baltimore: University Park Press.

Crane, J.; Anderson, B.; Marshjall, R.; & Harvey, P. (1981). Subsequent physical and mental development in infants with positive contraction stress tests. *Journal of Reproductive Medicine, 26,* 113–118.

Davidson, P. W.; Willoughby, R. H.; O'Tuama, L. A.; Swisher, C. N.; & Benjamins, D. (1978). Neurological and intellectual sequelae of Reye's Syndrome. *American Journal of Mental Deficiencies, 82,* 353–541.

Erickson, M. L. (1976). *Assessment and management of developmental changes in children.* St. Louis: C. V. Mosby.

Field, P. A. & Morse, J. M. (1985). *Nursing research: The application of qualitative approaches.* Rockville, Md.: Aspen Systems.

Fleming, J. (1981). An evaluation of the use of the Denver Developmental Screening test. *Nursing Research, 30,* 290–293.

Fox, R. N., & Ventura, M. R. (1984). Efficiency of automated literature search mechanisms. *Nursing Research, 33,* 174–177.

Frankenburg, W. K., & Dodds, J. B. (1967). The Denver Developmental Screening Test. *Journal of Pediatrics, 71,* 181–191.

Frankenburg, W. K.; Dodds, J. B.; Fandal, A. W.; Kazuk, E.; & Cohrs, M. (1975). *Denver Developmental Screening Test, Reference manual,* Rev. ed. Denver: University of Colorado, Medical Center.

Ganong, L. H. (1987). Integrative reviews of nursing research. *Research in Nursing and Health, 10,* 1–11.

Glaser, B. G. (1978). *Theoretical sensitivity.* Mill Valley, Calif.: Sociology Press.

Harper, D. C., & Wacker, D. P. (1983). The efficiency of the Denver Developmental Screening Test with rural disadvantaged preschool children. *Journal of Pediatric Psychology, 8,* 273–283.

International Nursing Index (1986). New York: American Journal of Nursing Company.

Jaffe, M.; Harvel, J.; Goldberg, A.; Rudolph-Schnitzer, M.; & Winter, S. T. (1980). The use of the Denver Developmental Screening Test in infant welfare clinics. *Developmental Medicine and Child Neurology 1980, 22,* 55–60.

Kirkconnell, S. C., & Hicks, L. E. (1980). Residual effects of lead poisoning on Denver Developmental Screening Test Scores. *Journal of Abnormal Child Psychology, 8,* 257–267.

Lichenstein, R. (1981). Comparative validity of two preschool screening tests:

Correlational and classificational approaches. *Journal of Learning Disabilities, 14*(2), 68–72.

McCloskey, J. C. (1981). The effects of nursing education on job effectiveness: An overview of the literature. *Research in Nursing and Health, 4*, 355–373.

Majeres, R. L., & Timmer, T. (1981). Imitation preference as a function of motor competence. *Perceptual and Motor Skills, 52*, 175–180.

Meier, J. H. (1975). Screening, assessment and intervention for young children at developmental risk. In N. Hobbs (Ed.) *Issues in the classification of children*, Vol. 2. San Francisco: Jossey-Bass.

Mercer, J. R., & Lewis, J. F. (1978). *SOMPA: System of multicultural pluralistic assessment*. New York: The Psychological Corporation.

Miller, V.; Onotera, R. T.; &, Deinard, A. S. (1984). Denver Developmental Screening Test: Cultural variations in Southeast Asian children. *Journal of Pediatrics, 104*, 481–482.

Moore, M. C.; Guenter, P. A.; & Bender, J. Hogan. (1986). Nutrition-related nursing research. *Image: Journal of Nursing Scholarship, 18*, 18–21.

Morrison, T. L., & Newcomer, B. L. (1975). Effects of directive vs. non-directive play therapy with institutionalized mentally retarded children. *American Journal of Mental Deficiencies, 79*, 666–669.

Morrison, D., & Pothier, P. (1972). Two different remedial motor training programs and the development of mentally retarded pre-schoolers. *American Journal of Mental Deficiencies, 77*, 251–258.

Newton, J. B. (1973). Screening the preschool and school child: The Leduc-Strathcona Health Unit Program. *Canadian Journal of Public Health, 64*, 374–379.

Nugent, J. H. (1976). A comment on the efficiency of the Revised Denver Developmental Screening Test. *American Journal of Mental Deficiencies, 80*, 570–572.

Olade, R. A. (1984). Evaluation of the Denver Developmental Screening Test as applied to African children. *Nursing Research, 33*, 204–207.

Pless, I. B., & Douglas, J. W. B. (1971). Chronic illness in childhood. Part 1. Epidemiological and clinical characteristics. *Journal of Pediatrics, 47*, 405–414.

Rothenberg, P. B., & Varga, P. E. (1981). The relationship between age and mother and child health and development. *American Journal of Public Health, 7*, 810–817.

Sandler, L.; DeLessen, O.; Cohen, L.; Emkey, K.; & Keith, H. (1971). Developmental test responses and test behavior of disadvantaged children in get-set programs. *American Journal of Orthopsychiatry, 41*, 324–325.

Sandler, L.; Jamison, D.; Deliser, O.; Cohen, L.; Emkey, K.; & Keith, H. (1970).

Developmental test performance of disadvantaged children. *Exceptional Children, 39*(3), 201–208.

Sandler, L.; Van Campen, J.; Ratner, C.; Stafford, D.; & Weismar, R. (1970). Responses of urban preschool children to a developmental screening test. *Journal of Pediatrics, 77,* 775–781.

Shapira, T., & Harel, S. (1983). Standardization of the Denver Developmental Screening Test for Israeli children. *Israel Journal of Medical Sciences, 19,* 246–251.

Solomons, G., & Solomons, H. C. (1975). Motor development in Yucatan infants. *Developmental Medicine and Child Neurology, 17,* 41–46.

Solomons, H. C. (1982). Standardization of the Denver Developmental Screening Test on infants from Yucatan, Mexico. *International Journal of Rehabilitation Research, 5*(2), 179–189.

Song, J.; Zhu, Y.; & Gu, X. (1982). Restandardization of the Denver Developmental Screening Test for Shanghai children. *Chinese Medical Journal, 95,* 375–380.

Sturner, R. A.; Horton, M.; Funk, S. G.; Barton, J.; Frothingham, T. E.; & Cress, J. N. (1982). Adaptation of the Denver Developmental Screening Test: A study of preschool screening. *Pediatrics, 69*(3), 346–350.

Ueda, R. (1978). Child development in Okinawa compared with Tokyo and Denver, and the implications for developmental screening. *Developmental Medicine and Child Neurology, 20,* 657–663.

Werner, E. E. (1972). Review of Denver Developmental Screening Test. In O. K. Buros (Ed.) *Seventh mental measurements yearbooks.* Highland Park, N.J.: Gryphon Press.

Whaley, L. F., & Wong, D. L. (1983). *Nursing care of infants and children.* St. Louis: C. V. Mosby.

Williams, P. O. (1984). The Metro-Manila Developmental Screening Test: A normative study. *Nursing Research, 33,* 208–212.

6

Research Design: Identification and Evaluation

INTRODUCTION

Simply stated, a research design is the set of logical steps taken by the researcher to answer the research problem. The design forms the blueprint for the study and determines the methods used by the researcher to obtain subjects, collect data, analyze the data, and interpret the results. The research design flows directly from the research question and the specific purpose of the study.

In this chapter, we will discuss the two broad types of nursing research design: experimental and nonexperimental.

OBJECTIVES

After reading this chapter, you will be able to

1. Identify common nursing research designs.
2. Discuss the relationship of the research design to the research question.
3. Identify common problems (risks to validity) inherent in the various types of research designs.
4. Evaluate the effectiveness (internal and external validity) of a design used in a nursing research study.

NEW TERMS

Levels of inquiry
Experimental design
Manipulation
Control
Randomization
Extraneous variables
Pretest-posttest control
  group design
Posttest-only control
  group design
Solomon four-group
  design
Factorial design
Factors
Hawthorne effect

Double-blind techniques
External validity
Mortality
Quasi-experimental
  design
Nonequivalent control
  group design
Time series design
History
Maturation
Testing effect
Multiple time series
  design
Nonexperimental design
Descriptive design

Ex post facto design
Informants
Subjects
Historical research
Evaluation research
Cross-sectional studies
Longitudinal studies
Retrospective studies
Prospective studies
Meaning
Subjectivity
Lack of context
Internal validity

HOW RESEARCHERS SELECT A DESIGN: LEVELS OF INQUIRY

The research design flows directly from the particular research question and the specific purpose of the study. The highlighted area of Figure 6.1 depicts this interrelationship. Often the reader of a research report or proposal can infer much about the design of the project by simply reading the stated question. Let us look at the following examples.

- ① What is the nature of the life experiences of elderly persons when they are relocating into a retirement home?

- ② What are the most common concerns expressed by elderly persons applying for relocation into retirement homes?

- ③ What is the relationship between expressed concerns of elderly persons applying for entry to retirement homes and their expressed level of self-esteem?

- ④ Does a pre-admission support program increase self-esteem in elderly persons upon entering a retirement home?

These four questions all deal with feelings and concerns of elderly persons relocating to retirement living. The questions are examples of various **levels of inquiry** that can be used in a nursing research study. The level of inquiry at which the question is stated corresponds with the level of sophistication of nursing knowledge concerning the variables in the study. All four questions above attempt to increase nursing knowledge. The best studies, from the clinical point of view, set the level of inquiry so that the results add to, or clarify, what is already known. Each question, however, requires different information to provide an answer.

The first question is used if very little is known about the concepts that are the focus of the study, or if little is known about the nature of the entire situation surrounding the concepts. This type of question is also asked when there is reason to suspect that current theories or beliefs about the phenomenon are not correct. The researcher may not even be sure of the precise variables involved in the study. For example, what are the variables involved in the experiences of elderly persons at the time of entering a retirement home? Could the variables be mobility, self-esteem, the ability to communicate, or the quality of their spousal relationships? A nonexperimental, qualitative study could help to ferret out possible variables and to uncover the meaning of these variables for future studies.

_____ Figure 6.1 _____

RESEARCH PROCESS FLOWCHART

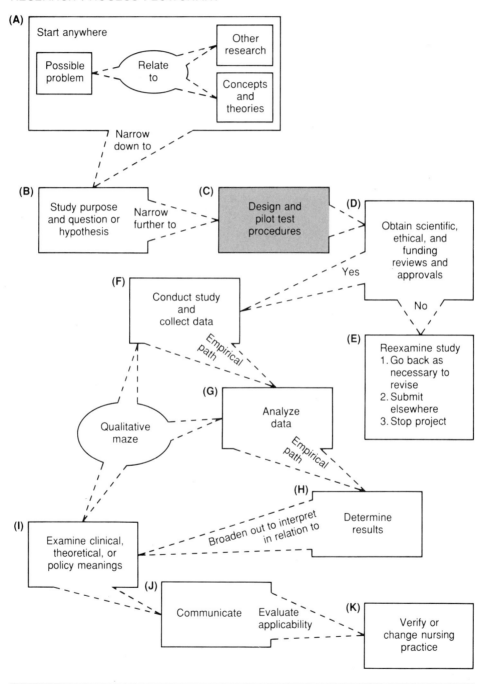

The second question seeks to uncover information about the kind and number of concerns expressed by elderly persons. Purely descriptive data is needed about one set of variables (concerns) to answer the question. For this type of study some knowledge of the situation, and of some of the likely concerns, is needed. This information might come from clinical knowledge, or it might be evident from a literature review.

The third question involves two variables—concerns and self-esteem—and asks if there is a relationship between them. If the researcher has sufficient information about concerns from a study of the second question, or from reviewing the literature, an examination can be done to ascertain whether concerns are in some way associated with self-esteem. At this level there would not be enough information actually to explain or predict the nature of the relationship between the two variables; however, the researcher can explore the existence of a relationship.

The fourth question assumes a more theoretical understanding of the topic. This question aims to explain the theoretical relationship between two variables—the presence of a particular support program and level of self-esteem. This kind of question can lead the researcher to a design in which predictions are made and hypotheses are tested.

In summary, the first three questions are seeking descriptive knowledge of the variables. The most appropriate study design would use nonexperimental or quasi-experimental methods. The last question assumes that a great deal of information is already known about the variables and the relationship between them. This question demands a more structured, experimental approach.

DETERMINING STUDY DESIGN BY LEVEL OF INQUIRY

There is a close interrelationship between the level of inquiry of a study's question, the state of nursing knowledge at the onset of the study, and the possible methods and type of study design. The two major complementary approaches to research—qualitative and quantitative—are both represented in Table 6.1. There are four somewhat arbitrary groupings of types of designs in the table. The state of development of the conceptual background and the relative quantitative/qualitative focus of the design form four levels (Brink & Wood, 1988) that exist along a continuum (Field & Morse, 1985). Thus, there can be some overlap between the rows of the table. For example,

_____ Table 6.1 _____ *See design tree in notes* _____

THE RELATIONSHIP OF RESEARCH QUESTION TO RESEARCH DESIGN

Level of Inquiry[2]	Stem of Question[3]	Number of Variables	Conceptual Background	Type of Design	Possible Designs
1	What is the nature of the phenomena?	(To be determined in the course of the study)	Little known about phenomena, possible bias in current theories	Qualitative[1]	Phenomenologic, ethnographic, ethnologic, and ethnoscientific designs
2	Who, what, how many, how much, etc.?	One or many	Little knowledge of specific aspects of the variable	Quantitative: Non-experimental	Descriptive and ex post facto survey designs
3	What are the relationships (if any) among the variables?	Two or more	Some knowledge, but action of variables not always predict-able. Usually there is a conceptual framework.	Quantitative: Quasi-experimental[3]	Nonequivalent control group; time series; one group, pretest-posttest designs
4	Does one variable cause the other?	Two or more	Conceptual framework or theory	Quantitative: Experimental[3]	Pretest-posttest and control group designs

_____

[1] Qualitative section based on Field and Morse (1985).

[2] Quantitative sections adapted from Brink and Wood (1988), who refer to our levels 2–4 as I, II, and III, respectively.

[3] Quasi-experimental and experimental sections are based on Cook and Campbell (1979).

Handwritten annotations: CAN BE VALID; "discover"; can be >1; LEAST VALID; Obj. + purpose; I.V. → to uncover new knowledge; one at a time; freq.; 2nd MOST VALID; at same time; e.v. how much listing about phenomena; may help to ferret out poss. variables for future studies; (manet but not enpeer grp); MOST VALID; assumes something; Cause & Effect; only one to look @ causality; SEE p146; Solomon; → life exper; → from subjects perspective; → theory specific; → socially; → how subjects view their world from way they talk about; → after the fact

the form the question takes, and the method actually selected for a study, may skip to the row above or below on the table and still be considered acceptable. However, it is more likely that the question and the design fit well with each other if they are at the same row of the table, or the same level of inquiry, and thus at the same place on the continuum. If all the elements of the study are not on the same row of the table, you will need to examine more closely whether the design is at the appropriate level.

Table 6.1 will help you to determine the design of the study you are reading and to make an initial determination of the fit between the level of the study question and the design that the investigator has chosen. Often the wording of the question in the study will be similar to the wording in Table 6.1 or to the examples given in the preceding section. Thus, you will be able to fit most questions into one of these basic groupings. As an additional clue, the level of development of the concepts and theories at the onset of the study and the number of variables will help you to determine the level of the question in the study. You may, however, have difficulty identifying the type of question and design you are reading about if synonyms are used and if the writer refers to less common terms that are not included in this table. If the study methods (the data collection and analysis plan) are not in the table, then check the terms in the Glossary at the back of this book for a synonym to help you determine the level of the question and design.

_____ *COMMON RESEARCH DESIGNS* _____

The sample questions, text discussion, and Table 6.1 provide an overview of frequently used nursing research designs. Each of the four types of design will be explained in more detail in the following sections, starting with the quantitative designs at the bottom of Table 6.1 and working up to the qualitative designs at the top of the table.

Experimental design is presented first because its characteristics are somewhat more distinct, and thus easier to identify as you are learning. Quasi-experimental design, probably the most commonly published type of design in nursing research, is described next. It has some, but not all, of the characteristics of experimental design. Next, quantitative, nonexperimental designs, which are also frequently published, will be described. Finally, qualitative, nonexperimental designs, which are increasingly found in the nursing research literature, will be discussed. Qualitative designs can easily be confused with the descriptive nonexperimental quantitative designs, but are differentiated by the very different philosophy from which they emerge.

Experimental Designs

Experimental design differs from nonexperimental approaches primarily in that the researcher can control the action of the specific variables being studied. In a study with an experimental design, the researcher controls or manipulates the action of the independent or causal variable(s) and observes and measures the action or outcome on the dependent variable(s). Until recent years, experimental designs were not prevalent in the nursing research literature because many research problems required the study of questions at the second (descriptive) and third (quasi-experimental) levels of inquiry in order to build more theoretical background before level four, hypothesis-testing questions, could be examined. However, experimental-type designs are beginning to take their place in the nursing research literature.

Experimental nursing research is often the most logically applicable to clinical practice. Many factors, however, limit the extent to which purely experimental approaches can be used in nursing research, most notably, the fact that the subjects and settings are human. Studying human beings usually limits the researcher's control over the variables involved. For example, it would be unethical for a researcher to control the amount of smoking in human subjects if smoking was to be the independent or causal variable in an experimental design.

Campbell and Stanley (1966), in their classic work on experimental and quasi-experimental design, provide an excellent discussion of this type of research. A true experimental design allows the researcher to have maximum control over the independent variable(s) in the study. In order to carry out a true experiment three conditions are necessary.

1. **Manipulation:** It must be possible for the researcher to manipulate the action of the independent variable.
2. **Control:** The researcher must be able to exercise control in the experimental situation by eliminating the actions of other possible variables beyond the independent variable. This control can be achieved through using control groups.
3. **Randomization:** The researcher must select subjects randomly from the population and randomly assign them to control and experimental groups.

Example 6.1 illustrates the concepts of manipulation, control, and randomization.

Example 6.1 shows that the researchers manipulated the independent variable—the health promotion intervention—by giving only one group of patients the special experimental treatment.

The use of a control group of patients who did not receive the experimental health promotion intervention provides the basis of comparison necessary to evaluate the outcome behaviors or dependent variable. If no control group had been used, the researchers could not be

___ Example 6.1 ___

EXPERIMENTAL DESIGN TO STUDY
HEALTH PROMOTION

In Ventura, et al. (1984) the conceptual framework is developed using a health promotion intervention based upon a process/outcome model of adult learning theory. This intervention was tested with subjects who attended a diagnostic and follow-up vascular laboratory. Eighty-six patients participated in the study. Forty-two patients were randomly assigned to an experimental group and received the special health promotion intervention. Forty-four patients were randomly assigned to a control group which did not receive the special intervention. All patients were assessed for certain health-related behaviors prior to the study, and at the conclusion of the study. Changes in behavior were measured, and experimental and control groups were compared.

See Ventura, M. R.; Young, D. E.; Feldman, M. J.; Pastore, P.; Pikula, S.; & Yates, M. A. (1984). Effectiveness of health promotion interventions. _Nursing Research, 33_(3), 162–167.

reasonably certain that it was the experimental treatment that had made a difference in the outcome variable. Subjects in the control group should be from the same population as those in the experimental group and thus be as similar as possible to the experimental group.

The random assignment to control and experimental groups assists in eliminating the effect of **extraneous variables** (those not under study) on the outcome. Random assignment can be done in several ways. The key factor is that each person (subject) in the larger group being studied (a representative group or population) has an equal chance of being selected to be in one of the study groups. The concept of randomization is discussed in more detail in Chapter 8 on sampling. Randomization is inextricably linked with experimental study design. It increases the chances that the sample is an unbiased, representative group.

In most nursing studies, circumstances do not permit the researcher to randomly select a sample from the entire population that is the focus of the study. Hence, a representative, convenience sample is chosen. However, the researcher can randomly assign this available portion of the population to experimental and control groups to promote the homogeneous composition of both groups for comparison purposes. Although rarely possible, the ideal situation in a true experiment occurs when subjects are randomly selected from the population and then randomly assigned to control and experimental groups. In Example 6.1, random assignment was to study groups from a clinic group. However, it was not clear in the report whether there was random selection of the sample from the entire population (that is, all persons with vascular problems), which should be done for a true experiment.

Campbell and Stanley (1966) identify three basic true experimental designs that we will discuss here briefly using their notation system:

— 0 = dependent variable measurement
— X = application of the independent variable
— R = random assignment

Figures 6.2–6.4 and Figures 6.6–6.8 are all represented with a left to right time line.

Pretest-Posttest Control Group Design   The classic **pretest-posttest control group design** is one of the most commonly observed in the literature and is the design used for the Ventura et al. experiment described in Example 6.1. This design is shown diagramatically in Figure 6.2.

____ *Figure 6.2* ____

PRETEST-POSTTEST CONTROL GROUP DESIGN

	TIME LINE OF STUDY EVENTS			
	Randomization	Pretest	Experiment	Posttest
GROUPS				
Experimental	R	O	X	O
Control	R	O		O

O = dependent variable measurement
X = application of the independent variable
R = random assignment to experimental or control group

Source: Based on Campbell, D. T., & Stanley, J. C. (1966). *Experimental and quasi-experimental designs for research.* Chicago: Rand McNally (pp. 8, 13).

Not all true experiments employ the use of pretests. Pretesting provides the researcher with information about the similarity of experimental and control groups on measures of the dependent variable before the independent variable is introduced. For example, Ventura et al. pretested health behaviors in experimental and control groups before introducing the health promotion intervention.

Posttest-Only Control Group Design   Campbell and Stanley (1966) maintain that use of pretesting is not always necessary when randomization is used since the inherent purpose of randomization is homogeneous composition of control and experimental groups. In many nursing studies it may be inappropriate or impossible to pretest before the independent variable is manipulated. Suppose a researcher wished to study the effect of a particular nursing intervention on the incidence of postoperative vomiting following hysterectomy. It would be difficult, and certainly inappropriate, to develop and induce a pretest of vomiting behavior. However, provided a random sample of hysterectomy subjects undergoing the same medical treatments and anesthesia that could be randomly assigned to control and experimental groups, the **posttest-only control group design** could be an appropriate design to use to study this problem. The posttest-only control group design is a true experimental design, which is diagramed in Figure 6.3.

Solomon Four-Group Design   Another experimental design that can be used by the researcher in studying particular problems where the pretest may influence the outcome of the dependent variable is called

Figure 6.3

POSTTEST-ONLY CONTROL GROUP DESIGN

TIME LINE OF STUDY EVENTS

	Randomization	Experiment	Posttest

GROUPS			
Experimental	R	X	O
Control	R		O

Source: Based on Campbell, D. T., & Stanley, J. C. (1966). *Experimental and quasi-experimental designs for research.* Chicago: Rand McNally (pp. 8, 25).

_____ Figure 6.4 _____

SOLOMON FOUR-GROUP DESIGN

TIME LINE OF STUDY EVENTS			
Randomization	Pretest	Experiment	Posttest

GROUPS

	Randomization	Pretest	Experiment	Posttest
1. Experimental	R	O	X	O
2. Control	R	O		O
3. Experimental	R		X	O
4. Control	R			O

Source: Based on Campbell, D. T., & Stanley, J. C. (1966). *Experimental and quasi-experimental designs for research.* Chicago: Rand McNally (pp. 8, 24).

the **Solomon four-group design.** This design allows the researcher to control for the effect of the pretest. Suppose a researcher wished to study the effect of a course designed to increase staff nurses' favorable attitudes toward using nursing research in practice. Administering a pretest on nurses' attitudes prior to the course may in itself have some influence on how nurses perceive the course and how they answer the posttest attitude questionnaire. By combining the pretest-posttest control group design with the posttest-only control group design to form the Solomon four-group design, the researcher can control the effect of the pretest. This design is diagramed in Figure 6.4.

In this experimental design, subjects are randomly selected from the population, then randomly assigned to four groups. Two groups receive pretests and two groups do not. The researcher can thus observe any interaction of the pretest.

Factorial Design   A fourth experimental design is classified as the **factorial design.** This design allows the researcher to test the effect of more than one independent variable in the same experiment. The independent variables are referred to as **factors,** and both the individual and combined effect of factors can be measured. This design incorporates the elements of a true experiment: randomization, control, and manipulation; it can also involve the use of a pretest. The researcher randomly assigns subjects to groups that receive various combinations of the independent variables. This design is frequently used in nursing research to study various combinations of interventions.

_____ Figure 6.5 _____

FACTORIAL DESIGN

TIME LINE OF STUDY EVENTS

| Randomization | Experimental factor combination | Posttest |

GROUPS
1.	R	X_{a1}	O
2.	R	X_{a2}	O
3.	R	X_{b1}	O
4.	R	X_{b2}	O

Source: Based on Campbell, D. T. & Stanley, J. C. (1966). *Experimental and quasi-experimental designs for research.* Chicago: Rand McNally (p. 26).

For example, Damrosch (1981) used a factorial design to examine how nursing students' reactions to rape victims are affected by a perceived act of carelessness. The students were randomly assigned to read four different versions of the circumstances surrounding a rape case. All information in the accounts was the same with the following exceptions: The first group read that the rape occurred at 10 p.m. and the victim's car door was locked. The second group read that the rape occurred at midnight and the car door was locked. A third group read that the rape occurred at 10 p.m., but the car door was unlocked; and the fourth group read that the rape occurred at midnight and the car door was unlocked.

This study employs two factors—X_a, time of rape and X_b, condition of the car door—with two levels (X_1 and X_2) tested for each factor. See Figure 6.5, where these combinations are represented with X_{a1}, X_{a2}, X_{b1}, and X_{b2}. With more factors, and more levels for each factor tested, more subject groups are needed to test the combinations. Therefore, experiments testing more than three or four factors are often not practical because of the large number of subjects required.

Strengths of Experimental Designs (2)

The major strength of an experimental design lies in the researcher's ability to manipulate the independent variable and control for the unwanted or unknown effects of variables on the outcome or dependent variable(s). The researcher can make predictions about the cause and effect with some assurance.

In Chapter 2 we examined the concept of *causality* as being central to the scientific method and the nursing research process. The level of research question and the design used to obtain answers to that question are closely related to the degree of cause that can be attributed to the results of a study. We identified four factors that scientists commonly identify as causal factors in interpreting events: <u>association, time priority, nonspurious relation, and rationale</u> (Labovitz & Hagedorn, 1981). These factors can be present in any level of inquiry, but are most often seen in experimental (level 4) designs.

(a) **Association** The concept of association in quantitative research is statistical in nature, and denotes the degree of relationship between two events. If two variables show a strong statistical relationship, in other words, if they vary together, the criterion of association is demonstrated. Level 3 questions attempt to show such associations.

An example is provided in the Burke et al. (1985) study of the use of the Denver Developmental Screening Test (DDST) with Cree Indian children. The following question was asked: Does the DDST produce developmental results that are similar to other measures of developmental status? One of the other measures of developmental status was the Minnesota Child Development Inventory (MCDI). Developmental scores for both the DDST and the MCDI were compared statistically and were found to be related to each other. In other words, children in the study sample with higher DDST scores tended to have higher MCDI scores and vice versa. The two developmental scores varied together.

(b) **Time Priority** For a causal relationship to exist between two variables, it is necessary to observe that one variable in a situation occurs, or changes, before the other. In some situations it is easy to observe this naturally. For example, if we look at the relationship between mother's smoking and low birth weight in infants, you can reasonably assume that mother's smoking occurred before the infant was born. The only sure way of establishing time priority of the variables is in the experimental situation, where the independent variable is manipulated by the researcher.

(c) **Nonspurious Relationships** To make causal statements about events, the researcher must be certain that changes in the dependent variable are the result of action of the independent variable, and not a third extraneous variable. If results can be explained by action of

variables other than the independent one, then the relationship is said
to be spurious. A nonspurious relation is most strongly assured in true
experimental designs. The ability to control for extraneous variables in
true experiments is maximized through randomization, control groups,
and manipulation.

ⓓ **Rationale** This fourth criterion relates to the conceptual or
theoretical underpinnings for hypothesized relationships. In Chapter 4
we discussed the purpose of theoretical and conceptual frameworks in
conceptualizing the problem and predicting how and why variables
should be related. All nursing research should be based upon sound
rationale; however, true experimental research most clearly demonstrates the predicted relationships between variables, the time priority
of variables, and the underlying mechanisms connecting the independent and dependent variables.

Problems with Experimental Designs ⟨2⟩

Although experimental designs are strong in explaining cause and
effect, the very controlled nature of the designs may present problems
for the nurse researcher in employing these designs in nursing practice.
①Ethical implications are involved when a researcher manipulates a
variable (see our discussion on maternal smoking and determining
causality in relation to low birth weight infants). From a practical
viewpoint, true experiments often require extra funds and are difficult
to conduct in natural settings such as hospitals.

The contrived nature of true experiments often sensitizes subjects and experimenters to hypothesized relationships and expected
behaviors. This sensitization is often referred to as the②**Hawthorne
effect.** Researchers attempt to control this effect through use of **double-
blind techniques** in which the subjects, and the researchers who
administer the experimental treatment, are both unaware of which
subjects are in the experimental group and which in the control. This
technique has been most effective in many pharmaceutical studies.

A second problem related to the contrived nature of true experiments is the difficulty of applying results to other populations and
settings. This concept of generalizability of research or③**external
validity** is discussed later in relation to all designs. However, there are
some particular implications for experimental designs. True experiments require rigid control, and it is often difficult to obtain and work
with large random samples in natural settings. A very small sample size,
coupled with contrived testing conditions, requires that results of true

experiments be interpreted with greater caution when implying causality to the larger nursing practice situation. Another danger that particularly threatens sample size, and therefore generalizability in true experiments, is loss of subjects from control and/or experimental groups. This effect is known as **mortality.** As used in research, this term does not necessarily mean death of subjects; it usually means that subjects have dropped out of the study for various reasons. This can have a devastating effect on generalizability for experiments running with an initially small sample size.

Quantitative, Quasi-experimental Designs (4)

Quasi-experimental designs are similar to experimental designs in that the researcher manipulates the independent variable. However, in a quasi-experiment the researcher omits some aspects of control that are observed in the true experiment. The researcher may omit a control group for comparison, or if a control group is used, the researcher may omit randomization in sampling and assignment to experimental and control groups.

Quasi-experimental designs are frequently used since nursing studies are usually conducted in natural, rather than laboratory settings, and therefore circumstances may not facilitate use of control groups and/or randomization. Referring to Table 6.1, you can see that quasi-experimental designs are usually at the third level of inquiry and are based upon a conceptual framework. However, because full experimental control is lacking, quasi-experiments do not provide the same assurance as true experiments in determining cause and effect between the independent and dependent variable(s).

There are a wide number of quasi-experimental designs outlined in the research literature. In fact, Campbell and Stanley (1966) present sixteen varieties. We have selected three of the most common types encountered in the nursing research literature to introduce you to the quasi-experimental type of design.

Nonequivalent Control Group Designs The most basic and most widely used quasi-experimental design in nursing research is the **nonequivalent control group design.** A nonequivalent control group can also be referred to as a comparison group. Upon reading a study employing this design, you may, at first, confuse it with the true experimental pretest-posttest control group design (see Figure 6.2). The nonequivalent control group design, however, does not use a control group with subjects from the same population as is done in experimental

_____ *Figure 6.6* _____

NONEQUIVALENT CONTROL GROUP DESIGN

TIME LINE OF STUDY EVENTS

| Pretest | Experiment | Posttest |

GROUPS			
Experimental	O	X	O
Comparison	O		O

Source: Based on Campbell, D. T. & Stanley, J. C. (1966). *Experimental and quasi-experimental designs for research.* Chicago: Rand McNally (p. 40).

studies. Furthermore, there is often no random selection or assignment of subjects to groups. In this design the researcher selects two samples from two similar available groups and, if randomization is done, it is within groups. The independent variable is administered to one group while the other group acts as a comparison. Figure 6.6 diagrams this design. Notice the absence of random assignment to groups as is shown in Figure 6.2. Measurements of the dependent variable before and after the introduction of the independent variable are compared for the experimental and control groups.

The study in Example 6.2 exemplifies the use of a nonequivalent control group design.

Campbell and Stanley (1966) point out that it is better to use a nonequivalent control group than no comparison group at all. Generally, the more similar the experimental and control groups, the less possibility there is of extraneous variables affecting the dependent variable. The similarity of groups can be assessed by comparing the pretest results. Lamontagne et al. (1985) note that both classes were selected from the same school to increase the chance of similarity in geographic area and socioeconomic status, and the initial pretest anxiety scores were very similar.

② **Time Series Design** The quasi-experimental **time series design** is an example of a quasi-experimental design that does not use either randomization or a comparison group. It is diagramatically represented in Figure 6.7. In this design the researcher collects data on the dependent variable from the experimental group at a set number

_____ Example 6.2 _____

USING A NONEQUIVALENT CONTROL GROUP
FOR COMPARISON

Lamontagne, Mason, and Hepworth (1985) studied the effect of a relaxation training program on anxiety reduction in young children. Children from two second-grade classrooms participated as subjects. Both classes were administered an anxiety pretest. Following this, one class received the relaxation training program while the other (comparison) class did not. Both classes were posttested on anxiety and results were compared. The researchers further strengthened this design by administering the relaxation program to the control group following the initial study, and then comparing anxiety levels with those obtained from the group while acting as a control. This can be diagramed as follows:

	Pretest	Program	Posttest	Program	Posttest
Experimental Class A	0	X	0		
Comparison Class B	0		0	X	0

See Lamontagne, L. L.; Mason, K. R.; & Hepworth, J. T. (1985). Effects of relaxation on anxiety in children: Implications for coping with stress. _Nursing Research, 34_(5), 289–292.

_____ Figure 6.7 _____

QUASI-EXPERIMENTAL TIME SERIES DESIGN

TIME LINE OF STUDY EVENTS

Pretests   Experiment   Posttests

GROUPS
Experimental   O   O   O   O   X   O   O   O   O

Source: Based on Campbell, D. T. & Stanley, J. C. (1966). _Experimental and quasi-experimental designs for research._ Chicago: Rand McNally (pp. 37, 40).

of periods of time, both before and after the introduction of the independent variable. No control group is used for comparison. The data collected prior to, and after, the introduction of the independent variable
are compared for differences in the dependent variable.

This design can be useful in many situations when no control
group is available. For example, suppose a nurse researcher wished to
study the effect of a primary nursing care system on the quality of
nursing care plans produced by nurses on a particular pediatric unit, and
no similar unit was reasonably available for comparison. The researcher
could design a time series study that would involve collecting data about
the quality of care plans completed at several points in time prior to the
introduction of the new system, perhaps monthly for a period of five
months. The new system then would be introduced and data on quality
of care plans examined at monthly intervals for the next five months
following its implementation.

The strength of this basic time series design lies in the repeated
data collection over periods of time before and after the independent
variable is introduced. Subjects act as their own "control," providing a
strong indication that the independent variable could be responsible for
observed change in the dependent variable.

The quasi-experimental time series design is considerably stronger than the one-group single pretest and single posttest, which is a
design classified by Campbell and Stanley as pre-experimental. In this
design only two observations of the dependent variable are carried out,
one before and one after the introduction of the independent variable.
Without randomization and the use of a control group, there is little
evidence to support the notion that the cause of change observed between the two observations is the result of the experiment.

Three possible problems surround the use of quasi-experimental
designs and the basic time series design in particular—history, maturation, and testing.

_a)_ **History** refers to extraneous variables that occur between the
testing periods and influence the action of the independent variable on
the dependent variable. In our example concerning the effect of primary
nursing on the quality of nursing care plans, many factors (extraneous
variables) are likely to be operating in addition to the change in method
of client care (independent variable). For example, staffing changes, new
administrative policies, or changes in client census could have profound
effects on quality of care plans. Two observations would present only a
very narrow picture. A time series design, covering extended periods of
time, helps to broaden the picture but, unfortunately, it does not totally
eliminate the threat of history.

b) **Maturation** is closely related to history. Maturation refers to those variables that affect change within subjects over time. For ex- △ *over* ample, subjects may change their perspective of events, or undergo *time* other emotional, intellectual, or biological change. The time series *eg IQ.* design, with repeated data collection times can reduce, but not eradicate, the possible impact of maturation on results.

The inherent strength of time-series designs, which resides in repeated measuring, can also prove to be a potential weakness. Repeated data collections from the same subjects over time can produce what is known as a **testing effect.** In this situation, repeated data collection or testing influences how subjects respond on subsequent tests. This is a special case of maturation where learning and sensitivity to experimental variables influence change in the dependent variable(s). The testing effect is similar to the Hawthorne effect that threatens true experiments. The testing effect is particularly threatening when subjects are required to answer the same questionnaire on several occasions. Familiarity and boredom, as well as any real changes over time, are apt to be reflected in the answers.

③ **Multiple Time Series Designs**   Campbell and Stanley present a more sophisticated version of the basic time series design, the **multiple** *sim to time* **time series design.** This design employs a nonequivalent control group *series z* that does not receive the independent variable. The group has similar *series z* characteristics to the experimental and control groups. All groups are *a control grp* tested at set time periods (O_1, O_2, etc.) as in the time series design, and results are compared, as diagrammed in Figure 6.8.

_____ *Figure 6.8* _____

QUASI-EXPERIMENTAL MULTIPLE TIME-SERIES DESIGN

TIME LINE OF STUDY EVENTS

	Pretests				Experiment			Posttests
GROUPS								
Experimental	O_1	O_2	O_3	O_4	X	O_5	O_6	O_7 O_8
Control	O_1	O_2	O_3	O_4		O_5	O_6	O_7 O_8

Source: Based on Campbell, D. T., & Stanley, J. C. (1966). *Experimental and quasi-experimental designs for research.* Chicago: Rand McNally (pp. 55–57).

If this design is feasible in a setting, it is considerably stronger than the basic time series design and the nonequivalent control group design, in that it allows the researcher greater control over the effects of history, maturation, and testing. This design could be used to great advantage in the hypothetical study of primary nursing and quality of care plans. A pediatric unit, closely resembling the experimental one in characteristics but not undergoing primary nursing, could be used as a control group for comparison of change in quality of care plans.

Quantitative, Nonexperimental Designs

Nonexperimental research is clearly distinguishable from experimental and quasi-experimental research in that there is no manipulation of the independent variable by the researcher. In **nonexperimental designs** the researcher observes the action of variables as they occur in the natural state. The major purpose of this type of research is to uncover new knowledge about the action of variables and to describe relationships between variables. These designs are used to answer level 2 and 3 questions (see Table 6.1). The lack of experimental control makes these designs weaker than experiments or quasi-experiments in determining cause and effect, but they are very useful in generating knowledge in a variety of situations where it would be difficult or impossible to employ an experimental approach. Similarly, a nonexperimental study may be a necessary step to generate knowledge before proceeding with an experiment.

Nonexperimental designs are frequently used in nursing research when it is unethical or impractical to manipulate variables in human subjects. We have already discussed the variable of smoking from an ethical standpoint. Other variables that are difficult or unethical to manipulate but frequently studied in nursing include pain, family support, fear, obesity, alcohol intake, drug abuse, grieving, and physical or emotional illness.

Classifications of Nonexperimental Designs Many types of nonexperimental designs are described in the literature, but basically there are two broad categories, descriptive and ex post facto. **Descriptive designs** are the simplest form of research since they are aimed at answering level 2 questions. For example, what are the concerns of clients following a heart attack? Or, what is the percentage of staff nurses who smoke at Valley View Hospital? These studies are relatively easy to conduct because only one variable is observed and measured, and relatively large samples can usually be obtained. Data are collected by observation of behavior, questionnaires, or interviews. *Exploratory research* is a term commonly used to describe this type of research; some authors refer to descriptive research as *survey research*. The term survey more accurately describes the method of data collection than the research design *per se*.

Rarely will you find purely descriptive nursing studies. Usually nursing studies with a descriptive element involve a study question that explores the relationship between variables. The questions in these studies are at level 3 (Table 6.1). This type of study is called **ex post facto** or *correlation research*.

The term *ex post facto* is derived from Latin meaning "after the fact." Data are collected on the dependent variable after change has already occurred naturally in the independent variable. For example, if a researcher wishes to study the relationship between maternal age and reported nausea in the first trimester of pregnancy, it would be impossible to manipulate maternal age. However, recording maternal reports of nausea in early pregnancy from a variety of age groups is feasible. The relationship between "age" and "reports of nausea" is determined statistically, usually through the use of a statistical test known as *correlation coefficient*.

Ex post facto research designs are usually stronger in meeting the causality criterion of association, but are often weaker in providing evidence for nonspurious relationships and time priority because the classical experimental control is lacking. However, this design has the advantage of using large samples from a given population in uncontrived settings, and it can provide meaningful information about how variables function in relation to one another.

Qualitative, Nonexperimental Designs

Qualitative designs are appropriate when there are no clear theoretical frameworks or nursing knowledge about the nature of the variables involved in a particular situation. This approach was first introduced in Chapter 2. An example of this level of inquiry is found in Stern's (1982) study of stepfather families, and her development of the theory that conflicting family cultures are an impediment to family integration. Stern used a qualitative design since the prior level of knowledge was sparse.

Qualitative designs are also appropriate when the existing theory is thought to be biased or incorrect. Hutchinson's (1984) study concerning stress among NICU nurses is another example of a qualitative study.

(See Example 2.1, which is an abstract of the study.) Her design was developed to challenge and expand on the current literature on the topic.

Qualitative designs emerge from a different philosophical perspective than do quantitative designs. (See Chapter 2, in which various ways of thinking are explored.) Pragmatically, the different perspectives and sets of designs and methods complement each other, and all are necessary at different stages in the development of nursing knowledge. In Table 6.2 the most commonly used qualitative design approaches are

_____ Table 6.2 _____

IDENTIFYING QUALITATIVE APPROACHES, DESIGNS, AND METHODS

Design	Research Approach and Question	Possible Data Collection and Analysis Methods
Phenomenology	Describes a life experience, using a variety of data sources and without a prior conceptual framework to find the essence of the experience: What is it like to experience certain life events?	Interviews, books, film Intuition without preconceived notions
Ethnography	Studies the phenomenon from the perspective of the subjects and within the context in which it occurs: What do the subjects in a particular setting think or do in relation to the phenomenon?	Observation, interviews, participant observation Grounded theory, constant comparative, and content analysis
Ethnology	Has goal of developing theories of culture or society rather than of the individual within a specific setting (ethnography); can be used cross-culturally: What are the norms and values of a particular group in relation to a specific topic? How do these compare with other groups?	Same methods as ethnography
Ethnoscience	Studies how the subjects view their world from the way they talk about it; elicits both questions and answers from subjects: From the perspective of the subjects, what are the significant factors in a particular situation?	Linguistic analysis for significant factors in written and spoken words Development of domains and taxonomy

Sources: Based on the methodological perspective of Field and Morse (1985) with expansion of the ideas from Bogdan and Biklen (1982), Miles and Huberman (1984), and Chenitz and Swanson (1986).

displayed, along with typical research questions and data collection and analysis methods.

The distinctions between qualitative and quantitative nonexperimental designs can be briefly summarized as follows. Qualitative designs usually deal with ideas that are collected and analyzed in the form of words, whereas quantitative designs deal with variables that are analyzed as numbers (Miles & Huberman, 1984). Considerable overlap between the two types of design is seen because words can be counted and thus analyzed as numbers, and variables can often be represented by words instead of numbers. For instance, the concept of gender could be categorized by a qualitative researcher into elaborate descriptions of the nature of maleness and femaleness; while a quantitative researcher would likely code the same data as 1 (female) and 2 (male). Both forms of viewing gender are correct: The important point is that they should fit the overall nature of the question and thus the selection of the design.

You will not find a consistent format or uniform use of terms in qualitative studies. While this initially will be confusing and frustrating, with the help of this chapter, Table 6.2, and the Glossary, you will be able to identify the essential component parts of the study, including the design.

Since more studies with quantitative designs are published, the terms common to those designs are used here whenever possible. Parallel concepts in qualitative research often are referred to by a wide variety of terms. The consistency in terminology will assist you to understand the parallels between methods. For example, qualitative researchers usually refer to the persons who supply their data as **informants,** whereas the quantitative researcher refers to the same persons as **subjects.** Bogdan and Biklen (1982, pp. 45–48) provide a table comparing the concepts and terms of qualitative and quantitative research. The Glossary provides additional synonyms for the various terms you may encounter in a qualitative study.

Qualitative Approaches   Qualitative approaches fall along a continuum from firm adherence to phenomenism, as in the phenomenology approach, to a type of phenomenism that leans toward the philosophical basis for most quantitative designs—which is positivism. The most common qualitative design approaches are presented in this order in Table 6.2 along with their related methods. These qualitative data collection and analysis methods are presented in the following chapters.

The differences in design and method are considerable within the wide variety of qualitative approaches. Nevertheless, it can generally be said that proposed qualitative designs are stated in a speculative way; indeed, the researchers will refer to the design as an "approach" to the study problem. During the conduct of the study the design will evolve, taking direction from the results that are emerging from the data. In Figure 6.1 the qualitative maze demonstrates the enactment of the design, which is an interplay between data collection, analysis, and the determination of the meanings from the study.

In Table 6.2 a distinction is made between the type of study design and the data collection and analysis methods that are chosen. Such a distinction is not always clear in a study report. Certain methods are often used with a specific design or approach, and these methods have come to be used almost exclusively. This usage is limited however, as it tends to exclude from consideration other suitable data collection or analysis methods. For example, Spradley's (1980) work on participant observation is presented exclusively as an ethnography approach. This has led to a consistent linking of the two—one a design (ethnography) and the other a method of data collection (participant observation). However, there are other data collection techniques that are suitable for ethnographers, and there are other designs that could benefit from the use of participant observation as a data collection technique.

One qualitative technique—grounded theory—has been popular in nursing research and has become almost synonymous with the entire scope of qualitative research (Chenitz & Swanson, 1986). However, Field and Morse view it as essentially a technique that can be used with several types of qualitative designs. Grounded theory, as an analysis technique, is discussed in Chapter 10. In the grounded theory study (Example 2.1) Hutchinson used an essentially ethnographic design, with participant observation as the primary data collection technique, and grounded theory as a data analysis method.

Other Designs — describe 1 aspect of the design

Several other techniques have come to be considered designs, but strictly speaking are not. They often describe one aspect of the design. For example, the *case study* more accurately describes the sampling technique and not the design. Campbell and Stanley (1966) refer to case studies as pre-experimental. They can be used as a qualitative data collection technique, but more and more the technique is replaced by small samples within which meanings can be compared.

Historical research describes the time frame and the type of data used by the researcher. It usually involves qualitative designs and methods, and it can employ any of the highly varied design approaches in Table 6.2. The purpose of this research usually involves the collection and analysis of data relating to past events in order to gain a better understanding of events in the present. It is unusual for such studies to have current clinical applicability; therefore, they will not be discussed in detail.

②**Evaluation research** refers not to the design itself, but to the type of study whose purpose is to examine the effectiveness or efficiency of the goals of a specific treatment or program. Qualitative, quantitative, or both types of designs, are often used in such studies. Any of the designs in this chapter would be suitable, depending on the nature of the study question (Green, 1977).

There are four types of studies that are used to examine changes over time. Such studies are referred to as cross-sectional, longitudinal, retrospective, or prospective.

Cross-sectional studies and **longitudinal studies** employ designs that allow the examination of a variable as it develops or changes over time. For example, in the Burke et al. study (1985), a cross-sectional design was used to examine the developmental status of a particular group of North American Indian children. The independent variable was the age of the child and the dependent variable was the developmental status of the child. One purpose of the study was to examine the relationship of age and developmental status over time. This was done by taking a cross-sectional sample of all babies and young children in the population. This covered the age range of interest to the researchers, who then tested the development status of all the subjects once at approximately the same time. A longitudinal approach with the same purpose would have sampled a smaller group of babies and tested their developmental status at regular intervals as they developed into preschoolers. The longitudinal and cross-sectional designs each have their own advantages. The longitudinal design allows the subjects to act as their own controls, in other words, each subject's changes over time can be compared with the same subject's earlier data. Early trends in the dependent variable might be more readily apparent in a longitudinal design. The long term relationships between the researchers and the subjects can provide more depth and meaning to the results. In contrast, the cross-sectional design lessens the possible effects of testing, maturation, and history risks to the results by testing each subject only once. Cross-sectional studies tend to be less costly and more manageable for the researcher.

Retrospective and **prospective studies** are terms commonly used to describe the time perspective within which the variables are viewed. Ex post facto designs are retrospective in that the researcher studies the association of events that have already occurred in the past. Suppose we wished to study the relationship between grades obtained in a statistics course, taken in the junior year of a nursing program, and grades obtained on a research methods course in the senior year. This could be easily done by selecting a sample of students who have completed the two courses and comparing their grades. This approach is retrospective since events have already taken place when data is collected and analyzed.

A prospective approach to studying a question involves selecting a sample that characterizes the independent variable and then waiting for the dependent variable to occur naturally within that sample. To study the above example prospectively, a researcher would select a sample of students in their junior year enrolled in a course on statistics, record their grades, and wait for this sample to complete a course in research methods in the senior year. This approach could be as effective as the retrospective approach in this situation, but problems can emerge if the occurrence of the dependent variable cannot be reasonably expected to occur. For instance, if students in our study are not required to take a course in research methods in the senior year, we may lose a large portion of our sample from the study using a prospective approach. This situation can be somewhat overcome through use of large samples, but this may be costly and impractical in some clinical studies. For example, waiting for lung cancer to develop in a group of smokers would be a difficult means to examine the relationship between smoking and lung cancer in human subjects. One major strength of prospective versus retrospective studies is the ability to determine time priority of the variables. Both approaches, however, are weak in determining causality because of the inability to use experimental controls.

EVALUATING RESEARCH DESIGNS

This chapter has presented considerable background about the purpose and methods used by researchers in designing the study to answer the research question. As we have noted, all of the designs discussed have definite strengths and a number of potential problems. In evaluating a published research report, you may experience a great deal of difficulty deciding which aspects of the design make the study useful and important, or which aspects imply serious flaws that would inhibit the use of findings in practice.

Table 6.3 summarizes the evaluation of a design for scientific

_____ *Table 6.3* _____

EVALUATING A STUDY DESIGN

Scientific Adequacy	*Clinical Applicability*
Is the design a logical one for the level of inquiry of the question?	Is the design one that is apt to address the clinical aspects of the study question?
Are the features of the designs that limit validity balanced with those that enhance it? (See Figure 6.9.)	

Qualitative Studies: Level 1 Only

Are the philosophical stance and research approach clearly stated? (See Table 6.2.)	Does the type of qualitative approach used logically fit the nature of the clinical phenomenon?
Are the steps of the study and strategies used clearly enough described so that, if you have been there, you know what the researcher would do next?	

Quantitative Studies: Levels 2–4 Only

Is the place in the design of each variable in the study question clear enough to draw a study events figure? (See Figures 6.2–6.8.)	Does the design "capture" the real world of the clinical nursing question fairly well, i.e., do the location, timing, sequence of data collection, and experimental maneuvers closely parallel the actual clinical setting?
- figures c̄ time line	Are there critical clinical features that have been ignored?

Meaningfulness[1]

If the degree of researcher subjectivity in the design is high, is that balanced with other ways to check the validity of the designs?	What is the likelihood that the design will yield results that are clinically important and meaningful to nurses?
Are there features of the design that are apt to bias the findings in a particular direction?	Is the design likely to yield findings that are out of context and therefore could be misconstrued if the researcher did not understand the nature of the clinical setting?

Internal Validity or Causality[1]

Are unwanted factors (extraneous variables) controlled or accounted for in some manner by the design?	Are there critical elements in the clinical setting or the subjects (patients or nurses) themselves that are not controlled or acknowledged in the design? In other words, what is the possibility of maturation or history?
Is the act of doing the study itself apt to change what is observed (the data and thus the findings)? In other words, is the Hawthorne effect or testing effect likely?	

(continues)

_____ *Table 6.3* _____

CONTINUED

Scientific Adequacy	Clinical Applicability
***External Validity or Generalizability*[2]**	
Does the design have some meaningfulness and a degree of internal validity?	Are the study concepts operationalized in a way that would permit the extension of conclusions at another time in the same clinical situations and/or in similar clinical settings?

_____

[1] See Chapters 8–10 on sampling, data collection, and data analysis for other aspects of meaningfulness and internal validity.

[2] See Chapter 12 on the interpretation of findings for a more detailed discussion of clinical generalizability.

_____

adequacy and, to a degree, clinical applicability. The real test of the clinical applicability of a design comes after it is operationalized with data collection and analysis (see Chapters 9 and 10) and the findings are produced. It is in the researcher's discussion and conclusions as well as your own conclusions about the findings that you can truly evaluate the clinical applicability of a design (see Chapter 12).

Identifying the Design

The first step in identifying design is to read the study report carefully and then go back to the introduction and reread the specific study question. Remember that the design should be carefully linked to the question; by identifying the level of inquiry of the question (see Table 6.1), you should be able to gain some clue as to the basic design of the study. An examination of the variables in the question may provide more clues. For example, if the independent variable(s) is impossible to manipulate in the stated population, then you know that the design must be nonexperimental, since both experiments and quasi-experiments involve manipulation of the independent variable. This status may be difficult to determine in situations where the independent variable can be manipulated, but the researcher chose to study the variables after change had already occurred. This situation can be demonstrated by the following study questions:

- Do younger clients express more concerns about body image than older clients following mastectomy surgery?

• Do students who participate in a preceptorship program in the fourth year of a baccalaureate program report more self-confidence on graduation than those students who have not participated in the program?

The first question can only be studied using a nonexperimental ex post facto approach, since "age" cannot be manipulated. The second question is more difficult because "participation in a preceptorship" can be manipulated, but circumstances may make this difficult. The researcher may study the question using a nonexperimental design to examine the relationship between variables on graduation. If the object is to study relationships, this should be made clear in the purpose statement; this is not always done in reality.

The study design is described in the researcher's report on methods or procedures for carrying out the study. Some research reports clearly state the type of design used to study the question(s); however, many researchers simply leave it to the reader to infer the design from the described procedures. The first decision you should make is whether or not the independent variable was manipulated before examining what methods were used to obtain subjects and collect data.

Evaluating Effectiveness of Design

In evaluating the effectiveness of the design, the likelihood of four critical factors must be considered:

— That the design will address the research question
— That the design will produce results that are meaningful
— That the design will demonstrate cause if implied in the study question
— That the results are generalize to other nursing situations if implied in the study question

The first factor refers back to the notion of a match between the level of the question and the design, as detailed in Table 6.1. There must be consistency in the level of inquiry between the question and the design. In the analysis chapter (10) you will see that this requirement of consistency of the level of inquiry also extends to how the data are analyzed. The second factor, meaningfulness, is primarily a qualitative concept, while the third and fourth factors, causation and generalizability, are primarily quantitative concepts. The last three all refer to validity. All four factors, however, are relevant to all the designs

_____ Table 6.4 _____

POTENTIAL FOR VALIDITY OF RESEARCH DESIGNS

Validity Factor	Type of Design			
	Qualitative	Quantitative		
	Nonexperimental	Quasi-Experimental	Experimental	
Meaningfulness (content validity)	High potential	Some potential	Some potential	Some potential
Causality (internal validity)	Low potential	Low potential	Some potential	High potential
Generalizability (external validity)	Potential difficult to determine	Low potential	Some potential	Some potential

Sources: Ratings are abstracted from the work of Field and Morse (1985) for qualitative designs, and from Cook and Campbell (1979) for quantitative designs.

discussed in this chapter. Table 6.4 illustrates the potential for the various designs to demonstrate these relatively meaningful, causal, or generalizable results. These factors also come into play in the methods of implementing the design, that is, data collection tools, study procedures, and sampling.

Evaluating Meaningfulness

Meaning   One of the major goals of qualitative nursing research is meaning, which has definite implications for quantitative research as well. Meaning is present when implicit knowledge gained from the study setting and sample is conveyed explicitly to the readers of the report (Field & Morse, 1985). In reading a report for meaning, the reader examines the design for evidence that the subjects, setting, and theory are representative of the phenomena being studied, and of the results obtained from the study. Subjectivity and lack of context are two main threats to the meaningfulness of research design.

Subjectivity   The subjectivity of the design is a risk to the meaningfulness of the results. Field and Morse (1985) point out that this risk is a concern when the researcher is directly involved in the collection of data. The quality of the data and the analysis hinge on the skill of the researcher. The source of the data, as determined by the design, can yield subjective results unless care is taken. This type of risk to validity is also referred to as *bias*. When you read a report for meaningfulness, question the possible biases that could come into play from the researcher, the data collection instruments, and the subjects.

Lack of Context   There will be a risk to the meaningfulness of design in a given clinical setting in many of the studies that you read. Since the topics studied by nurses are complex, researchers must narrow the boundaries of what they actually study. Statements taken out of context can often give the opposite impression of what was intended. Practicing nurses with experience in a particular area are better equipped than a researcher to judge whether or not the study design is likely to lead to results that lack context. For example, a maternal and child nurse would clearly see the lack of context evident in a study of self-esteem in hospitalized children if only the mothers were asked for data, or if the data were collected from the children immediately prior to a stressful procedure.

Validity of the Study Design

Causality or Internal Validity   **Internal validity** refers to the truth or falsity of the relationship between the variables in terms of causality as implied by the study question. We have already discussed the criteria for causality in terms of quantitative research designs. True experiments have the capacity to be most internally valid; quasi-experiments have potential for less internal validity; and nonexperimental designs have the potential to be the least internally valid. We have observed that means of control over unwanted variables and statistical methods to determine association between variables are more possible in some designs than in others.

Qualitative research can demonstrate a similar type of validity without the use of statistics, if checks are made of more than one type of data, and if care is taken to select the subjects who are most likely to have and share the knowledge of the phenomenon under study (Chenitz & Swanson, 1986). The use of both qualitative and quantitative data and of systematic comparisons (termed triangulation) has been demonstrated to provide additional evidence for internal validity, for example, in historical research where separate oral history accounts are compared with one another and with letters written at the time (Burke, Maloney, & Baumgart, 1986; Jick, 1979).

Throughout the chapter we have discussed a number of possible risks to the internal validity of specific designs. For example, history, maturation, testing, and the Hawthorne effect are particularly evident in some experimental and quasi-experimental designs. The lack of randomization and control over the experimental variable are particular problems in nonexperimental designs. Specific problems related to sampling, setting, procedures, instruments for data collection, and analysis of data will be discussed in future chapters.

External Validity or Generalizability   **External validity** has to do with generalizing the results of the study to a particular set of persons or settings or generalizing across persons or settings. This concept is dealt with in more breadth in Chapter 12 where the interpretation of findings is discussed. Earlier, we briefly introduced the concept of generalizability as one possible problem with some experimental designs. Several factors in the design of the study can effect generalizability of study results. First, the design must hold a degree of internal validity and meaningfulness as a prerequisite for external validity. Therefore, it is important to consider if the researcher has adequately controlled the experiment for the effect of extraneous variables on the outcome variable(s). Second, the size of the sample of subjects used to test or observe the action of variables is a consideration. Even in a highly controlled randomized study, if the sample of subjects tested is very small, the generalizability of findings may be in question. The issue of sample size will be discussed in more detail in Chapter 8.

One other factor that influences the external validity of the study findings and is specifically related to the design involves how the researcher operationalizes the concepts to be studied. In nursing research we study a number of complex concepts that are often difficult to operationalize. Consider the concepts pain, anxiety, client's recovery, satisfaction, and well-being. If, for example, we chose to measure clients' well-being using only physiological measures, can we say these measures alone represent the concept?

Making Decisions About Validity   Estimating the validity of the results, based on the design of the study, is a deductive process in which the research consumer systematically thinks through and weighs both the evidence for the possible validity of the results from the

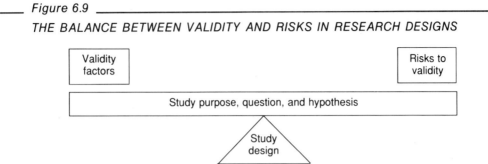

_____ *Figure 6.9* _____

THE BALANCE BETWEEN VALIDITY AND RISKS IN RESEARCH DESIGNS

particular design, and the possible effect of each of the risks to validity (Cook & Campbell, 1979). Figure 6.9 illustrates these relationships. In the best studies the researcher has accomplished this and included it in the discussion and conclusion sections of the report. This does not mean that you should rely on the researcher's judgments, but rather that you can add the researcher's evaluations to your own.

One common problem shared by many beginning consumers of nursing research is the tendency to over-criticize. It is literally impossible to design the perfect study of human behavior. A careful evaluation of all aspects of a study should be carried out before decisions are made about application to practice. The design of a study is an essential component in determining validity of the findings, and this design must be based upon a well-conceptualized, sound, researchable nursing problem (see Chapter 4). Data must be collected (Chapter 9), analyzed (Chapter 10), and interpreted (Chapter 12) appropriately for findings to be useful and meaningful in practice. It is imperative that all aspects of the study be communicated clearly by the researcher to the reader.

_____ **SUMMARY** _____

This chapter has presented an overview of the most common designs found in nursing research. Experimental designs are the strongest in determining cause and effect between variables, but may be difficult to use in natural settings because of the degree of experimental control required. True experiments in particular may suffer from problems associated with generalization to other populations and settings, as well as sensitization of subjects and experiments to experimental hypothesis(es).

Quasi-experiments are more suitable for use in natural settings, but sacrifice some experimental control and are less convincing in determining causality. Particular strengths and disadvantages are discussed in relation to nonequivalent control group design and time series designs.

Nonexperimental descriptive and ex post facto designs are viewed as least causal in nature, but may be necessary in uncovering needed information before a more controlled study is undertaken by the researcher. In addition, many situations in nursing research make it impossible or unethical for the researcher to manipulate the independent variable.

Qualitative approaches are particularly useful in describing the nature of variables and the determination of meaning of phenomena. The most common methods found in nursing research are described.

The final sections of the chapter deal with evaluation of research design. Validity (meaningfulness, causality, generalizability) is discussed in general terms for each design type, and the balance between risks and clinical validity is summarized.

EXERCISES

1. From the following research questions and summary of procedures for data collection,
   a. Identify and diagram the basic type of experimental, quasi-experimental, nonexperimental, or qualitative design used in the study.
   b. Determine the appropriateness of this design to answer the level of question asked (see Table 6.1).
   c. Identify possible risks to meaningfulness and internal validity. See Table 6.3 for the questions to ask yourself, and the likely risks to meaningfulness and internal validity.

Recovery Time Following Activities of Daily Living in Post-Myocardial Infarct Clients*

Purpose

To investigate the minimum recovery time required by uncomplicated MI (myocardial infarction) clients following activities of daily living.

Quota Sampling

---

* Adapted from unpublished research proposal by S. Bendicks et al. (1986). Queen's University School of Nursing. Kingston, Ontario.

Research Question

Will younger clients demonstrate shorter recovery times than older clients following the same activities of daily living?

Will clients' perceptions of recovery time be shorter than that indicated by physiological parameters?

Procedure

Forty-five male clients between the age of 40 and 70 years, 8–10 days post MI, were selected by the researchers from two general hospitals. Subjects were selected on criteria indicating clinical stability. Subjects were assigned to one of three age groups, 40–49 years, 50–59 years, 60–70 years. The study was carried out over a one-year period until fifteen subjects were tested for each age group.

Baseline physiological data about heart rate, blood pressure, and electrocardiogram was obtained by the researcher from each client (in sitting position) before activities began.

Each subject performed the same activities in exactly the same sequence, showering, dressing, shaving, teeth brushing, and hair combing. Each activity was carried out according to a specific protocol which included time limits. The same physiological measurements taken prior to activity were retaken at two minute intervals until the readings returned to baseline. Subjective data on how each subject felt was also recorded along with each reading. The subjects moved on to perform the next activity when physiological data returned to baseline and when each subject stated he felt comfortable with proceeding.

Effects of Fathers' Attitudes on Breastfeeding Success*

Purpose

To determine whether or not fathers' attitudes affect success of breastfeeding in first-time mothers.

Research Question

Are first-time mothers more likely to successfully breastfeed their infants if the father reports a positive attitude toward breastfeeding than if the father reports a negative breastfeeding attitude?

---

* Adapted from unpublished research proposal by D. McMillan et al. (1986). Queen's University School of Nursing. Kingston, Ontario.

Procedure

Two hundred voluntary new parent couples (primiparous mothers) whose infants were born through uncomplicated vaginal births at a large teaching hospital served as subjects for the study.

On the first or second day post-partum all fathers were asked to complete a demographic questionnaire about age, socio-economic status, and source and quantity of pre- and post-natal information received about breastfeeding. Families were then randomly assigned to two groups. One group of fathers was asked by staff nurses to respond to a breastfeeding attitude scale to which they indicated degree of agreement with twenty statements about breastfeeding. The second group of fathers did not respond to the scale. Eight or nine weeks following discharge all mothers were contacted by the researcher and were interviewed about breastfeeding success over the phone. The study took place over a six-month period.

*The Effect of Structured Visual Stimulation Upon the Development of Eye Tracking Abilities in Hospitalized Preterm Infants**

Purpose

To determine the relationship between the amount of visual stimulation received by preterm infants when in hospital and the normal development of eye tracking.

Research Question

Will preterm infants that receive a structured visual stimulation program show faster development of eye tracking than preterm infants who receive only normal visual stimulation?

Procedure

Sixty preterm infants were selected over a twelve-month period from admissions to the Neonatal Intensive Care Unit of a general hospital. Subjects were selected for the study if gestational age was less than 35 weeks, birth weight was between 10th and 90th percentile for gestational age, if baby was single birth with no malformations, not dependent on mechanical ventilation, breathing room air, not demonstrating neurological abnormalities, and parents visiting 0–4 hours daily. Infants were assigned to two groups of 30, one experimental and one control group.

---

* Adapted from unpublished research proposal by M. Cronin and S. MacKenzie (1986). Queens University School of Nursing. Kingston, Ontario.

Upon admission, the Brazelton Neonatal Behavioral Assessment Scale (BNBAS) (Brazelton, 1985), was administered by a trained examiner to the preterm infants meeting the criteria to be included in the study.

The amount of unstructured stimulation (nursing care) was calculated through an observation checklist. The NICU staff was observed on all three shifts over a two-week period and observations averaged. The control group received stimulation from "normal nursing care" and parental visits, which were timed. They were tested specifically for eye tracking, using the BNBAS section referring to orientation response—inanimate visual, at one-week intervals until discharge.

The experimental group received a structured stimulation program in addition to the unstructured stimulation that both they and the control group received. This structured visual stimulation program was presented to the infants randomly, three times daily, five minutes at a time from the second day of admission until discharge. This group was measured with the same specific section of the BNBAS at one-week intervals until discharged.

2. Example 2.2 (p. 39) is a brief abstract of a qualitative study by Hutchinson (1984). Identify and describe the possible risks to internal validity and meaningfulness of results. Use Table 6.4 to help you.

REFERENCES

Benedicks, S.; Empson, S.; Hulbert, M.; Lum, D.; Mescal, S.; & Schonmaier, E. (1986). The minimum recovery time required following activities of daily living carried out by uncomplicated post-myocardial infarct patients. Unpublished research proposal. Year IV students. Queen's University School of Nursing. Kingston, Ontario.

Bogdan, R., & Biklen, S. K. (1982). *Qualitative research for education: An introduction to theory and methods*. Boston: Allyn and Bacon.

Bowen, M. (1978). *Family therapy in clinical practice*. New York: Jason Aronson.

Brazelton, T. B. (1985). *Neonatal behavioral assessment scale,* 2nd ed. New York: Lippincott & Crowell.

Brink, P. J., & Wood, M. J. (1988). *Basic steps in planning nursing research from question to proposal*. Monterey, Calif.: Jones and Bartlett.

Burke, S. O.; Sayers, L. A.; Baumgart, A. J.; & Wray, J. G. (1985). Pitfalls in cross-cultural use of the Denver Developmental Screening Test: Cree Indian children. *Canadian Journal of Public Health, 76,* 303–307.

Burke, S. O.; Maloney, R.; & Baumgart, A. J. (1986, May). Activity value orientations among nurses and mothers: Interactive analysis of transcultural qualitative and quantitative data. Paper presented at the International Nursing Research Conference in Edmonton, Alberta.

Campbell, D. T., & Stanley, J. C. (1966). *Experimental and quasi-experimental designs for research.* Chicago: Rand McNally.

Chenitz, W. C., & Swanson, J. M. (1986). *From practice to grounded theory: Qualitative research in nursing.* Menlo Park, Calif.: Addison-Wesley.

Cook, T. D., & Campbell, D. T. (1979). *Quasi-experimentation: Design and analysis issues for field settings.* Boston: Houghton Mifflin.

Cronin, M., & MacKenzie, S. (1986). Structured visual stimulation: Its effect upon the development of eye tracking abilities in hospitalized preterm infants. Unpublished research proposal. Queen's University School of Nursing. Kingston, Ontario.

Damrosch, S. P. (1981). How nursing students' reactions to rape victims are affected by a perceived act of carelessness. *Nursing Research, 30*(3), 168–170.

Field, P. A., & Morse, J. M. (1985). *Nursing research: The application of qualitative approaches.* Rockville, Md.: Aspen Systems.

Fishbein, M. (1967). *Readings in attitudinal theory and measurement.* New York: John Wiley.

Green, L. W. (1977). Evaluation and measurement: Some dilemmas for health education. *American Journal of Public Health, 67*(2), 155–161.

Hutchinson, S. A. (1984). Creating meaning out of horror. *Nursing Outlook, 32,* 86–90.

Jick, T. D. (1979). Mixing qualitative and quantitative methods: Triangulation in action. *Administrative Science Quarterly, 24,* 602–611.

Labovitz, S., & Hagedorn, R. (1981). *Introduction to social research,* 3rd ed. New York: McGraw-Hill.

Lamontagne, L. L.; Mason, K. R.; & Hepworth, J. T. (1985). Effects of relaxation on anxiety in children: Implications for coping with stress. *Nursing Research, 34*(5), 289–292.

Leininger M. N. (Ed.). (1985). *Qualitative research methods in nursing.* New York: Grune and Stratton.

LoBiondo-Wood, G. (1986) Introduction to design. In G. LoBiondo-Wood & J. Haber (Eds.), *Nursing research: Critical appraisal and utilization.* St. Louis: C. V. Mosby.

McMillan, D.; Fletcher, B.; MacKenzie, A.; Stevenson, S.; Blackburn, W.; & Dickenson, J. (1986). Effects of fathers' attitudes on breastfeeding success. Unpublished research proposal. Year IV students. Queen's University. Kingston, Ontario.

Miles, M. B., & Huberman, A. M. (1984). *Qualitative data analysis: A sourcebook of new methods.* Beverly Hills, Calif.: Sage Publications.

Spradley, J. P. (1980). *Participant observation.* New York: Holt, Rinehart and Winston.

Stern, P. N. (1982). Conflicting family culture: An impediment to integration in stepfather families. *Journal of Psychosocial Nursing and Mental Health Services, 20*(10), 27–33.

Ventura, M. R.; Young, D. E.; Feldman, M. J.; Pastore, P.; Pikula, S.; & Yates, M. A. (1984). Effectiveness of health promotion interventions. *Nursing Research, 33*(3), 162–167.

7

Ethical Considerations for the Research Consumer

INTRODUCTION

Clinical nursing research must study human beings in order to discover meaningful knowledge for changes in nursing practice. Because nursing research has matured relatively recently compared to research conducted in other fields, nurse researchers have available a wealth of guidelines for the protection of the rights of human subjects and all other project participants.

The nurse researcher's work is strictly directed by established ethical guidelines. The researcher must act within such guidelines at all phases of the research process. Furthermore, it is the responsibility of every professional nurse who participates as a research subject, a research consumer, a member of an ethics review committee, a research team member, or a caregiver in a research setting to be aware of the professional human rights guidelines and to ensure that they are maintained.

OBJECTIVES

After reading this chapter, you will be able to

1. Identify steps taken by the researcher to ensure that the subjects participating in a study have been protected from any violation of human rights.
2. Identify key sources for ethical guidelines in carrying out human subject research.
3. Discuss what is meant by informed consent and the key elements that should be included in an adequate informed consent.
4. Identify high-risk groups in human subject research and the appropriate steps that must be taken by the researcher in working with these groups.
5. Evaluate circumstances that might compromise a subject's informed consent to participate in clinical nursing studies.
6. Cite factors involved in the balance between ethical research and scientific research.
7. Evaluate the ethical implications of a research report.
8. Discuss the clinical nurse's accountability to client subjects participating in nursing or other research.
9. Discuss the accountability of research team members in maintaining ethical standards of research.

NEW TERMS

Ethics

Human rights

Informed consent

Ethics review board

PROFESSIONAL ETHICS RESEARCH _GUIDELINES_

Before the advent of World War II, few written guidelines were available to researchers to ensure the protection of human subjects participating in research. As a result of the postwar Nuremberg Trials, which exposed the atrocious acts conducted in the name of science, a group under the direction of the American Medical Association developed a code of ethics to judge scientific research. This code outlined a number of important articles that provided the foundation for numerous ethical research guidelines developed by government and professional organizations involved in the conduct of research on human subjects. The Nuremberg Code mandated voluntary consent, justification of research for the good of society with appropriate balance of risk and benefit, adequate protection of subjects from risk or harm, subjects' right to withdraw from experimentation, and adequate scientific qualifications for researchers (Katz, 1972).

In the 1960s, the World Medical Association formulated the Declaration of Helsinki to guide medical research. It outlined two categories of research: that aimed directly toward therapeutic value for the client, and that aimed toward building a knowledge base that will not have direct therapeutic value for the client. This document stated that client subjects participating in such experiments must be informed of expected self-benefits before giving consent to participate. The Declaration of Helsinki further reiterated the earlier statements of the Nuremberg Code and emphasized the importance of written consent (World Medical Association, 1964).

The articles of the Nuremberg Code and the Declaration of Helsinki are strongly reflected in ethical research guidelines set out by professional nursing organizations. The American Nurses' Association has developed two documents to provide guidance for nurses engaged in research. _Guidelines for the Investigative Function of Nurses_ (1981) outlines the rights of professional nurses, with various levels of research preparation, to participate in research. A summary of these guidelines was presented in Chapter 3. _Human Rights Guidelines for Nurses in Clinical and Other Research_ (1985) is directed toward the protection of clients who participate as subjects in nursing research. The Canadian Nurses' Association came forth with a similar document, _Ethical Guidelines for Nursing Research Involving Human Subjects_ (1983). In the United Kingdom, the Royal College of Nurses (1977) has also produced ethical guidelines for engaging in research with human subjects. In addition to subject protection, all three documents address practical and ethical issues found within clinical nursing research settings. The above professional guidelines provide the basis for discussion in this chapter and are summarized in Table 7.1.

_____ *Table 7.1* _____

SUMMARY OF PROFESSIONAL GUIDELINES FOR NURSES FOR THE PROTECTION OF HUMAN SUBJECTS' RIGHTS

American Nurses' Association[1]	*Canadian Nurses' Association*[2]	*Royal College of Nurses, United Kingdom*[3]
1. Types of activities involved If research participation (medical, nursing, or other) is a condition of employment, nurses must be informed in writing of the nature of activity involved in advance of employment and if this is not done, nurses must be given the opportunity of not participating in research. Potential risks to others must be clarified in advance of research as well as ways to identify risks and counteract potential harm. 2. Guidelines for the protection of human rights of subjects Freedom from risk of injury or harm. Researchers must estimate risk and benefit involved, and subjects must be informed of any potential mental or physical risk as well as personal benefit and procedures or activities	1. Scientific merit of research must be demonstrated. Scientifically unsound research is unethical to implement. 2. There must be assurance of human subject's voluntary, informed consent and protection of confidentiality. Sufficient knowledge must be given for consent to be informed; guidelines are presented. Subjects must consent freely, involving appropriate advocate for disadvantaged or incompetent groups. Consent should be written or verbal. Only written is legal in some provinces. Consent should be obtained from others involved or affected by research, i.e., staff nurses or spouses. This may be informal in some situations and involve sharing information. All research data must be handled in such a way to protect subjects' confidentiality and	1. Research must demonstrate necessity and a contribution to body of knowledge. 2. Subjects must be informed in detail about expected participation and explicitly informed that participation is voluntary and they may withdraw at any point in the project. 3. Informed consent must be obtained from all subjects or appropriate legal representative. 4. Subjects must be protected from physical, emotional, mental, or social harm. 5. Confidentiality of data and anonymity of subjects must be assured and maintained. 6. Researchers must be qualified investigators and are obliged to publicize outcomes of projects investigated and

(continues)

Table 7.1

CONTINUED

American Nurses' Association[1]	Canadian Nurses' Association[2]	Royal College of Nurses, United Kingdom[3]
which extend beyond personal need. Nurses must carefully monitor sources of potential risk of injury and protect subjects who are particularly vulnerable as a result of illness or members of captive groups—i.e., prisoners, students, institutionalized patients, and the poor. Right to privacy and dignity. All proposals, instruments, and procedures involved in the research activity must be discussed with prospective subjects and others participating in the project so that individuals may make an informed decision to take part or not. Right to Anonymity. The researcher must outline to prospective subjects methods which protect the identity of subjects and information obtained under privileged conditions. 3. Guidelines for the protection of human rights apply to all individuals involved in research activity. The use of subjects with limited civil freedom can usually only be justified when there is predicted benefit to them or others in similar circumstances. 4. Nurses have an obligation to protect human rights as well as a professional responsibility to support	anonymity. Specific guidelines are given for storing and retrieval of information from data banks. Subjects must be protected from mental, emotional, moral, or physical injury. Potential benefit to subject should outweigh potential risks. 3. Guidelines involving the setting for research. Agency must provide mechanism for scientific and ethical review of projects. Investigator must provide adequate information and protocol including roles and ethical considerations of those involved in research. The rights of staff members to choose to participate or not in research must be respected and be spelled out as a prior condition of employment in areas where research activity is continuously carried out.	prevent misuse of findings. 7. There should be a clear delineation of duties and protocol in contracts between an investigator and a sponsoring agency for research. 8. Guidelines for commissioned research within organizations are presented with emphasis on securing individualized informed consent from prospective participants. 9. Practicing nurses are obliged to ensure the protection of client rights and safety in settings where research is conducted. 10. Nurses who participate in research projects maintain the same ethical codes as the researchers in respecting confidentiality of data and human rights of subjects.

_____ Table 7.1 _____

CONTINUED

American Nurses' Association[1]	Canadian Nurses' Association[2]	Royal College of Nurses, United Kingdom[3]
research to broaden the nursing scientific knowledge base for practice and delivery of service. 5. Voluntary informed consent to participate in research must be obtained from all prospective subjects or their legal representatives. 6. Nurses have an obligation to participate on institutional review boards to review ethical implications of proposed and ongoing research. All studies involving data gathering from humans, animals, or charts should be reviewed by health care professionals and community representatives for the protection of subject's rights. 7. Practical guidelines for conducting research. a) Content and function of institutional review boards b) Institutional sponsorship of outside investigators, i.e., graduate students c) Subject recruitment process.		

[1] Adapted and summarized from *Human rights guidelines for nurses in clinical and other research* (1985). American Nurses' Association.

[2] Adapted and summarized from *Ethical guidelines for nursing research involving human subjects* (1983). Canadian Nurses' Association.

[3] Adapted and summarized from R. Schrock (1984). "Moral issues in nursing research" in *The research process in nursing*. D.F.S. Cormack (Ed.), London: Blackwell Scientific Publications.

_____ WHAT IS ETHICAL RESEARCH? _____

The **ethics** of nursing research can be defined as those aspects of the project that impinge upon the moral and social aspects of society (Arminger, 1977). Given this broad definition, the nurse researcher is faced with an enormous responsibility and challenge to generate knowledge that is directed toward better client care within a framework that respects a wide range of individual human values.

Earlier in this text we stressed that the investigator must pursue the keystones of causality and objectivity in developing knowledge that can have implications for a large number of societal groups. We might ask, however, whether these scientific concepts of causality and objectivity are in conflict with ethical concepts that emphasize sensitivity to the individual. This question may spark considerable philosophical debate, but from a professional and humanitarian viewpoint, research that is insensitive to human values cannot be accepted as a basis for positive changes affecting the human condition. The researcher who engages in human subject research is constantly challenged to provide and demonstrate a balance between scientific and human values without infringement on human rights.

The professional guidelines in Table 7.1 provide nurses involved in research with principles that are intended to safeguard human rights. The nurse researcher must consider these guidelines at every stage of the research process—from the conceptualization of the problem, the design of the study, and the collection and analysis of data, to interpreting and publishing results.

_____ WHAT HUMAN RIGHTS ARE PROTECTED? _____

A number of common concepts underlie human rights guidelines. **Human rights** is a term that is frequently discussed in the literature dealing with the protection of human subjects and participants in research. Basically, the term refers to three rights outlined in the ANA guidelines (1985, pp. 6–7).

—Right to freedom from intrinsic risk of injury
—Right to privacy and dignity
—Right to anonymity

These rights apply to everyone involved in a research project, including team members who may be involved in data collection and practicing nurses involved in the research setting, as well as the participating subjects.

Freedom from Intrinsic Risk of Injury

The right to freedom from risk of injury is the primary concern of the researcher in conceptualizing the research question and designing the project. Injury includes physical, emotional, mental, and social consequences to individuals involved. If the research problem is one that involves a potentially harmful intervention, the research problem may have to be abandoned or restated to allow investigation within ethical guidelines. For example, it would be unethical to control the amount of smoking and alcohol intake in pregnant subjects in order to observe infant outcomes. Without intervention, a researcher could ethically observe the relationship between smoking or alcohol intake in pregnancy and infant birth weight retrospectively in a population of mothers who chose to continue smoking and drinking during pregnancy. This research question cannot be stated in causal terms, but it can be stated in terms of an existing relationship, and as such the design of the study must be descriptive, ex post facto rather than experimental (Level 2 or 3 rather than Level 4; see Table 6.1).

In making the decision concerning potential risk involved in planning nursing research, the researcher and reviewers must consider a number of factors. In balancing scientific principles and humanitarian values, the degree of potential benefit to those involved and to society as a whole must be estimated. In the above example, the potential risk to subjects would be overwhelming in an experimental study. However, a well-designed descriptive study, although of little benefit to those clients being studied, would likely provide important information for other pregnant women in society.

Weighing risk and benefit in many nursing research studies is not always clearcut. Few nursing studies hold the potential for physical harm. However, we commonly study variables, such as anxiety and stress, that may hold highly individualized significance for subjects and require more complex decision making in weighing risk/benefit. Sadly, in nursing we can benefit from some earlier behavioral studies that inadvertently miscalculated the risk/benefit ratio. A famous example frequently quoted in the literature is the Milgram (1963) experiment. This psychological experiment involved the study of destructive obedience in the laboratory. Naive subjects were ordered to administer varying degrees of shocks to actors masquerading as real victims. The subjects were unaware that the victims were actors not receiving the shocks, and as a result many subjects suffered extreme emotional stress. It seems unlikely to think such a situation could occur in nursing research. However, as more nurses become involved in research, and as the preparation of nurses to carry out research in a wide variety of areas becomes more sophisticated, the danger remains ever present.

A second factor which must be considered in calculating risk of injury is the vulnerability of potential subjects. In clinical nursing research, potential subjects are nearly always clients within the health care system; they are already stressed by physical or emotional illness and require special considerations for risk of injury. All professional guidelines caution against the use of such captive groups as minors, prisoners, the mentally retarded, the mentally ill, students, the poor, the unborn, the dead, the elderly, and the dying. ANA guidelines (1985) justify the use of such captive groups only when the research can demonstrate future benefit to them or similar groups.

Because risk of injury is of great individual significance, and because of the need to assure that individual freedom is protected, all potential subjects must be informed of the expected activity required of them in a research project, and all potential risks and benefits to self or others must be carefully explained so that an individual may make an informed choice to participate or not in proposed research.

Right to Privacy and Dignity

Privacy and dignity are individual values that have far-reaching consequences for everyone involved in research, and they cannot be determined solely by the researcher. In nursing research we often use methods of data collection that may be highly sensitive to the privacy and dignity of certain subjects as well as to those collecting the data. Many questionnaires and interviews require subjects to provide data, such as income, marital status, and personal habits, that may be a source of embarrassment for the subject as well as for the interviewer. Many methods of observation used to collect behavioral data may easily be construed as an invasion of privacy. The use of cameras, tape recorders, and one-way mirrors are common examples. The collection of physiological data—for example, the use of indwelling rectal temperature probes—often involves discomfort and embarrassment.

Participant observation is a frequently used method of data collection in qualitative nursing research studies in which the researcher participates actively in the research setting while collecting data. When this approach is not clearly understood by subjects, the researcher may elicit data without full subject consent. This is a culturally sensitive issue in some anthropological studies. Field and Morse (1985) stress that researchers should remind subjects of the study and ask ongoing permission to use sensitive data if the subject seems unclear about what information will be used in the research.

The researcher can reduce the possibility of risk to privacy and dignity when designing the study by

— Ensuring the objective wording of questions
— Avoiding intrusive observation techniques when possible
— Building into the study appropriate mechanisms to ensure confidentiality of data

However, only those who are potential participants in the study, whether subjects or research assistants, can decide whether aspects of the research are a violation of their own privacy or dignity. The researcher is obligated to ensure that prospective participants clearly understand all procedures, data-collection methods, and activities in the study so that an informed decision can be made to participate or refrain from involvement.

Right to Anonymity

Closely tied to the protection of privacy and dignity is the right of individual subjects to remain anonymous. This requires careful planning on the part of the researcher and other members of the research team for the handling, reporting, and storage of data. Data should be coded and provisions made for storage of all data in such a way that any identifiable documentation associated with the research is not easily traceable by persons other than the research team. The researcher must inform subjects of plans to protect anonymity and of persons with access to data. If results are to be published, subjects must know what safeguards will be taken to protect individual identity. The latter concern is particularly important when the number of study subjects is small and the research setting is easily identified.

The use of computers in the research process poses a special set of risks to anonymity, privacy, and confidentiality. The nature of these particular ethical risks are discussed in Chapter 11 on the use of computers in nursing research.

PROCEDURES FOR PROTECTING _____ _HUMAN RIGHTS_

There are a number of procedures that are used in the course of a study to ensure that human rights are protected. These include procedures for obtaining informed consent and independent review of the study protocols by an ethics review committee, which is often referred to as an Institutional Review Board (IRB).

Informed Consent—Key Elements

Implicit in the protection of human rights is the idea that individuals make a free choice to determine whether or not to participate in any or part of a research study. In order to make this choice, decisions must be based upon adequate information. All professional guidelines emphasize that researchers are required to obtain **informed consent** from all prospective subjects. Although most guidelines acknowledge that consent may be verbal or written, written consent provides sounder evidence of informed consent, and in some parts of North America it is the only form of consent considered legal (see C.N.A. Guidelines, 1983).

The format for written consent can vary somewhat, but essentially it must contain adequate information for subjects to make an informed decision as to protection of their rights, explicit assurance that participation is voluntary, and that subjects may withdraw at any time without risk of negative consequences. The language and format of the consent is best kept as simple as possible to ensure understanding by all proposed subjects. Misleading statements should be avoided. A narrative letter using concise paragraphs, and clearly printed, is one of the best approaches. As a research team member, subject, caregiver to a subject, or ethics review committee member you will see such informed consent forms. The following practical guidelines will help you evaluate the adequacy of a written consent.

1. _Title:_ A title should indicate that prospective subjects are consenting to participate in a research project. For example,

   Subject Consent to Participate in the Research Project: First Time Mother's Concerns about Breastfeeding.

2. _Purpose:_ A simple introductory statement should include the purpose of the study, why particular subjects are being

approached, and who will be conducting the research. For example,

Joan Smith, R.N., Master of Science Student, Lakeview University, School of Nursing, under the direction of Professor M. Brown, R.N., Ph.D.

3. *Subject participation:* A concise but clear explanation of how subjects will be involved must be given. This should include a complete description of a procedure, the length of time required to complete the procedure, and whether comparison groups will be used. If experimental and control groups are part of the design, subjects must be informed that they may be chosen as members of either group, and procedures for both groups should be described.

4. *Risks:* A complete description of any possible risks or discomforts to the subject should be presented. These include any risk affecting the physical, emotional, mental, or social well-being of the individual. Discomforts such as loss of time should be indicated.

5. *Benefits:* A complete description of potential immediate or long-term benefits to the subject or others must be disclosed.

6. *Alternative treatments:* If the research involves an intervention or treatment, subjects should be informed of alternate, available procedures that may benefit the subject.

7. *Compensation:* If subjects are expected to be exposed to any significant risk as a result of the research, any plans to compensate the subject should be explained. For example, if any physical, emotional, mental, or social injury may result, subjects must be informed as to the researcher's plans for assistance or intervention that will counteract any injury received. If subjects are to be paid for their time, this should be carefully outlined.

8. *Confidentiality:* Plans for protecting subjects' anonymity and confidentiality must be explained. This includes an explanation of how the data will be handled and stored and who will have access to the data. If results of the research will be published, subjects should be informed as to how individual anonymity and confidentiality will be maintained.

9. *Free choice:* Subjects must be assured that participation is completely voluntary and that they may refuse to participate or may withdraw from the project at any time without any risk to well-being or care.

10. *Sources for information:* Phone numbers and addresses of individuals who may provide further and ongoing information to subjects about procedures, risks, benefits, compensation, and the like should be stated.

11. *Signature of consent:* If the informed subject agrees to participate, the consent form must be signed by the subject and dated. Witnesses are not always necessary but do provide evidence that the subject concerned actually signed the form. (The use of a witness to a consent signature may be required by some granting agencies.) In situations where the subject is physically or mentally incapable of signing the consent, a legal representative must sign. In these situations every effort should be made by the researcher to inform the subject and representative as fully as possible. In the case of minors, parental consent or consent of the legal guardian must be obtained. However, it is generally advisable to have children sign in addition if they are old enough to do so. Similarly, the researcher must inform the child about the research and human rights in a manner appropriate for age level. The investigator should also sign the form to indicate commitment to the agreement.

12. *Language:* Informed consent assumes that the form will be read by or to the potential subject in a language with which the subject is comfortable. It must also carefully balance full explanation with avoidance of technical research language. If the form was read or translated for the subject, the details should be written on the form.

A sample of an informed consent form is seen in Figure 7.1.

Process of Obtaining Informed Consent

The process of obtaining an informed consent has some definite implications for promoting an ethical and trusting relationship between the researcher and potential subjects. The research consumer as well as the research team member should be aware that the researcher's letter of consent as well as the process of obtaining consent have been implemented with the utmost concern for protection of human rights. The

_____ *Figure 7.1* _____

PATIENT INFORMATION AND CONSENT FOR PARTICIPATION IN AMBULATORY SURGERY RESEARCH STUDY

Dr. Sandra Stone, R.N., and Dr. Martha Smith, R.N., Faculty of Sun Vale University School of Nursing in cooperation with Sun Vale Hospital are doing a research study about patients' recovery and those who care for patients at home following day surgery. As more people are having minor surgery done in a clinic rather than in hospital, they would like to find out more information about how people feel when they go home and how this affects the family or other people helping them. They are also interested in asking patients about how happy they are with the care and information given in the day surgery unit.

This study will try out questionnaires and interviews for getting information about patients and those who help them. Also we will ask some questions about how you and the person who helped care for you while you were recovering felt during the first day after surgery. Other questions include some personal information such as your age, occupation, and income. If you agree to participate, a trained research assistant will make an appointment to visit you in your home, two to five days following your surgery. That person will also ask that your caregiver be present at this time. If this is not possible, arrangements can be made to visit the caregiver at a better time, if the caregiver is willing to provide us with a phone number to make necessary arrangements. The caregiver will be given a sheet like this one and asked to participate in the study.

The interviewer will ask you to do two short questionnaires and have a brief interview. Your caregiver will also be requested to answer the same two short questionnaires. To assure your privacy during the interview, your caregiver will be asked to complete the questionnaires in a separate room during your interview, and then you will fill out the questionnaires after being interviewed. The entire visit should take about forty-five minutes.

Although this study will not benefit you directly, we are asking you for a little of your time to help in this project. In the long run it is hoped this information can be used to improve our services to others and those who help care for them at home. Whether or not you agree to help is entirely up to you and will in no way affect your care now or in the future. If at any time you decide not to continue in the project or any part of it, you are free to refuse without any disadvantage to you.

No ill effects or stress are expected for you, the caregiver, family, or others. All information will be numbered and your name will not be used. All information is confidential and will be seen only by members of the project team. If a report of results is published, only information about the total group will appear.

If you have any questions relating to this study, you should contact either of the following people:

Name _____   Name _____

Phone Number _____   Phone Number _____

Position _____   Position _____

Consent

_____

Patient (Please Print Name)

I have read and/or had explained to me the contents of this form, understand, and agree to participate in this study. I understand that I am free to refuse to answer any of the questions and that I can end my participation at any time, without this affecting my care now or in the future. This form is being signed in duplicate and I am retaining a copy for my information.

Signed: _____   Witness: _____   Date: _____

ANA guidelines (1985) discusses five stages for recruiting potential research subjects. These stages, which are taken from an earlier article by Scott (1982), are useful guides in obtaining informed consent. The stages are introductory-informative stage, consent stage, demographics stage, testing stage, and termination-debriefing stage. The following paragraphs consider some of the ethical issues surrounding each of these stages.

Introductory-Informative Stage During the introductory-informative stage the potential subjects are identified, and the groundwork is laid in preparation for the informed consent. When approaching potential subjects to invite participation, several factors need sensitive consideration. Most important is the avoidance of any kind of coercion. Coercion is sometimes not easily identified. For example, certain groups within society may feel compelled to participate by virtue of their role or position. We have already discussed this problem in dealing with such captive groups as the elderly, minors, mentally retarded subjects, students, and prisoners. In clinical nursing research the most frequent subjects are institutionalized clients, and investigators may be professional nurses. Under these circumstances the client may easily become confused as to the investigator's roles as nurse and as researcher. May (1979) addresses this issue and expresses concern that clients may not truly give informed consent when clarification is lacking between the roles. Clients' expectations about the caring, protective nurse are likely to be different from expectations concerning an investigator in a research project. Since clients may know little about the role of nurse researchers, they may be consenting to the nurse rather than the researcher.

May emphasizes that, when approaching potential subjects, nurse researchers must be sensitive to the issue of consent for nurse as opposed to consent for research to ensure high levels of informed consent. The role of nurse as researcher should be clearly evident to subjects, and research activities easily distinguished by the client. This is often a difficult dilemma for the staff nurse/research team member who may be asked by the researcher to obtain subject consents. The most important consideration is that the subjects be informed that they are being asked to participate in a research project, and the research activities and roles of nurses involved be carefully explained as they relate to regular caregiving roles and activities. An alternate approach is to have the investigator, or a research team member who is not involved in direct client care and therefore out of uniform, invite participation from clients.

The timing of invitations to subjects to participate and consent is also an important factor in producing ethical research. In clinical nursing research client subjects, who are frequently confronted with the physical and emotional stressors of illness, are often asked to participate in research at critical times. Consider the client who is anxious about impending surgery and is confronted with a research consent an hour or so before surgery. If it is at all possible, the researcher should plan to avoid highly critical times and approach such a client at an earlier, less stressful time so that an unbiased, informed decision can be made.

Consent, Demographic, and Testing Stages The consent, demographic, and testing stages of the recruitment process involve actually informing subjects, obtaining consent, and describing the contract between subjects and investigator as the project proceeds. During the data-collection stage the researcher must maintain normal human relations with subjects. He or she must abide by the agreements in the informed consent with particular concern for any subject's wish to withdraw. One of the biggest concerns of researchers and team members is maintaining the balance between protecting human rights through informing the subjects and, at the same time, maintaining a scientifically valid project.

In Chapter 6 we discussed a number of risks to validity of research findings and the impact of subject sensitivity on the researcher's expected outcomes. Considering this and our earlier discussion concerning ethical and scientific research, it is rarely acceptable to practice deception with subjects and is usually unnecessary in a well-designed project. However, there may be rare occasions when such deception will be condoned in a very significant and beneficial project where full disclosure of information to subjects at the consent stage could unavoidably jeopardize results. When any form of deception is used, subjects must be informed that full information cannot presently be given and why, and that a complete explanation will be provided at the finish of the project. Deceptions about risks to subjects or expected participation activities are never justified.

Termination-Debriefing Stage In the termination-debriefing stage all subjects should be given an opportunity to express feelings about their experience in the project. The termination-debriefing stage is an important aspect of research that often is not followed through because it is time consuming and often expensive in large projects. However, a brief statement to subjects about the findings of the project and a letter of appreciation go a long way toward encouraging respect and trust in the subject-investigator relationship. If any deception was used, it should be explained at this time. Subjects who are convinced that their participation is appreciated and has made a significant contribution to knowledge are more likely to consider giving their time to future research.

Ethics Review Boards or Committees

In addition to the researcher's responsibility to ensure that potential subjects give informed voluntary consent to participate in a research study, most institutions and funding agencies that sponsor research submit the research proposal to a separate and independent ethics review. The composition of **ethics review boards** is variable, but generally consists of a committee of the researcher's peers, specialists in the content area of the research, and often one or two members of the public who can identify with the proposed subjects.

The researcher is required to submit to the review board a fairly detailed proposal of the research that includes a description of the procedures to be used for data collection and sampling as well as detailed descriptions of methods to be employed for protection of human rights. The decision of the review board is based upon the adequacy of the research in meeting guidelines for a scientifically sound, ethical study (see Figure 6.1, Cell D). Figure 7.2 is a list of questions that are considered by the researcher and ethics review committee members in examining proposed research for protection of human rights at Queen's University School of Nursing, Kingston, Ontario. These guidelines provide detailed questions about the ethical implications of research that can be helpful to you as a reviewer and consumer of published research, as well as a guide in evaluating research in which you may be participating as a team member.

Consent or Approval of Others Involved in Research

In addition to potential subjects who may be minors or individuals unable to sign their own consent to participate, there may be other situations where the researcher may need to seek consent from a third party. For example, suppose a researcher proposes to collect data from mothers about the father's support during the birth experience. It may not be necessary to secure a formal consent from the fathers because they will not be contributing data directly; however, given the closeness of the relationship, it would certainly be wise to share information about

_____ Figure 7.2 _____

QUEEN'S UNIVERSITY SCHOOL OF NURSING: ETHICS REVIEW CHECKLIST

(To be completed prior to commencement of a research study involving human subjects.)

Name of Principal Investigator: _____

Title of Project: _____

Type of Subjects: _____

Date: _____ 19_____

Questions:

1. Is the study scientifically sound and of value to society?   YES   NO
2. Will the subjects be informed—prior to their actual involvement in the collection of data—of all features of the research that reasonably might be expected to influence willingness to participate?   YES   NO
3. Will the subjects be told that they can discontinue their participation at any time?   YES   NO
4. Does the study involve concealment and/or deception of the subject?   YES   NO
5. Will deception be used in order to obtain agreement to participate?   YES   NO
6. Will it be clear to the participants in your study that they are subjects of investigation?   YES   NO
7. Will information on your subjects be obtained from third parties?   YES   NO
8. Is any coercion exerted upon subjects to participate?   YES   NO
9. Is confidentiality of the subject's identity positively guaranteed?   YES   NO
10. In case there is a possibility that a subject's identity can be deduced by anyone other than the experimenter, is the participant's right to withdraw his/her data respected?   YES   NO
11. Will the researcher fulfill all his/her promises to the subjects?   YES   NO
12. Does the study involve physical stress (or the possibility of the subject's expectation thereof; examples: fatigue, pain, sleep loss, deprivation of food and drink, drugs, alcohol)?   YES   NO
13. Does the study involve the induction of mental discomfort to the subject (examples: fear, anxiety, loss of self-esteem, shame, guilt, embarrassment, becoming aware of personal weaknesses)?   YES   NO
14. Does the study involve subjects who are legally or otherwise not in a position to give their valid consent to participation (example: children, prison inmates, mental patients)?   YES   NO
15. Is information obtained on individual subjects disclosed to third parties?   YES   NO
16. Could publication of the research results possibly interfere with strict confidentiality?   YES   NO
17. Could publication of the results possibly harm the subject—either directly or through identification with his/her membership group?   YES   NO
18. Are there any other aspects of this study that may interfere with the protection of the well-being and dignity of the subject?   YES   NO

(continues)

_____ Figure 7.2 _____

CONTINUED

19. Will the experimenter make all efforts to ensure a normal human relationship between subject(s) and experimenter after the collection of data has been terminated?   YES   NO

20. In cases in which a subject is dissatisfied or complains about the research procedures, will the experimenter explain to the subject(s) that they may express their feelings to the Head of the Department?   YES   NO

21. Is the importance of the objective of the study in proportion to the inherent risk to the subjects?   YES   NO

22. Is there any hazard to the safety of the research personnel (professors, students, research staff, etc.)?   YES   NO

Signed: _____
Date: _____ 19____

Revised and approved,
Faculty Board, October 23, 1985

_____

Source: Queen's University School of Nursing. Kingston, Ontario. Used with permission.

the project with the "significant other" and gain the father's consent in order to maintain professional trust within the research relationship. The CNA *Ethical Guidelines* (1983) speak particularly to this issue.

Other situations involve sponsoring agencies, staff nurses, and physicians who may be directly involved in treatment and care of potential subjects. Some institutions may require a formal consent or contract to be signed with the researcher following an ethics review. In the case of nurses, physicians, and other health care professionals who are caring for or treating proposed subjects, it is usually not necessary for a formal consent to be signed unless the proposed research may interfere with, or is closely associated with, treatment or care being provided by others. However, it is very important to gain support of other health care workers in the research setting to ensure cooperation and respect throughout the project. It is also necessary for the researcher to share information and obtain verbal or written support for the project from these individuals. If others in the research setting are actually involved in the conduct of research (that is, in selecting subjects or collecting data) they must be fully informed and should sign a consent or contract to participate.

In certain situations the cultural, political, or social affiliations of subjects may require informing special groups to obtain approval or permission to conduct a project. For example, Burke's studies (Burke, Sayers, Baumgart, Wray, 1985) using native Indian children as subjects required the approval of the Chief and Band Council.

ACCOUNTABILITY OF PRACTICING NURSES AND RESEARCH TEAM MEMBERS

Today, nurses are more active in research than ever before. This fact is well recognized in the American, Canadian, and British professional guidelines for ethical research. Frequently nurses are invited to participate in nursing as well as medical and other clinical research. Like subjects, nurses' human rights must be safeguarded; participation must be voluntary, with the right to withdraw without penalty, and adequate information must be provided by the researcher to ensure protection of the nurse as well as client subjects. In many settings where research is conducted frequently, participation is outlined in the terms of employment.

Too often, nurses are requested to take part in medical experiments in which they are dispensing investigative drugs, the effects of which are not fully known. Creighton (1977) warns nurses that they may be placing themselves and clients in great jeopardy if they are not informed as to action, use, mode of administration, and side effects of such treatments in order to assess client reactions adequately. Nurses have an obligation to know the ethical review process of the study design, the intent and nature of the research, and whether the investigator is scientifically and clinically qualified. In addition, every nurse should be knowledgeable about the nursing profession's guidelines for ethical research.

If the nurse is satisfied that ethical guidelines have been met and consents to involvement in research, then he or she is similarly accountable to participate in producing valid, scientific findings. Data that are collected haphazardly and not according to protocol are a waste of valuable time, subjecting clients to unnecessary inconvenience or stress and in this sense are an unethical practice. Similarly, the researcher who uses these data unknowingly is producing invalid findings that may have long-term effects on clients if used in clinical situations.

Formal recognition for participation is often a concern of those who are involved in research projects. Everyone who contributes actively to a research project deserves a formal thank you; ideally, this should be placed in an acknowledgement if the study is published. The inclusion of names as co-investigators involves a high level of participation and usually encompasses involvement in conceptualization, planning, and development of specific instruments for the project. If such credits are to be given upon publication, this should be agreed upon in a contract with the researcher prior to onset.

Research assistants are often hired to conduct certain aspects of the project under the direction of the principal investigator or director of a project. Nurses, graduates, and undergraduate students frequently work in this capacity. Essentially the same guidelines for ethical and scientific research apply to protect the rights of research assistants. An employment contract between the researcher and assistants should completely inform the prospective assistant of the purpose and nature of the project and outline expected activity for assistants as well as payment and formal acknowledgment upon publication. The research assistant can then make an informed decision as to whether or not to accept the appointment. If the assistant agrees to involvement, he or she then becomes accountable for maintaining scientific and ethical behavior throughout the investigation.

_____ EVALUATING ETHICAL ELEMENTS OF A _____ RESEARCH REPORT

When reading a published nursing research report to evaluate the evidence for the protection of subjects' human rights, often very little information is provided except for a sentence or two concerning consent. Generally, most refereed scholarly journals examine the ethical implications before the article is accepted for publication, but that does not constitute an absolute assurance that no weaknesses exist which can be improved through future research. Ethical implications are extremely important if you are considering adopting research findings into practice because avoiding possible risk to clients is of primary importance.

The "Ethical Review Checklist" (Queen's University School of Nursing, 1985) is an excellent guide to use when you have a complete research report or proposal to review that contains an example of informed consent and an in-depth account of how the researcher protected the human rights of subjects. However, without a detailed description of data-collection instruments and a consent form in a published report, there are still a number of factors in a single article that you can critique from an ethical point of view. Table 7.2 will help you assess the ethical acceptability.

_____ Table 7.2 _____

GUIDELINES FOR CRITIQUE OF PROTECTION OF HUMAN RIGHTS

Criteria for Critique	*Comments*
1. Is the research problem a significant one for nursing? Is the design scientifically sound?	If an answer to the problem will not benefit clients or contribute to nursing knowledge, it may not be ethical to involve subjects.
2. Is the research designed to maximize benefit to human subjects and minimize risk?	If subjects are subjected to undue risk and the benefits or knowledge generated are low, there are ethical problems. Risky interventions have serious implications for clinical adoption.
3. Is the selection of subjects ethically appropriate to study the research problem?	It would be ethically inappropriate to use captive subjects such as prisoners, minors, elderly clients, and students when they are not the groups who would reap the benefit of the results.
4. Is there evidence of voluntary, informed consent?	Any evidence of subject coercion to participate and lack of information about the study purpose and subject participation violates human rights.
5. Is there evidence of subject deception?	Deception should be avoided if at all possible. The researcher must inform subjects about any deception and the reason(s) for that deception prior to subjects' consent. Subjects must be debriefed about deception at finish of study.
6. Have subjects been invited to consent when under high stress?	Consent under stress should be avoided if possible. Timing of invitations should not add to already stressful periods such as immediately prior to surgery or other complex procedures. Timing invitations well in advance is preferable.
7. Is informed consent given by a legal guardian or representative of a subject incapable of giving own consent?	This must be done in the case of minors or subjects who are physically or mentally incapacitated.
8. Is there evidence in the report that individual subjects can be identified?	The researcher must take precautions that publication of setting, data collection, and analysis will protect anonymity of subjects.
9. Is there evidence of an independent ethics review by board or committee?	Ethics review should be mentioned in the report. It provides more evidence for assurance of human rights' protection in the study.

_____ *SUMMARY* _____

This chapter has presented in some detail the need for professional, ethical guidelines for the conduct of clinical nursing research. The concept of risk/benefit ratio is discussed within the framework of ethical, scientific research in formulating and designing a project. The accountability of staff nurses, other research consumers, and research team members is stressed in assuring that the human rights of client subjects have been maintained throughout a project. Specified steps for ensuring the protection of human subjects' rights are described. The role of institutional review boards is briefly outlined, and a sample set of guidelines for a nursing ethics review of proposed research is presented. A briefer set of guidelines is provided for the consumer evaluating the ethical implications of a completed research report.

EXERCISES

1. The following is an abstract and consent form for a proposed research study. From the information provided
   a. Discuss the ethical implications of conducting this study.
   b. Using the guidelines in Table 7.2 for evaluating a written informed consent, critique the proposed consent form.
   c. Describe the procedure you would use as a research assistant to invite subjects to participate in this study and to obtain cooperation of the hospital and health care professionals directly involved in the care of these clients.

The Effects of Touch on Intracranial Pressure*

Abstract

This research study will be conducted using a time series, quasi-experimental design to determine the effects of procedural and nonprocedural touch on intracranial pressure (ICP). Literature shows that touch has an effect on blood pressure and heart rate, which in turn affects cerebral perfusion pressure and thus ICP. A non-random convenience sample of comatose patients with a catheter in place to monitor ICP who are at risk for (or have) increased ICP will be selected from the neurosurgical services

_____

* From unpublished research proposal by L. Baker et al. (1985). Queen's University School of Nursing. Kingston, Ontario.

in a large metropolitan hospital. All three of the variables—procedural touch, non-procedural touch, and control—will be randomly selected, two of which will be performed during each shift. Examples of types of touch to be used are: holding, stroking, squeezing, or patting the hand; giving a bedbath; providing mouth care; and carrying out passive range-of-motion exercises. Potential nursing implications will include reducing the frequency of any touch found to increase ICP and increasing the frequency of any touch found to lower ICP.

Information and Consent for Participation in Research Study:
The Effects of Touch on Intracranial Pressure

The purpose of this study is to look at how unconscious patients respond to certain kinds of touch. We know patients respond to touch through changes in blood pressure and heart rate. We want to find out how certain kinds of touch change pressure in the head. The pressure in the head is already being measured by the monitor. Several times each day for about one week, we will record these measurements.

The kinds of touch your family member will receive are: holding, stroking, squeezing, or patting the hand; giving a bedbath; giving mouth care; and exercising the arms and legs.

Each of these, except touching the patient's hand as described, must be done regularly by the nurse whether or not the patient is a part of this study. Therefore, touching the hand is the only possible risk in this study. If, for some reason, we find that pressure in the head rises too high, touching the hand will be stopped right away. We feel that touching the hand may help the patient by lowering pressure in the head, and by giving a feeling of safety and comfort.

Your family member may or may not directly benefit from this study; however, in the long run, we hope that any information we learn will help us to give better care to similar patients. Whether you agree to participate is your decision and will not change the care given to your family member now or in the future. If at any time you no longer want your family member in the study, you may withdraw your consent.

All names and personal information will be kept private, even if a report of the study's results is made public.

If you have any questions about this study, you may contact any of the following:

Investigators: Linda Baker   Lori Langille
               Vanessa Daniel   Dawn Wright
               Cheryl Kind
                    (Year IV Nursing Students)

Supervisor: Professor A. Brown

Queen's University School of Nursing, Kingston. Phone: 545-2668.

    I have read and/or have had the information in this form explained to me and agree to having my family member _____ be a part of this study. I can have the study stopped at any time without affecting the nursing care my family member will receive.

Date   Signature   Witness

2. The following consent form was developed by two students who proposed to study the effects of environmental sound on stress reduction in female prisoners.
   a. Evaluate the adequacy of the information to be provided about the project to this disadvantaged group of subjects.
   b. Suggest ways in which you might improve this letter of information and consent form for the proposed study.

*Environmental Sound Therapy for Stress Management Project Information and Consent Form**

We are fourth year nursing students, doing a study about stress management under the direction of Professor Carol Roberts at Queen's University. The study will involve listening to a tape of environmental sounds, which are sounds found in nature. One example is ocean sounds, such as waves breaking on the shore and sea gulls.

    The prison environment can be very stressful and it is known that high amounts of stress can have harmful effects on the body. If the way a person copes with stress can be improved, then a healthier individual may result.

    Those who give consent to take part in the study will be divided randomly into two groups. Both groups will be asked to fill out a questionnaire. One group will be asked to listen and relax to the environmental sound tape for 1/2 hour every evening for four weeks. The other group will not participate in the sound therapy. After four weeks, both groups will be asked to complete the

---

* From a proposal by G. Barton and V. Jozefowicz (1987). Queen's University School of Nursing. Kingston, Ontario.

questionnaire again. The questions will address the number of times you experienced certain symptoms over a two-week period. Some of the symptoms are linked to stress.

There are absolutely no known risks to you if you decide to participate; however, if you are assigned to the group which will listen to the environmental sounds, you will be giving up 30 minutes of your evening for four weeks.

In the long run, it is hoped that the results of the study can be used to benefit you and other inmates by reducing the stress-related sickness you experience.

Whether or not you agree to participate is entirely up to you. Your decision will in no way affect the kind of care you receive, or how you are treated in the prison. It will have no effect on your length of sentence.

If at any time you decide not to continue in the project, you will be free to refuse without any disadvantage to you.

All of the information received will be confidential and your name will not be used. If the results of this study are published, your name will not be used.

If you have any questions relating to this study, please contact Vivian Jozefowicz or Gwen Barton by leaving a note at the Prison hospital. Please inform us that you have questions, and we will get in touch with you.

REFERENCES

American Nurses' Association. (1985). *Human rights guidelines for nurses in clinical and other research.* Kansas City, Mo.: American Nurses' Association.

American Nurses' Association, Commission on Nursing Research. (1981). *Guidelines for the investigative function of nurses.* Kansas City, Mo.: American Nurses' Association.

Arminger, B. Sr. (1977). Ethics of nursing research: Profile, principles, perspective. *Nursing Research, 26*(5), 330–336.

Baker, L.; Daniel, S.; King, C.; Langille, L.; & Wright, D. (1987). The effects of touch on intercranial pressure. Unpublished research proposal. Year IV students. Queen's University, Kingston, Ontario.

Barton, G., & Jozefowicz, V. (1987). Environmental sound therapy for stress management. Unpublished research proposal. Year IV students, Queen's University, Kingston, Ontario.

Burke, S. O.; Sayers, L. A.; Baumgart, A. J.; & Wray, J. O. (1985). Pitfalls in cross-cultural use of the Denver Developmental Screening Test: Cree Indian children. *Canadian Journal of Public Health, 76,* 303–307.

Canadian Nurses' Association. (1983). *Ethical guidelines for nursing research involving human subjects.* Ottawa: Canadian Nurses' Association.

Creighton, H. (1977). Legal concerns of nursing research. *Nursing Research, 26*(5), 337–341.

Field, P. A., & Morse, J. M. (1985). *Nursing research: The application of qualitative approaches.* Rockville, Md.: Aspen Systems.

Katz, J. (1972). *Experimentation with human beings: The authority of the investigations, subject, professions and state in the human experimentation process.* New York: Russell Sage Foundation.

May, K. A. (1979, January). The nurse as researcher: Impediment to informed consent? *Nursing Outlook,* 36–39.

Milgram, S. (1963). Behavioral study of obedience. *Journal of Abnormal and Social Psychology, 67*(4), 371–377.

Queen's University School of Nursing. (1985). *Ethics review checklist.* Kingston, Ontario: Queen's University School of Nursing.

Royal College of Nursing of the United Kingdom. (1977). *Ethics related to research in nursing.* London: Royal College of Nursing of the United Kingdom.

Schrock, R. (1984). Moral issues in nursing research. In D.F.S. Cormack (Ed.), *The research process in nursing* (pp. 193–204). London: Blackwell Scientific.

Scott, D. W. (1982). Ethical issues in nursing research: Access to human subjects. *Topics in Clinical Nursing, 4*(1), 74–83.

World Medical Association. (1964). *Declaration of Helsinki: Recommendations guiding doctors in clinical research.* New York: World Medical Association.

8

Sampling and Its Effect on the Study

The match of the sampling procedures to the purpose and the design of the study is a critical factor in assessing the meaningfulness, internal validity, and external validity of the study findings. (For a review of these linkages, see Table 6.4.) For the research team member, a clear understanding of the rationale behind the sampling protocols helps to ensure the correct selection of the subjects. For the research consumer, an understanding of the rationale behind the researchers' sampling design and a conceptual understanding of how the sampling procedures affect the findings will help in making more logical decisions on the applicability of the findings to practice.

OUTLINE

Population, Setting, and Sample

Types of Samples

A General Critique of
  Probability and
  Nonprobability Samples

Determining the Adequacy of
  a Sample

OBJECTIVES

After reading this chapter, you will be able to

1. Identify a study's population, setting, and type of sample.
2. Evaluate the appropriateness of the type of sample for the study's purpose and design.
3. Assess the quality of the sampling process.
4. Determine the impact of the sampling on the applicability of the results to your practice.

NEW TERMS

Sampling

Population

Site or setting

Sample

Nonprobability sampling

Probability sampling

Case study

Purposive or theoretical
  sampling

Convenience sampling

Quota sampling

Snowball sampling

Network sampling

Matching

Random sampling

Simple random sampling

Systematic sampling

Stratified random sampling

Cluster sampling

Representative sample

Sampling error

Sampling bias

Sample size

Power analysis

Figure 8.1

RESEARCH PROCESS FLOWCHART

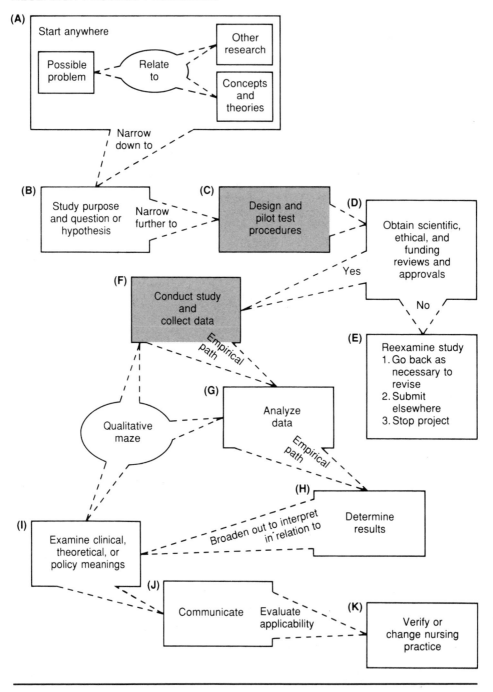

_____ POPULATION, SETTING, AND SAMPLE _____

You will usually find a section of the study report that describes its sample, setting or site, or population, or some combination of these terms. These research concepts are an integral part of the process called sampling. **Sampling** is the process by which researchers select the subjects to whom a study question will be addressed, or on whom a study hypothesis will be tested. The plan for the sampling procedures is developed during the design phase of the research process (Figure 8.1, Cell C) and is carried out during the conduct of the study (Cell F). Figure 8.2 shows how these research terms are related to each other. Which terms are used will depend on the type of study.

As implied in Figure 8.2, the target **population** is the entire group to whom the researchers expect to be able to generalize the study results. The **site** or **setting** is where the population or the portion of it that is being studied is located and where the study is carried out. The **sample** is the small portion of the population that the researchers are studying in the particular site or setting.

For example, in an article entitled, "Determination of Normal Variation in Skin Blood Flow Velocity in Healthy Adults" (Huether & Jacobs, 1986), the population (healthy adults) can be deduced from the title. Following the purpose and review of the literature sections of the report is the method section, in which the first subsection is entitled "Sample." The authors do not use the terms *site* or *setting*, but clearly describe the location where the subjects were and where the data was

_____ Figure 8.2 _____

THE RELATIONSHIP OF THE STUDY POPULATION, SETTING, AND SITE TO THE SAMPLE

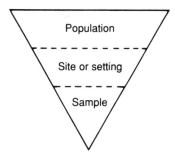

collected. This is the usual format for the written report for a quantitative study. In this example, the site was the College of Nursing at the University of Utah and the setting was the Physiological Nursing Laboratory. The sample, or those members of the population of healthy adults who were actually the subjects in the study, was 51 nursing students.

Qualitative studies are more likely to emphasize the setting and the site in the report of the study. For example, Kus (1986) did an ethnographic study of gay men and women. Under the methods section of the report, he uses three paragraphs to describe his subjects and the settings. This is typical of the written report for qualitative studies.

Occasionally you will come across a study of an entire population. This is likely to occur in qualitative or quantitative descriptive studies when there are only a few persons who have the characteristics in which the researcher is interested. For example, if the purpose is to describe a particular care-seeking behavior that is known to be present only among persons of a small ethnic group, it might be possible to study the entire population. This type of study also occurs when a data base is used that includes (at least theoretically) all the members of a population. Sheps (1985) followed this format when he used a computerized registry of all severely handicapped children in British Columbia as the source of data.

Many types of samples are used in nursing research. Each has a different purpose and is best suited to a specific type of study design. The optimum number of subjects varies with type of sample used. Table 8.1 gives an overview of the relationships between study design, type of sample, and sample size.

You will recall from Chapter 6 that study design is inextricably linked to the level of inquiry of the question or hypothesis, and to the degree of development of nursing knowledge on the topic under study. (For a quick review of these relationships, see Table 6.1.) By extension, the sample also should fit with the level of knowledge and study question. For example, in the case of a researcher studying an area in which little knowledge had accumulated, the researcher would be correct in selecting a level 1 question and a qualitative design. The choice of sample would flow from this decision, and the researcher would select a suitable sample, ranging from a single case study to a convenience sample. Table 8.1 shows that a stratified random sample would not be suitable in this example. Conversely, if a study employed an experimental design, the nonrandom samples would be suitable.

_____ Table 8.1 _____

RELATIONSHIPS BETWEEN SAMPLE TYPES AND STUDY DESIGNS

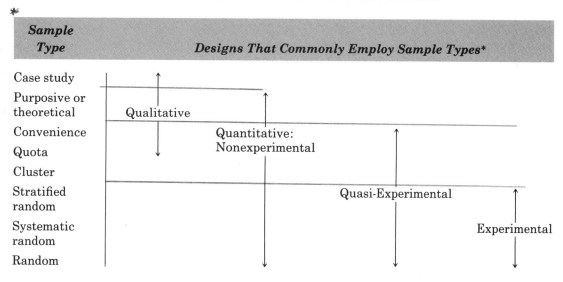

* The suitability of a particular type of sampling for a particular type of design can be more controversial when there is an overlap among possible types of designs.

_____ TYPES OF SAMPLES _____

All types of samples can be categorized under two major groupings—nonprobability and probability sampling. They each strive to be representative of the population and/or the phenomenon under study, but employ entirely different methods to do so. Both have their strengths and weaknesses. **Nonprobability sampling** uses the judgment of the researcher to select those subjects who know the most about the phenomenon and are able to articulate and explain nuances to the researcher. The nonprobability sampling plan is constructed from an objective judgment of a likely starting point, and the direction the sampling takes will be a decision made by the researcher as the study progresses (Field & Morse, 1985). **Probability sampling** requires that every person or element of the population have an equal chance of being selected for the sample. This equal chance is obtained through the use of randomization. A very specific sampling plan is made at the onset of the study and only rarely are departures made from this plan. Four of the most common types of nonprobability and probability samples are discussed below.

Nonprobability Sampling (5)

(1) **Case Studies**   Case studies by definition use either one or very few subjects. The phenomenon under study is examined with an extreme rigor and thoroughness. The subjects or cases are selected using clearly stated criteria that are consistent with the purpose of the study. Field and Morse use the term *opportunistic sample* to describe the selection of subjects who are willing and able to discuss and explain the phenomenon to the researcher. They use the term *judgmental sample* to refer to the selection of subjects because of their special knowledge of the topic. Kus (1986) used both of these sampling techniques to select the cases in his study of the clinical implications for nurses when caring for gay men and women.

(2) **Purposive or Theoretical Samples**   Purposive sampling is designed to select subjects who are most likely to facilitate further development of the emerging nursing knowledge, concepts, or theory (Field & Morse). This approach is used in both qualitative and quantitative studies. Theoretical sampling is the term applied to a somewhat more elaborate process used in tandem with the analysis of the data in grounded theory studies. As the analysis proceeds to unravel the relationships between the elements of the emerging theory, new subjects are sought to clarify, extend, and refute these findings (Chenitz & Swanson, 1986). This is the type of sampling Wilson (1983) used in her study of the "dispatching process" for clients moving from the hospital to the community mental health system. As her study progressed and the key elements of the concept of a dispatching process emerged, she purposefully sought subjects and observations that would help to further elaborate or refute the elements of the process.

(3) **Convenience Sampling**   Convenience sampling takes advantage of a group of subjects that fall within the population of interest and are conveniently located or readily accessible to the research team. This type of sample is also referred to as an *accidental sample*. Used without the direction of a theoretical sample, a convenience sample can be the same as the population of the study. In the first example used in this chapter, Huether and Jacobs (1986) studied the population of healthy adults and used a convenience sample of student nurses. As a research consumer reading this particular study, you would have to decide whether or not the convenience sample truly represents the population or, at the other extreme, if the study was only of the population of student nurses at one school of nursing. Specifically, if

your clinical setting deals with healthy adults, to what extent are the student nurses in the study similar to your clients?

④ **Quota Sampling**   Quota sampling uses sampling methods such as those described above and below to fill one or more groups with a predetermined number or proportion of subjects with particular characteristics. This is done so that the researcher will later be able to compare these particular characteristics of the subjects in the analysis of the data. The characteristics of the subjects that will have quotas imposed on them become variables that the researchers have predetermined to be important components of the phenomenon under study. For example, if a researcher decides that a process will be different for men and women, then a quota of 50% of each might be set. After this number of members of one sex is reached, sampling stops for subjects with that particular characteristic, but continues for persons of the other sex until that quota is filled.

⑤ **Special Techniques**   Several techniques are used in nonprobability sampling. **Snowball sampling** is a technique wherein each current subject suggests the names of others who might be willing to participate. **Network sampling** is a related technique that can be used when there are limited formal lists or ways of reaching potential subjects. For example, Burke, Maloney, and Baumgart (1987) used networking and snowballing to obtain the names of recent native Indian immigrants to a large city. **Matching** is a special technique used to construct a comparison group by filling it with persons who are similar to each subject in the other group by predetermined variables. Ideally, any variable, other than the independent variable that could affect the dependent variable, should be matched. Practically, however, the more variables matched the more difficult it is to obtain an adequate sample size. Thus, only a few variables are usually matched. Sex, age, and social class are frequent matching variables. In the Burke (1978) study, for example, a comparison group of two parent families with all normal children was needed for comparison with two parent families with handicapped children. Each family was matched by neighborhood to obtain a group of families with similar socio-demographic characteristics.

Probability Sampling and Randomization — used in all quant research

Probability samples all use the process of random selection of the subjects within a population. In random selection all the persons in the

population have an equal and independent chance of being chosen to be
sampled. **Random sampling** is used in all types of quantitative research
to increase the odds that a representative sample is selected, thereby
increasing the chances that any generalizations from the study results
will actually apply to the target population.

The process of randomization can be used for the selection of the
entire sample or within a sample selected by other means, such as a
purposive or convenience sample. For example, the concept of randomization was introduced in Chapter 6 in conjunction with experimental
designs, where random assignment to study groups was discussed.
However, random selection of subjects from a population, and random
assignment of subjects from a sample of convenience to groups within
the study are separate processes, and the use of randomization for one
does not necessarily mean that it is used for the other. The use of
randomization wherever feasible within the design usually strengthens
a quantitative study. Strictly speaking, however, probability sampling
refers to the randomization in the initial procedures used to select
subjects from the population.

Simple Random Samples Simple random sampling is commonly referred to as random sampling. Random sampling may be difficult to achieve in many clinical studies, but it offers the clearest way
of describing the sampling processes since other types of probability
sampling all use the same randomization procedures.

To clarify the concepts in probability theory that are behind the
process of randomization, imagine the following procedure. Suppose
you want to select 10 subjects randomly from a population of 100 clients
within a unit for an in-depth survey of a particular aspect of their
nursing care. You could do this by writing each of their names on a
separate slip of paper, placing them all in a paper bag, selecting one,
noting the name, replacing that name, shaking the bag and selecting a
second, and so on. Note that you must replace each name after each
selection to keep the odds of being selected at 1 in 100, not 1 in 99, then 98,
and so forth. If someone is selected twice, then you repeat the process
until you have 10 unique names. This is an example of random selection
with replacement.

Researchers apply the same principles but are more likely to use a
table of random numbers (see Table 8.2) or a computer-generated list of
random numbers. To use a table of random numbers such as Table 8.2,
close your eyes and place a pencil on the table. The number closest to the
tip is the number selected. To use a table of random numbers for the
example above, you must first give each potential subject a unique

_____ Table 8.2 _____

A TABLE OF RANDOM NUMBERS

83 82 19 63 47	61 54 77 13 93	01 29 14 13 49
11 69 00 30 23	58 21 92 70 52	18 74 32 78 62
13 40 82 66 65	07 00 85 43 53	12 76 05 46 47
38 79 17 09 85	90 46 54 51 43	42 59 36 20 46
92 96 58 86 29	13 49 90 63 19	58 30 03 39 64

number between 1 and 100. (Note that these will be read as 01 to 00 on the table.) Then you could repeat the process with the pencil ten times to get the ten subjects needed. Alternatively, you could select the first number and then move across the row to the right (or down, just as long as you are consistent and have determined the pattern ahead of time) to select the next number until you have the 10 subjects needed. For example, if your pencil landed on 92 (second block, second line, third number) that becomes the first subject; progressing along that line, the next numbers would be 70, 52, 18, 74, 32, 78, and 62. Next you might move down one line and select 13 and 40 to make up the needed number of subjects.

Systematic Sampling   When a lengthy list of the population exists, systematic sampling is often used. It is easier to select a single random number (by one of the methods described above) and then to systematically select, say, every tenth person on the list after that random start. If the initial list is of the entire population, then systematic sampling is a type of probability sampling; however, if this is not the case, then the result is a nonprobability sample. Nonprobability samples result when systematic sampling is used to select a smaller sample with a minimum of bias, for example, from a list obtained as a convenience sample.

In Burke's (1978) study, the sample of two-parent families with a handicapped child was selected using systematic sampling. An unnumbered, alphabetically arranged list of about 300 families, which constituted the population within the site of the study, was obtained. Then, using some of the procedures discussed in the sample size section of this chapter, it was determined that 20 of the families were needed for the sample, or one in every 15 of those on the list. Next, a table of random numbers (see Table 8.2.) was used to randomly select the starting number within the 01 to 15 range. In this example the number was 07. So the first subject selected was the seventh one on the list; and since one in 15 families on the list were needed, every fifteenth family was selected after this random start. Thus, the 22nd, 37th, 52nd, etc. through to the 292nd families were selected until there were 20 families.

There can be problems with the representativeness of this method if the entire list is not used and if there is some known or unknown order in the list. For instance, if Burke had used every fifth family, thus sampling only the first portion of the list, and if the list had been arranged so that those families with the more severely handicapped children were listed first, the sample would not have been representative. It would have been biased toward more severely handicapped children. Other types of bias are discussed below.

Stratified Random Sampling When the researcher, for theoretical reasons, wants to ensure that certain characteristics of the population are represented in the sample, a stratified random sample can be more efficient than either the simple or systematic random sample. To expand on the example of Burke's study, differences between single and two-parent families were one of the foci of the study. Since simple or systematic random sampling would have resulted in more two-parent families than single parent families, strata or groupings of the members of the population were made by the number of parents. Samples were then selected from each strata. Separate lists of single and two-parent families (two strata) were each sampled using systematic sampling.

Cluster Samples Cluster sampling uses another type of grouping. This procedure is followed to reduce the cost of data gathering when the population is large and far flung. Suppose a researcher wanted to study all adults undergoing surgery on an out-patient basis in a particular state. Other types of random sampling would involve obtaining a list of all possible subjects and randomly selecting from this list. This would be time consuming, and the data-collection process from such a sample would be complex and expensive. To illustrate what is involved in cluster sampling, imagine that there are a hundred sites in the state where such surgery is done. The patients within each site would be called a cluster. Ten clusters could be randomly selected and all the patients, or a random selection of patients within each cluster could be done.

Since only the clusters, and not the subjects, are truly randomly selected, it is possible that the sample might not be representative. Specifically, the major risk to representativeness is that the subjects themselves may not echo the characteristics of the population. Some researchers check the clusters along key variables such as social class and city size, before proceeding with data collection. However, this process can introduce bias if, for example, a new sample is drawn because one of the clinics is presumed to be uncooperative rather than because the sample was deemed to be unrepresentative.

Samples and Generalizability

As a research consumer you are concerned, first, with how **representative** the sample is of the population and the phenomenon that it purports to study. Second, you will have to decide whether or not the findings from the particular sample can be generalized to your particular setting. Two factors implicit in all sampling procedures commonly limit the generalizability of the results—sampling error and sampling bias.

Sampling Error Every study will contain error to the extent that results will never be 100% representative of the entire population; every sample will be slightly different from the next sample of the same population. Sampling error is more likely to occur if the population or sample size is relatively small. When careful probability sampling is used, it is possible to estimate the degree of error statistically. Nonprobability sampling leaves the question of error open and unpredictable.

Sampling Bias In contrast to sampling error, which is random, sampling bias occurs when the sampling plan or procedure introduces some sort of systematic distortion of the eventual sample. Sources of sampling bias can be the time of day or year when the data were collected; the place the data were gathered; the languages used; and the social circumstances of the subjects (Field & Morse, 1985). Further bias can be introduced by the person collecting the data, to the extent that personal views color the data collected or the actual responses of the subjects who might tend to wish to hurry, please, or displease the person collecting the data. For example, when Huether and Jacobs (1986) undertook a study of healthy adults and then used a convenience sample of nursing students, several biases were introduced. The sample was biased to the extent that it did not represent the population of healthy adults in terms of gender and age. However, given the nature of the physiological measures used, it is not likely that time, place, language, and so on were sources of bias. To the extent that this sample was biased, the generalizability of the results is limited.

In general, probability samples will contain less bias than non-probability samples. However, the procedures used in either type of sampling can inadvertently introduce bias. For example, in Burke's (1978) study where lists of families with handicapped children were used for the sampling procedures, a bias existed in the original lists. The lists included only those families that obtained services from the formal health care system; families that chose alternate health care, such as a healer, or no health care at all, were excluded. Thus there was a bias in the sample toward families who used the formal health care system. Generalizability to the entire population of families with handicapped children was limited by this bias.

A GENERAL CRITIQUE OF PROBABILITY AND NONPROBABILITY SAMPLES

An overview of the strengths and weaknesses of the two general types of samples will help you assess the applicability of the findings to your clinical practice. This is done by examining error and bias. Further considerations include the quality of the population and the selected sample that were available to the researcher.

Probability Sample Critique

The strength of the probability sample resides in the reduction to a known minimum of the sampling error and sampling bias. The chances of a representative sample, and therefore generalizable results, are much higher with a probability sample than with a nonprobability sample of the same population.

Problems arise when the entire population is not accessible, as seen in the example above (Burke, 1978). A second problem concerns the availability of the sample once it is selected. Even when the entire population is accessible for sample selection, portions of the sample will not be available for reasons such as a move out of town or a refusal to participate. When both of these problems occur, as they often do, the biases and error in the sampling are compounded.

A further criticism of random samples emerges from the nature of our subjects, who are individual and unique human beings. Phenomenologists and qualitative researchers argue that no matter how a sample is selected, it cannot represent the entire population, but only those particular persons at that particular time and place. While acknowledging this concern, most consumers of nursing research do not take such a conservative view. Whether or not this is a problem for a study must be judged by determining the degree of difference between subjects, and whether such differences seriously limit generalizations.

Nonprobability Sample Critique

For the local, practical, and/or economic reasons discussed above, most nursing research uses nonprobability sampling. This places a much greater burden of judgment on you, the research consumer, as you attempt to gauge the degree of generalizability of study results. The extent of error due to sampling will be unknown, and therefore should be conservatively estimated to be high. Bias will be present, but it might be better identified because the researcher should be aware of this threat to the generalizability, and should explain possible bias in the report. The quality of the data obtained has the potential to be high if the researchers are dealing with willing and able subjects. The meaningfulness of the results has the potential to be high depending on the logical and theoretical direction that the researcher can impose on the sampling process.

In summary, when evaluating probability samples, the quality might initially be seen as either high or low—black or white—with some shades of gray emerging as the sample design and procedures are examined more closely. However, evaluation of the quality of the nonprobability sample usually begins with an assessment of it as perhaps adequate but having limitations, and thus appears to be a mid-gray. Later in the evaluation process the research consumer will often modify this judgment of the quality and assess it as a relatively lighter or darker shade of gray.

_____ DETERMINING THE ADEQUACY OF A SAMPLE _____

Sample Size

The number of subjects in a study constitutes the size of the sample; this is commonly referred to as **sample size.** The shorthand notation for sample size is n for number. You will read that "$n = 100$," meaning that the sample size was equal to 100, or "to increase the $n \dots$," meaning that in order to increase the size of the sample such and such was done.

Sample size is determined on scientific grounds, but is achieved within the pragmatics of the real world. There is a human tendency to be more likely to believe results from studies that have larger sample sizes. While it is often desirable to have such a size, the ultimate criterion for the adequacy of the samples is the representativeness of the meanings, relationships, or causes as stated in the study purpose. A larger sample size with a poor design or protocol can inflate error and bias.

Selecting the appropriate size and obtaining the size needed are major concerns for the researcher. As a research consumer, you will assess the adequacy of the logic behind the selection of the sample size as well as the actual size of the sample. The rationale used to determine an adequate size for the sample is logically linked to the type of sampling used, which is in turn linked to the purpose and design of the study. Sample size is also linked to the type of analysis to be used on the data collected and the ethical consideration of confidentiality.

Pragmatically, the best sample size from the scientific perspective is subject to limitations related to access to the population as well as the limitations of the personnel and fiscal resources available to the researchers. These factors can be of concern if they result in serious error or bias in the sample. As a research consumer, you usually have to deduce what these limitations were and then assess their effect on the sample. For example, in the Huether and Jacobs (1986) study you would probably deduce that there were only so many students who volunteered to be subjects, only so many months in which to complete the project and only so many dollars available to pay for equipment and data collection. All these factors taken together could have limited the size of the sample to the 51 subjects in the study.

The scientific and pragmatic factors that influence sample size vary with the purpose, design, and type of sample used. In qualitative studies where the purpose is to explore meanings and phenomena, an adequate sample size is one that is large enough to accomplish this goal. The exact number often cannot be determined in advance because the researcher will continue until the meanings are clear. Often the number of subjects is smaller than in quantitative studies. The proposition that a larger sample size is always better does not apply in studies where the type of sample is usually purposive or theoretical. Too many subjects would serve to cloud the issues and overcomplicate the complex analysis process. For these types of studies, the sample size is adequate when the meanings are clear and the data are fully explored (Polit & Hungler, 1987; Field & Morse, 1985). There has been a trend away from the single case study toward n's of 5 to 20 or even 30 in qualitative studies. Sample

_____ Table 8.3 _____

TOTAL NUMBER NEEDED WITH FIVE PER CELL AND FOUR TYPES OF SUBJECTS

	Females	*Males*		
Older persons	5	5		
Younger persons	5	5		
			Total	20

sizes smaller than this make it more likely that the meanings are idiosyncratic and, furthermore, make it difficult to obscure the identity of subjects as is required in most ethical consent forms. Larger sample sizes would be impossible to analyze given current methods and probably would be best left to quantitative methods.

Quantitative nonexperimental and quasi-experimental studies that use nonprobability samples can be assessed using rough guidelines. One set of rough guidelines is related to how the data will be analyzed. Most researchers agree that there should be at least 5 of each type of subject in the sample, and recommend at least 10, with 20–30 per type of subject preferred (Polit & Hungler, 1987). For example, Tables 8.3 and 8.4 show how quota sampling would be used if researchers wished to study both older and younger men and women. Four types of subjects would result—older men, younger men, older women, and younger women. To apply the minimum number of 5 per type (or 5 per cell of the table that would eventually be in the results section of the report), there would be a total $n = 20$ (4 cells × 5 subjects). Similarly, if a more generous number per cell of 20 was used, then the total n would be 80 (4 cells × 20 subjects).

_____ Table 8.4 _____

TOTAL NUMBER NEEDED WITH TWENTY PER CELL AND FOUR TYPES OF SUBJECTS

	Females	*Males*		
Older persons	20	20		
Younger persons	20	20		
			Total	80

In these types of studies the larger numbers will produce results that are more stable; that is, if the same procedure were repeated, the researcher would be more likely to obtain similar results the next time if larger numbers were used.

A similar type of logic is behind some very large sample sizes when the incidence of the type of subject or variable is relatively rare. For example, a very large number of subjects would be needed if a survey was being done of all children who had been hospitalized to determine whether or not they had some specific, relatively rare problem. This is because a small sample might not contain any subjects or too few to analyze. Whenever the researchers can estimate the rate of probable occurrence of the variable of interest, it is possible to calculate the total sample size needed. In this example, if the rate of occurrence was estimated to be 5%, then a sample of 100 should result in the minimum of 5 of this particular group of subjects. A sample of 600 would be needed to obtain about 30 of the children with the variable of interest. The researcher must decide on the relative cost/benefits of the larger and smaller sample sizes. The research consumer must decide if the resulting sample size is representative enough to apply the findings to a particular setting.

When probability sampling is used in quantitative studies, it is possible to calculate the exact number of subjects needed using a statistical procedure called **power analysis.** (Technical terms associated with this are alpha, beta, and effect size.) The researcher uses the following information along with a specific power analysis formula and tables (Cohen, 1977) to determine in advance the number of subjects needed. The following estimates and parameters are entered into the formula:

1. The relative acceptable chance that the hypothesis might be wrong, but accepted
2. The relative acceptable chance that the hypothesis might be right, but rejected
3. The degree of variation that can usually be expected in the dependent variable
4. The number of groups of subjects under study

Depending on how accurate each estimate used in the formula is, it is possible to determine the sample size with some precision. It would be easier for the research consumer if power analyses were always reported, but often they are not done or not reported. A consumer might have to write to the researcher and/or obtain the technical assistance necessary to have such an analysis conducted if the results of such a study are being given serious consideration for implementation in a clinical setting.

In studies that use probability samples, the larger the sample the greater the chance that the sample is representative of the population. Looking at the elements that enter into a power analysis, you might be able to deduce that the larger the sample the greater the chances that the hypothesis is correctly accepted or rejected.

Evaluating a Sample   *2 steps*

Evaluating the quality of a sample is a two-step process. First, the research consumer must determine the adequacy of the sample from the perspective of the researchers. Some modifications may be necessary because you will not have all the technical expertise. Using the questions in the first column of Table 8.5 and the content of this chapter you will be able to make these judgments.

The second step is to evaluate the clinical applicability of the results obtained with the sample. This must be done in the light of your evaluation of the scientific adequacy of the sample. Thus, you will examine each aspect of a sample first from one perspective, and then from the clinical perspective. The background that you will need to answer the questions in the second column of Table 8.5 is your own clinical experience, that of your colleagues, and information from textbooks and other reference materials within your own clinical field.

_____ *SUMMARY* _____

The sampling procedures used in a study must match the purpose and design of the study in order to assure the meaningfulness and validity of the study findings. The strengths and weaknesses of the two major types of sampling—nonprobability and probability sampling—are described; and questions of generalizability of results, including sampling error and sampling bias, are explored.

——— *Table 8.5* ——

EVALUATING THE ADEQUACY AND APPLICABILITY OF THE SAMPLE

Scientific Adequacy	*Clinical Applicability*

Population

Is the intended population clearly stated?
Is there any bias in the way that the population was accessed?

Is the population similar to that in your clinical area?
Is there any bias of a type that would limit applicability to your setting?

Setting

Is the setting clearly described?
Is there any bias in the way that the setting was selected?
Is there any bias in the way in which the setting was accessed?

Is the setting similar to your clinical setting?
Is there any bias of a type that would limit applicability of the results to your clinical setting?

Fit with Purpose and Design

Does the type of sample fit with the type of design?
Does the type of sample fit with the level of inquiry and purpose of the study? (See Table 6.1.)

Does this type of sample produce results that have clinical meaning in your setting?

Qualitative Studies Only

Does the sampling strategy have the potential to enhance knowledge and meaning?

Does the sample yield results that add needed knowledge and/or meaning?

Quantitative: Nonexperimental Studies Only

Does the sampling strategy have the potential to enhance knowledge of specific aspects of the variables studied?

Does the sample yield results that add needed knowledge of clinically significant variables in your setting?

Quantitative: Quasi-experimental Studies Only

Do the sampling plan and procedures have the potential to enhance knowledge of the nature of the relationships between the variables under study?

Does the sample yield results that add needed knowledge about relationships between clinically significant variables?

Quantitative: Experimental Studies Only

Do the sampling plan and procedures have the potential to enhance knowledge of causes and effects between the variables under study?

Does the sample yield results about the causes of variables that are significant to your clinical setting?

Sample Size

Is a methodological or theoretical rationale

Would a nurse with experience with the type

_____ *Table 8.5* _____
         CONTINUED

Scientific Adequacy	Clinical Applicability
for the sample size clearly explained? Is the sample size similar to those in similar studies? For qualitative studies, do there seem to be enough subjects to describe the phenomenon, but not so many as to cloud the issues? For studies with a probability sample, was a power analysis done? For quantitative studies, are there enough subjects of each type so that there will be at least five in each cell for the analysis?	of clients under study think that the size is appropriate?

Sample Design and Selection Procedures

Scientific Adequacy	Clinical Applicability
Is the most rigorous sampling design applicable to the particular study design used? If not, or if diversion from the design is made, is the rationale clearly stated? Is enough information given so that another researcher would be able to replicate the sampling procedures? Is any attrition of subjects clearly described? Does the actual sampling procedure employ the stated sampling design?	Does the actual sample still fit well with the study design and purpose? Does the actual sample still compare with your clients?

Sampling Bias

Scientific Adequacy	Clinical Applicability
Are known and probable sources of bias noted by the researcher? Are these biases reflected in the interpretation of the results section of the report? Are there other biases which the researcher has not noted?	Are the biases critical in your clinical situation? Based on clinical experience, are there other sources of bias?

Sampling Error

Scientific Adequacy	Clinical Applicability
Have sources of sampling error been controlled or minimalized? Are the comparison or control groups similar in all but the dependent variable?	Does the actual sample seem to represent the clinical group that the study purports to examine?

EXERCISES

From the two abstracts below answer the following questions. In some instances it may be that the question cannot be answered fully with the information provided. If this is the case, then state what is clear, what can be deduced, and what is not known.

1. What is the population sampled in the study? Hint: Look at the titles of the articles.

2. What is the site or setting of the sampling for the study?

3. What type and level of inquiry is the design for each study?

4. What is the sample size?

5. How was the sample selected?

6. Based on your answers to Exercises 1–5, you now have the basic information needed to answer the questions in Table 8.5, which evaluate the scientific adequacy and implications for clinical applicability of the samples. Use Table 8.5 to answer those questions that are applicable to each of the abstracted studies.

A Qualitative Study*

The focus of the study was the children's perceptions of themselves as well as the manner in which they explain themselves to their peers. The dilemmas were the focus of the article. Eight boys, aged 7–13, were studied using qualitative methods. Participant observation was used over a five year period. The article does not state the duration of the observation with each child. Data were collected in interviews with the child, siblings, teachers, and parents in their homes, schools, and camps.

Field notes from interviews and observations were sorted according to categories and themes as they were collected. As themes emerged, the data were analyzed for linkages with other categories. Data were placed in categories until they were saturated, that is, until new information revealed only more of the same type of data.

The results are presented in some detail in the article and the following conclusions were drawn. There was a paradox in that at the same time that the children were becoming increasingly independent in the management of their own care, they

---

* Abstracted from E. K. Oremland (1986). Communicating over chronic illness: Dilemmas of affected school-age children. *Children's Health Care* (14), 218–223.

became less and less able to speak about it to their peers. Smaller peer groups were found to be more accommodating to the special needs of these children. Parents were found to play an advocacy role for these children. The author argues that if we accept the importance of social interactions with peers, then we should support the enabling work of parents in this regard.

A Quantitative Study*

The purpose of the study was to determine the effects of a personal control intervention on the reported pain, disruption and emotional upset, amount of pain medication used, and desire for control. One hundred and forty patients admitted to a large university hospital for cardiac surgery were asked to participate. For reasons of refusal, problems with the post-operative course, etc., 64 subjects were studied for the first two data periods and only 58 for the repeated measures analysis.

Subjects who consented were randomly assigned to either a self-administered or nurse-administered pain medication group. = control grp The groups were stratified by sex, number of incisions, and surgeon. Results of the measures for the dependent variables are reported in means and standard deviations and tested for differences between groups with analysis of variance. There were few significant differences between groups. However, the experimental group initially reported higher levels of pain.

7. For more practice, critique the sampling procedures used in the studies in the Appendix at the end of the book.

8. Imagine that you are studying the concept of self-esteem among student nurses. Use your class as the site or setting of the study. Examine the sampling bias and error relative to the potential meaningfulness of the results of a study with the following particular types of sampling.
   a. How would you go about selecting a purposive or theoretical sample?
   b. Select a random sample.
   c. Select a stratified random sample. Stratify by age (those above and those below the age of 23) and gender.

---

* Abstracted from B. K. King et al. (1987). Patient management of pain medication after cardiac surgery. *Nursing Research* (36), 145–150.

REFERENCES

Burke, S. O. (1978). *Familial strain and the development of normal and handicapped children in single and two parent families.* Doctoral dissertation. Toronto: University of Toronto.

Burke, S. O.; Maloney, M.; & Baumgart, A. (1987). Four views of childbearing and child health care: Northern Indians, urban natives, urban Euro–Canadians and nurses. Final Report of grant #6606–2748–42. Ottawa: Health and Welfare Canada.

Chenitz, W. C., & Swanson, J. M. (Eds.) (1986). *From practice to grounded theory: Qualitative research in nursing.* Menlo Park, Calif.: Addison Wesley.

Cohen. J. (1977). *Statistical power analysis for the behavioral sciences.* New York: Academic Press.

Field, P. A., & Morse, J. M. (1985). *Nursing research: The application of qualitative approaches.* Rockville, Md.: Aspen Systems.

Huether, S. E., & Jacobs, M. K. (1986). Determination of normal variation in skin blood flow velocity in healthy adults. *Nursing Research, 35,* 162–165.

King, B. K.; Norsen, L. H.; Robertson, R. K.; & Hicks, G. L. (1987). Patient management of pain medication after cardiac surgery. *Nursing Research, 36,* 145–150.

Kus, R. J. (1986). From grounded theory to clinical practice: Cases from gay studies research. In W. C. Chenitz & J. M. Swanson (Eds.), *From practice to grounded theory: Qualitative research in nursing* (pp. 227–240). Menlo Park, Calif.: Addison-Wesley.

Oremland, E. K. (1986). Communicating over chronic illness: Dilemmas of affected school-age children. *Children's Health Care, 14,* 218–223.

Polit, D. F., & Hungler, B. P. (1987). *Nursing research: Principles and Methods,* 3rd ed. Philadelphia: J. B. Lippincott.

Sheps, S. (1985). The use of a registry to estimate prevalence of "severe handicap" among children in British Columbia. *Canadian Journal of Public Health, 76,* 326–332.

Wilson, H. S. (1983). Usual hospital treatment in the United States community mental health system: A dispatching process. *International Journal of Nursing Studies, 20*(2) 75–82.

9

Understanding and Evaluating Methods of Data Collection

INTRODUCTION

The purpose of this chapter is to provide an overview and evaluation of the methods used by researchers for data collection in the conduct of quantitative and qualitative nursing research. Data collection is a major part of research design: It provides the information for researchers to analyze when formulating answers to the research problem, and the quality of data collection influences the internal and external validity of the research study. Although many of the methods used for data collection are the same for both qualitative and quantitative research, the factors determining the selection of methods are sometimes different. In addition, there are a number of methods that are unique to qualitative research.

OBJECTIVES

After reading this chapter, you will be able to

1. Identify factors that affect the selection or development of data collection methods used in quantitative and qualitative research.
2. Discuss the common instruments and methods used for data collection in quantitative and qualitative research.
3. Discuss the reliability and validity of data-collection methods used in qualitative and quantitative research.
4. Evaluate the strengths and weaknesses of data-collection methods used in a research study.

NEW TERMS

Data collection methods
Closed-ended questionnaires
Open-ended questionnaires
Likert scale
Bipolar scales
Response set bias
Social desirability response set
Acquiescence response set
Extreme response set
Interview schedule
Interviewer bias

Counterbalance approach
Interview guide
Q sorts
Projective tests
Direct observation
Structured observation
Observer bias
Subject sensitization
Participant observation
Life history
Content validity
Criterion validity
Predictive validity
Concurrent validity

Construct validity
Known group method
Triangulation
Internal consistency
Split-half technique
Stability
Test-retest method
Equivalence reliability
Interrater reliability
Parallel forms
Low-inference descriptors
Sensitivity
Pilot test

_____ FREQUENTLY USED METHODS FOR _____
DATA COLLECTION

Data collection methods are the procedures or instruments used by the researcher to observe or measure the key variables in the research problem. The methods used are planned as part of the study design to answer the research question. These methods must be appropriate for the study design and the proposed study population. Figure 9.1 depicts the relationship of data collection to the nursing researcher's process. At cell C, the data collection methods are selected, designed, and pilot tested. At cell F, the data is collected using the selected method.

Self-Report Techniques

The most common methods for data collection in nursing research are self-report techniques where the investigator requests subjects to verbally report information about the research variables. Usually this involves asking individuals to respond to a questionnaire or participate in an interview.

Questionnaires   A questionnaire can take several forms. The most common format found in nursing research literature is the **closed-ended questionnaire** in which a set of questions is presented to the respondent to read and then choose one response from a set of answers provided for each question. This technique is often used in large surveys when questionnaires are mailed to prospective subjects. Questionnaires can also be read to subjects while an investigator records the subject's choice of answer.

Open-ended questionnaires are less frequently found in nursing research, particularly when quantitative methods for data analysis are planned. In this situation the researcher has less control over respondents' answers because there are no fixed choices provided for each question. The following examples of questions about alcohol intake illustrate the difference between open-ended and closed-ended questions:

Open-Ended: How often do you drink alcoholic beverages?

Closed-Ended: How often do you drink alcoholic beverages?
(Choose the answer which best applies)

1	2	3
Not at all	On special occasions only	Once a week

4
More than once a week

_____ Figure 9.1 _____

RESEARCH PROCESS FLOWCHART

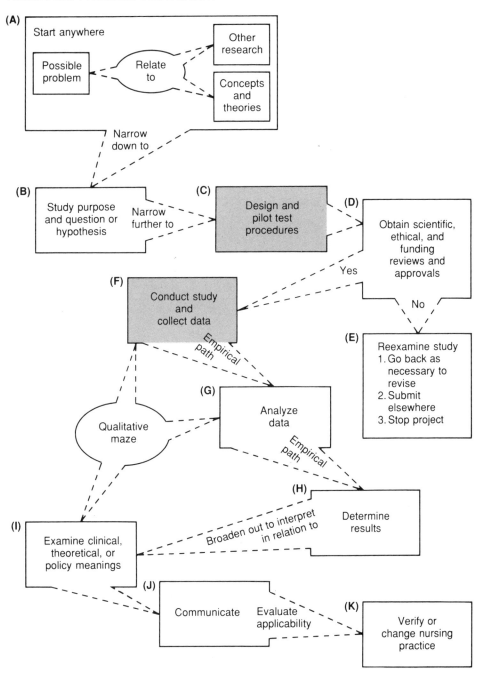

From this example you can imagine the variety of answers that might be given to the open-ended format, ranging from a specific "never" or a vague "sometimes" to a complex description of drinking patterns. The choice of format in this example would depend largely upon the research question, purpose, and design of the study. The open-ended format can be used to elicit meaningful data about the nature of drinking patterns in qualitative research most effectively when a skillful interviewer is present to encourage elaboration on vague responses. The closed-ended format can provide more measurable, specific answers about the frequency of drinking behavior, but the individual meaning of responses can be limited by the structured nature of the questionnaire.

The format of closed-ended questionnaires can vary depending on the variables being measured and how the data will be analyzed. Items on a closed-ended questionnaire are usually arranged in a scale format that provides for rating a variety of fixed responses. Each response on the instrument is assigned a numerical value for analysis purposes.

A **Likert scale** is frequently used to test attitudes or feelings and is summative in that item scores are added to obtain the final result. The respondent is presented with a statement and is asked to indicate degree of agreement with the statement by checking one of five alternative responses.

I am satisfied with my care.

Strongly agree	Agree	Uncertain	Disagree	Strongly disagree
1	2	3	4	5

Fixed alternative responses also can be presented to respondents in a matrix format. This approach is easily read and completed by subjects and can be useful in testing a number of characteristics related to a particular concept.

Please check the category that best describes your nightly sleeping pattern.

	Always	Frequently	Seldom	Never
1. Difficulty falling asleep				
2. Sleep is uninterrupted through night				

	Always	Frequently	Seldom	Never
3. Take sleeping medication				
4. Feel rested upon awakening				
5. Sleep lasts five or more hours a night				

Bipolar scales are another common questionnaire format found in nursing research. These scales are often referred to as graphic rating scales. Subjects are requested to rate certain attributes of a concept placed on a continuum falling between two extremes. Bipolar scales are two types: those that use number categories and those that use verbal categories.

Continuum

Please check (x) your degree of satisfaction with your care on the following scale.

Poor – – – – / – – – – / – – – – / – – – – / – – – – / – – – – / – – – – Excellent
          1   2   3   4   5   6   7

This type of scale can be similarly constructed using words instead of numbers to identify the categories. Usually these scales contain 5, 7, or 9 categories.

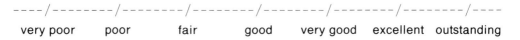

very poor   poor   fair   good   very good   excellent   outstanding

Questionnaires administered to subjects without the presence of an interviewer can be a relatively easy, effective, and inexpensive means of data collection. However, questionnaires, particularly the closed-ended format, can be expensive, time consuming, and difficult to construct. Questionnaires must be carefully worded to ensure meaningful responses from subjects.

One common problem researchers must consider when using closed-ended questionnaires is the possibility of **response set bias.** This occurs when subjects tend to respond in a set way to alternatives on the questionnaire although these may not accurately reflect the real situation. Questionnaires dealing with attitudes about psychological or social issues are particularly vulnerable to response sets. For example, subjects who are asked to agree or disagree with a set of statements may tend to respond in a socially desirable way (**social desirability response set**), or to respond in agreement with the questionnaire (**acquiescence response set**), or to respond in an extreme manner (**extreme response set**). In order to avoid the possibility of response sets biasing the end results of the study, the researcher must consider this possible effect when constructing the questionnaire. Frequently little can be done to ensure the absence of response biases as they are often an intricate part of the respondent's personality. However, balancing the occurrence of positively and negatively worded items on a questionnaire can reduce the tendency for respondents to agree or disagree in a set way.

A more global problem with self-administered questionnaires is that they can be used only with subjects who can read and write. For example, in some studies, particularly those investigating problems among lower socioeconomic groups, sampling may need to exclude important representatives of the population who would be unable to read and answer a self-administered questionnaire. In all situations where questionnaires are used, the researcher must consider such factors as educational level, physical capabilities, language, and cultural identity of subjects in order to construct a questionnaire that will provide meaningful data.

Not only must a questionnaire be understandable and answerable by subjects; it should be practical in length. Length is particularly important when questionnaires are mailed to respondents and the return rate at best is low (often less than 50%). This means large numbers of questionnaires need to be distributed in order to secure a reasonable return rate. A long questionnaire may not encourage a response, and it may prove costly for the researcher.

Interviews: Schedules and Guides   An **interview schedule** is essentially a very loosely structured or open-ended questionnaire that is administered to respondents by a skilled interviewer. The presence of the interviewer allows for probing of responses given by subjects and decreases the possibility of vague answers. This technique is used most often in qualitative studies, but may be used in quantitative studies in combination with other methods for data collection. This approach can yield a great deal more data than a questionnaire, but analysis of the data can be a long and complex task.

The very presence of the interviewer, however, introduces a possible risk to the study's internal validity because the interviewer's presence may inadvertently sensitize subjects to respond in a certain manner. The interviewer's preconceived notions about the research problem, age, sex, and personality of the subject, can contribute to what is known as **interviewer bias.** This effect can be equated with the Hawthorne effect discussed in Chapter 6, a particular risk associated with experimentally designed studies. Several measures can be taken by the researcher to reduce the possibility of interviewer bias.

Interviewers require careful training and practice in techniques of interviewing. This can be very time consuming and expensive for the researcher. Data collection procedures must be carefully planned and a set protocol established for everyone involved in the collection. Ideally, all interviews should be conducted by one trained person so that the effects of personal characteristics will be similar on all study subjects. Realistically, the ideal may be impossible in large studies. In studies where control or comparison groups are used, and two interviewers are needed, a **counterbalance approach** may be used in data collection. This can be done by having one interviewer collect data from one half of the experimental subjects and one half of the control or comparison subjects. The second interviewer then interviews the remaining half of each group. In this way the characteristics of both interviewers can be balanced between the two comparison groups of subjects.

An **interview guide** is simply a list of topics used by the interviewer to guide discussion during an interview. This approach to interviewing is much less structured than using an open-ended questionnaire or schedule. The quality of data collection depends largely upon the skill of the interviewer and his or her ability to record meaningful information for data analysis. This approach to interviewing is similarly subject to the risk of interviewer bias if interviewers are not carefully trained in the skills of interviewing subjects.

Q Sorts Q sorts or Q methodology is a technique for data collection that traditionally was not used frequently in nursing research, but recently its use has become more common. This approach involves distributing a set of cards to each subject. Each card contains a statement about the concept being studied. Subjects are then asked to sort the cards according to a scale determined by the researcher. For example, suppose a researcher wished to investigate what events clients perceive as most stressful following open heart surgery. The researcher would develop a set of cards, each containing a statement about an event that would normally occur following open heart surgery, for example, being on a respirator, having a tube in my chest, being in the ICU, and so on. The research question is the determining factor in the number of cards to be sorted, but best results are obtained when using 60 to 100 cards. Each subject is asked to evaluate each statement and assign it to a place on the scale. The scale would usually contain 9 or 11 categories, ranging from most stressful to least stressful. The researcher, however, determines the number of cards that should be placed in each category. The method is designed so that the majority of responses are placed in the middle and not the extreme categories.

	Most Stressful							Least Stressful		
Scale categories	→	1	2	3	4	5	6	7	8	9
Number of cards to be placed in each category as determined by researcher	→	3	5	8	11	15	11	8	5	3

The use of Q-sort methodology is time consuming and may be difficult to use with large numbers of subjects. However, it is a very useful method to investigate research questions about self-perceptions or opinions. Because the researcher can control the number of responses in each category, this method can reduce the possibility of extreme response set bias.

Projective Tests   Projective tests are seldom used for data collection in nursing studies. They are most commonly associated with psychological evaluation. However, they have been shown to be useful in studying certain variables and populations in nursing research. These techniques require subjects to respond in an instructed manner to some ambiguous stimulus. The subject's response and self-interpretation are observed by the researcher as outward projections of the subject's inner feelings, attitudes, and personality characteristics. Some common projective tests include word association, sentence completion, and methods to encourage various types of self-expression such as role modeling or constructing pictures or models. These approaches to data collection are highly subjective and encourage a great deal of creativity and imagination on the part of respondents, which render their responses difficult to analyze objectively. However, projective tests are particularly useful in nursing studies investigating children's attitudes and

Seldom used in nsg
¿used assoc

feelings. For example, Jerrett (1985) investigated children's views of pain by asking them to draw pictures of their pain experience, and then asked each child to provide a description of the picture created.

Observation Methods

Direct Observation Observation of behavior is another approach used to collect data about nursing research problems. Direct observation or **structured observation** is the commonest method of observation used in quantitative studies where an investigator or other trained observer simply observes and records certain aspects of subjects' behavior. For example, suppose a researcher wished to study the effect of prenatal classes on fathers' coaching behavior towards mothers during delivery. The researcher can prepare a checklist of coaching behaviors taught in prenatal classes along with those generally observed to be used by fathers in the delivery room. The researcher can then observe the subject fathers' behavior and record the occurrence and frequency of coaching behaviors on the checklist. The data can be analyzed and compared for fathers who attended prenatal classes and fathers who did not attend the classes.

Direct observation can be a useful method of data collection if the behavior or event to be observed can be clearly identified and objectively recorded. The behavior must be operationally defined before data collection, and the observer must be skilled. All forms of human observation are subjective to some extent, and this introduces the possibility of **observer bias** influencing results. Using a structured checklist as part of the research protocol can enhance objectivity.

A further source of bias associated with direct observation is **subject sensitization.** This is likely to occur when the observer's presence is clearly evident to the subject and, as a result, the subject's behavior changes from what would likely occur under usual circumstances. This problem is difficult to control when studying human subjects since it would be unethical to observe their behavior without the subjects' informed consent. Under certain circumstances, steps can be taken to minimize this bias. Keeping observations as unobtrusive as possible in a spacious, active environment where subjects are less inclined to focus on the observer may be possible in some studies. Often observers can remain outside of the direct line of subjects' vision. For example, in the above study concerning fathers' coaching behaviors in the delivery room, it may be possible to make observations from a special observation room overlooking the delivery room if one is available in the setting.

Participant Observation   A second observation method used for data collection in nursing research and social science or ethnographic research is known as **participant observation.** In contrast to direct observation this approach is less structured and objective in its application. The observer collects data through involvement with the study subjects and participation in activities with them in their environment. Through participation the observer collects data in an unstructured manner, and usually records events and behaviors in a descriptive manner after the fact, using a set of field notes or journal.

This method of data collection is commonly used in qualitative nursing research studies that are directed toward examining the nature of phenomena and where results are to be qualitatively analyzed. This approach can yield a great deal of data, but the quality of data collected is highly dependent upon the judgment, observation, and recording skills of the participant observer. Also, the observer must rely on a trained memory to recall important events and conversations for later recording.

The key element in participant observation is involvement with the subjects in their environment and the development of a trusting relationship. Spradley (1980) provides an excellent discussion of techniques used to collect and record data using this method. He outlines five types of participation, ranging from nonparticipation—simply observing—to complete participation—total involvement with subjects and environment (see Table 9.1). Spradley emphasizes the concept of "introspection" or the ability to use one's own feelings to understand experiences. The researcher who engages in participant observation experiences the subjective feelings of being an insider, but alternately sees himself or herself as an objective instrument observing outside events. The researcher's ability to observe behavior or events as an insider and outsider alternately and simultaneously contributes to the quality of data obtained from participant observation.

Other Methods

Life History   Life history is a qualitative data collection approach used with informants (a qualitative term for subjects), in order to understand circumstances that contribute to present or past events.

_____ *Table 9.1* _____

DEGREE OF INVOLVEMENT AND PARTICIPATION IN OBSERVATION RESEARCH

Involvement	Participation	Examples
High	Complete	Studying nursing behavior on a unit while working as a nurse on that unit doing active patient care
	Active	Studying nursing behavior on a unit in the role of nurse researcher, with considerable involvement in providing nursing care and day-to-day interaction with nurses
	Moderate	Studying nursing behavior on a unit in the role of nurse researcher through interaction with nurses, but less involvement in nursing care
Low	Passive	Studying nursing behavior through unobtrusive observation of nurses' behavior with clients, with little interaction or involvement with nurses
None	Nonparticipant	Studying nursing behavior in situations removed from the subjects' immediate environment, for example, from a viewing gallery or one-way mirror; no interaction, only direct observation

Source: Adapted from J. P. Spradley (1980), *Participant observation*. New York: Holt, Rinehart and Winston. Copyright 1980 by Holt, Rinehart and Winston, Inc., reprinted by permission of the publisher.

The researcher conducts in-depth interviewing with selected individuals who represent the topic of interest. Subjects are guided by the interviewer to recount certain aspects of their lives in detail so that patterns surrounding a particular theme can be identified. For example, a career history taken from nurses of various ages may reflect changing patterns in nursing education, which may in turn explain current practices.

In their discussion of life history, Field and Morse (1985) caution that this approach requires a great deal of depth in order to gain sufficient information, and informants may require a long time commitment to the project. Given the nature of this method, sample size is often small and loss of informants can be crucial to the outcome of this type of research.

Documents, Photographs, and Audio and Video Recordings Physical evidence such as personal and public documents, photographs, and audio/video recordings are sometimes used as methods of data collection in nursing research to enhance interviews, observations, and life histories. Such methods can enrich the accuracy of data collection; sometimes these techniques are used as the sole method of data collection. Because of the personal nature of much of this evidence, it is extremely important that the researcher gain the subjects' informed consent to use these data. Photographs and recordings in particular can easily identify individuals, and careful plans must be made to protect anonymity. When recordings are used to complement interviews, the researcher must also consider the possibility of subject sensitization to the presence of the equipment, for this may affect responses given. Field and Morse suggest that nurse interviewers often are skilled in doing process recording, and this may be a very feasible method for recording the subject's own words in sensitive situations.

Biophysical Measures Biophysical measures are being used more frequently to collect data in clinical nursing research examining physiological variables. Recent technology has resulted in the development of a variety of monitoring techniques to measure vital signs and other physiological data. These devices yield quantitative data that can be easily analyzed and, if properly used, these instruments can provide valid results. However, many sophisticated devices are costly and require specialized training to operate. Some devices may require invasive techniques and therefore can only be used in nursing studies where clients are already being monitored for medical purposes. For example, direct arterial blood pressure or intercranial pressure can be most easily measured as research variables by a specially trained nursing investigator who selects a group of subjects in an intensive care setting where they are being monitored clinically for these variables.

Indirect measures of biophysical variables may be less precise. However, newer models of sphygmomanometers and electronic thermometers are easy to use when available in the clinical environment, and they can provide fairly accurate results. Reliability and validity of results obtained from biophysical measures are important considerations for the researcher. We will elaborate on these concepts later in the chapter.

Summary of Methods

In this section we have attempted to provide an overview of some of the commonest methods used for data collection in quantitative and qualitative nursing research studies. A crucial issue for the researcher in selecting a method to collect data centers on the ability of the method to provide meaningful and valid information about the research problem. Recently, a new computer data base, the Health Instrument File (HIF), has been developed at the University of Pittsburgh (Purloff, 1988). This on-line data base provides easy access to a wide variety of nursing and health-related data collection instruments. Many times a combination of methods is used, which may require both quantitative and qualitative analysis. Feasibility is another factor that must be considered by the researcher when selecting the method for data collection. Table 9.2 provides a summary of some practical considerations for the selection of data-collection methods and possible advantages and disadvantages that may affect the researcher's selection of the method used.

_____ Table 9.2 _____

POSSIBLE PRACTICAL ADVANTAGES AND DISADVANTAGES OF METHODS USED FOR DATA COLLECTION

Method of Data Collection	Potential Advantages	Potential Disadvantages
Closed-ended questionnaire	Is easy to administer; can be mailed or presented to subjects Can be analyzed using quantitative means; is less time consuming than qualitative analysis Can be easily administered to large samples	May be expensive and difficult to develop May be susceptible to response set bias Respondents must be able to read and write if self-administered Responses are limited to choices provided on the instrument
Open-ended questionnaire Interview schedule Interview guide Life history	Can be fairly inexpensive and easy to construct Allows subjects to elaborate on responses; large, meaningful data base may result	Expensive and time-consuming procedure; requires a trained interviewer and high commitment of informers/subjects Interviewer bias and subject sensitization may be a problem

(continues)

_____ Table 9.2 _____

CONTINUED

Method of Data Collection	Potential Advantages	Potential Disadvantages
		Method may be very time consuming and difficult to use with large samples
		May be time consuming to analyze qualitatively
Participant observation	Can collect a large amount of subjective and objective data from subjects in the natural environment	Very time consuming; may require a lot of preparation and training
	May reduce subject sensitivity by prolonged contact with observer and build up of mutual trust between subject and observer	Memory of observer may be a problem when recording events later
		Qualitative analysis often a long process when data base large
Direct observation (using structured tool)	Can collect large amount of data that can often be easily analyzed using quantitative methods	Training observers may be expensive and time consuming
		Too much structure may mean important behavior is missed
		Subject sensitivity and observer bias may be a problem
Q-sort method	Can be very useful in investigating self-perceptions and opinions	Time consuming to develop and administer
		Difficult to use with large samples
	Can usually be analyzed easily using quantitative measures	Subjects require considerable instruction and time to grasp sorting—usually fairly high intelligence necessary
Projective tests	Has creative approach to study inner feelings and attitudes with certain groups of subjects	Highly subjective nature of method questioned, particularly when used without other evidence

_____ Table 9.2 _____

CONTINUED

Method of Data Collection	Potential Advantages	Potential Disadvantages
	Stimulates imagination; may be particularly useful with children	Some tests difficult to analyze and require much time and expertise using qualitative methods
		Time consuming to administer to large sample
Audio and audio/video recordings	Is excellent source of subjective data to enhance interview or field notes	Subjects may have ethical objection to use
		Subject sensitivity is possibility
Biophysical measures	Can provide precise, valid measurements of physiological data	Highly sophisticated instruments may be expensive to obtain or difficult to use without special training
	Can be easily analyzed quantitatively	

_____ FACTORS AFFECTING DATA COLLECTION _____

The concepts of validity and reliability are important considerations for the researcher when selecting or developing a method for data collection. They are the best assurance that the data collected by the researcher will provide the information needed to investigate the problem. In Chapter 6, we discussed the concepts of internal and external validity in evaluating the overall research design. The validity and reliability of data collected have an integral effect on both of these broader issues.

It should be noted that in this text, as in other texts and research reports, we sometimes refer to validity and reliability of research methods or instruments. In reality these two concepts can only be applied to data obtained from using the instruments.

Assessing Validity of Quantitative and Qualitative Data

The concept of validity applies to both quantitative and qualitative research in the sense that the findings of the research represent reality. However, as Field and Morse (1985) point out, the criteria for assessing the validity of data collected using qualitative methods are different from those applied to quantitative research. The objective nature of quantitative data enables the researcher to use statistical means to establish measures of validity. For example, results of a closed-ended questionnaire can be quantitatively analyzed using statistical measures to determine validity. Qualitative approaches to data collection, such as interviews or participant observations, cannot be easily subjected to statistical analysis. Such factors as the conditions under which data were collected, the focus of the data collection, the accuracy of the investigator in making observations, and recording the data are more important in assessing the validity of qualitative methods (Field & Morse, 1985).

Content Validity   Content validity is a very basic strategy a researcher can use to provide some evidence for validity of a data collection method. Usually this approach is used in the development of a questionnaire, interview schedule, or interview guide. The instrument is constructed using concepts from the literature to reflect the range of dimensions of the variable being measured in the problem. The completed instrument is then placed before a panel of judges who have some degree of expertise concerning the research topic. The judges evaluate each item on the instrument as to its degree of representation of the variable to be tested, as well as the instrument's overall appropriateness for use in examining the variable within the proposed study population. No statistical measurements are performed to evidence this type of validity. The basis of the method lies in expert judgment and validation from the literature. In quantitative research this validation strategy may be used in addition to statistical approaches. An example of content validity can be demonstrated as follows: In the construction of a questionnaire to test knowledge about labor and delivery in pregnant first-time mothers, a researcher would develop a questionnaire to test knowledge based on concepts found in the obstetrical literature and would ask a group of nurse clinicians in maternal child nursing to determine if answers to each of the questions would actually provide data reflecting first-time mothers' knowledge about labor and delivery. Following this appraisal by clinicians, the researcher should omit items that are not considered valid content for the study sample.

It should be noted that content validity (sometimes referred to as face validity) is the weakest form of validity testing. It is a good first step, but should be used in combination with other methods if possible, particularly in quantitative research.

When researchers use data-collection methods that allow for quantitative analysis of the data, statistical measures can frequently be used to determine instrument validity. In nursing research, the most common types of validity testing that employ both logical and empirical approaches fall under two categories: criterion validity and construct validity.

Criterion Validity Determining criterion validity involves comparing the results obtained through use of an instrument with a particular population sample to the results of some criterion measure believed to be valid for that population. Criterion validity testing can be further classified under two categories, predictive validity and concurrent validity. **Predictive validity** involves comparing the research instrument results obtained from a particular population to some event or measure (criterion) that is expected to occur within that population in the future. In other words, predictive validity of an instrument refers to the ability of the researcher accurately to predict events based upon results obtained from use of the instrument. The statistical degree of association between the research instrument results and the criterion measure is calculated to determine the predictive validity of the instrument (these statistical measures are discussed in Chapter 10). Example 9.1 demonstrates the concept of predictive validity.

_____ *Example 9.1* _____

DETERMINING PREDICTIVE VALIDITY

Burke, Sayers, Baumgart, and Wray (1985) tested the predictive validity of the Denver Developmental Screening Test with Cree Indian children. The authors questioned the use of this instrument with these native children because mixed results were reported for other cross-cultural studies. To test the predictive validity of the DDST, a group of native children were tested with the instrument and followed by the researchers for a three-year period to determine the number of health and developmental problems occurring in these children. When evidence from health records over the three-year period was compared with scores on the DDST, there was little statistical evidence for predictive validity.

———

See Burke, S. O.; Sayers, L. A.; Baumgart, A. J.; & Wray, J. G. (1985). Pitfalls in cross-cultural use of the Denver Developmental Screening Test: Cree Indian children. *Journal of Public Health, 76,* 303–307.

Concurrent validity differs from predictive validity in that the results of a data collection instrument are compared to those of a criterion measure at the same point in time. In the above example, concurrent validity testing of the DDST was carried out by concurrently administering another developmental screening test to these native children. Results of the Minnesota Child Development Inventory (Ireton & Thwing, 1974), along with developmental status chart summaries and mothers' current developmental ratings of their children, were compared with DDST results to determine concurrent validity.

Researchers often have difficulty establishing criterion validity of instruments with particular populations unless there is considerable observable behavior occurring in the population to serve as a criterion measure. Often, when other instruments are chosen for use as a criterion, the researcher must assume that the concepts being tested by the criterion and comparison measures are indeed measuring conceptually related outcomes. A second problem involves finding a criterion instrument that has been already validated with a similar research population. For example, an instrument measuring stress that has been validated with a study population will not necessarily provide valid results when used with hospitalized adults. Often the best assurance the researcher has in determining both predictive and concurrent validity is that two similar measures are compared in the same population with statistically significant results. How well concepts can be measured through use of a research instrument cannot be determined through tests of criterion validity.

Construct Validity Construct validity testing is the best method that the researcher can use to determine the ability of an instrument actually to measure the research concepts. Construct or concept validation is a time-consuming task but is considered well worth the effort when very complex concepts are being measured in nursing research. This type of validity testing is aimed toward examining the theoretical foundations of the research problem and how well the researcher has translated the abstract concepts from the research problem and theoretical framework into valid measures on the research instrument. Most researchers agree that the process for obtaining sound construct validity is a long one that requires the use of an instrument in a number of successive but different studies that employ various techniques for testing construct validity.

The approaches taken by researchers toward determining construct validity are varied, as reported in the literature. A number of research texts report specific, pragmatic, and empirical steps in the process (Holm & Llewellyn, 1986; Burns & Grove, 1987; Polit & Hungler, 1987). Our discussion will focus on an overview of the most common concepts involved in approaches to construct validity found in the nursing research literature rather than on specific steps in the development of these approaches.

The **known group method** is one of the most basic approaches to determining construct validity. It draws on the idea that the abstract construct in question is more likely to be observable in certain situations or groups than in others. Let us suppose the researcher uses the instrument with a known group expected to demonstrate the construct, and with a group not expected to demonstrate it. If the results obtained indicate a statistical difference in the expected manner, the instrument is deemed to have a level of construct validity.

For example, if a researcher develops an instrument to measure concerns about the aging process and tests the questionnaire with a group of teenagers and a group of adults over age fifty, it would be reasonable to expect different results from each of these groups. Although many teenagers would likely indicate some concerns about aging, and a few adults over fifty show little concern, the key issue in determining the validity of the instrument would be a statistical difference between the scores of both groups as expected.

A more comprehensive approach to testing the construct validity of an instrument involves using the concepts of convergence and discrimination. Convergence and discrimination form the basis of the multitrait-multimethod matrix approach developed by Campbell and Fiske (1959). Simply, *convergence* involves demonstrating that an instrument constructed to measure a concept yields results that are similar to several other known measures of that concept when tested with the same subjects. *Discrimination validity* can be determined by the researcher through testing the ability of an instrument to provide distinctly different results from other instruments testing slightly different but related concepts using the same subjects. The multitrait-multimethod approach is a complex but important method for determining construct validity requiring multiple measures and careful statistical analysis. A complete explanation of this matrix method is not discussed here but can be found in Campbell and Fiske (1959) and other nursing research texts that focus in more detail on the conduct of research, for example, Polit and Hungler (1987). Example 9.2 provides a basic overview of a nurse researcher's approach to determining construct validity of an instrument using convergence and divergence.

Example 9.2

DETERMINING CONSTRUCT VALIDITY

Rees (1980) developed three instruments to measure first-time mothers' feelings of motherliness (FOM), conception of the fetus as a person (CFP), and appropriateness of fantasies about the baby to be (AFB). She tested these three scales with a sample of 34 first-time pregnant mothers over a 3 week period. Rees postulated that her three scales represented three different aspects of the construct maternal identification and therefore should show a positive statistical relationship among one another to support convergent validity of the construct maternal identification. Results indicated that scales for FOM and CFP were positively, statistically related to each other, however the AFB scale results were not statistically related to FOM and CFP, providing only some evidence for convergent validity. In order to test discriminate validity the results of the three scales were compared to results obtained from two scales from a parental attitude research instrument developed by Schaefer and Bell (1958), measuring a similar but somewhat different construct. The statistical association was calculated and showed a more positive than negative relationship between the instrument scales, thus discriminate validity was not established.

See Rees, B. L. (1980). Measuring identification with the mothering role. *Research in Nursing and Health, 2,* 49–56.

Validity of Qualitative Data—Special Considerations

The very nature of qualitative research methods does not lend to statistical or empirical calculations of validity. However, a number of authors focusing on qualitative research methods have suggested strategies the researcher can employ in data collection to enhance the truthfulness or validity of qualitative results. Our overview includes approaches suggested by Miles and Huberman (1984), Field and Morse (1985), and Sandelowski (1986). Since participant observation and other unstructured interviewing and observation techniques represent the most common forms of data collection used in qualitative nursing studies, the ideas discussed here relate primarily to these methods.

Risks to Validity of Data

Collecting Representative Data Frequently, in qualitative studies the nurse researcher works alone in gathering large amounts of data from a small group of subjects or informants in order to gain intimate experience for the interpretation of meaning and later theory development. These factors can pose a number of risks to validity of data collected.

If the selection of informants is not well planned, the data collected may represent extreme viewpoints of a group and may not be accurate. For example, information given by a nurse administrator about the nature of stress in the workplace is likely different from that given by a staff nurse. Both viewpoints may be important to the question; however, the researcher should carefully consider contrasting views in determining the meaning of data to the research problem and theoretical context. Replicating data collection from various sources and planning sampling to identify representative "key informants" are important checks that can be used to promote the collection of valid data. Checking out extreme viewpoints and exploring and confirming the meaning of the data with informants can avoid later misinterpretation.

The social context where data are collected may represent another risk to the representativeness of the data. Individuals may behave differently and reveal different information under differing social circumstances. A researcher who is mindful of this will often interview the same informants and make observations of behavior in a variety of settings to make comparisons of similarities and differences before attributing meaning.

This process for verifying commonalities within data collected from subjects using various methods is known as triangulation. This technique is very important in determining the validity of data in qualitative research. It is also a useful approach that the researcher can employ when applying both quantitative and qualitative methods to collect data about the same research concept (Field & Morse, 1985). For example, quantitative data about pain experience can be collected from subjects using closed-ended questions, while qualitative data from the same subjects can be collected using an interview and a projective test.

Avoiding Researcher Effects The subjective involvement of the researcher in qualitative studies increases the risk that the data collection may be biased by the researcher's own values. Nurse researchers should examine their own values in light of the research situation and undergo extensive training as interviewers and observers before undertaking qualitative approaches to data collection.

As mentioned earlier, the very presence of the researcher may affect the validity of the data provided by subjects in some situations. Field and Morse suggest that in field studies the researcher should plan to spend sufficient time in the setting prior to the actual data collection to allow both the researcher and subjects to feel comfortable with each other.

Reliability of Data Collection Methods

Reliability of the research instrument is a second major concern of the researcher when collecting data. Reliability refers to the ability of a research method to yield consistently the same results over repeated testing periods. In essence, reliability is very much a part of validity in that an instrument that does not yield reliable results cannot be considered valid. Therefore, it is important for the researcher to determine both the reliability and validity of a method. It is possible that an instrument can be used to collect reliable data, but reliability of the method does not guarantee that the data collected are valid measures of the research concepts. For example, an instrument may consistently be used to measure anxiety levels time after time but if the research concept to be measured is depression, the instrument cannot be considered valid.

Estimating the reliability of data is of particular importance to the nurse researcher doing quantitative research, and a number of empirical tests can be used to estimate the reliability coefficient. In qualitative studies, where the researcher acts as the primary instrument, it is more difficult to calculate reliability. Strategies discussed under validity similarly affect the reliability of the data collected. In addition, several other strategies, which enhance the reliability of results, can be introduced at the data analysis stage in qualitative studies.

Quantitative Strategies Reliability testing of quantitative data collection methods falls under three basic categories. Internal consistency involves estimating the internal potential of an instrument to yield reliable results. Stability and equivalence testing provide evidence for the external reliability of results.

Internal consistency refers to the degree of homogeneity of items on a closed-ended questionnaire designed to measure a single research concept. For example, if a researcher developed a question-naire to measure assertiveness among staff nurses, the researcher would analyze the items on the instruments to estimate the extent to which all of the items measure the concept of assertiveness. The common method employed to estimate internal consistency is known as the **split-half technique.** Using this approach the researcher admin-isters the questionnaire to a group of subjects similar to the study population. The responses to items on the instrument are then split into two equal numbered groups or half-tests and scored independently. The scores are then statistically analyzed to estimate the correlation coefficient or the degree of relationship between the scores of the two half-tests. (A more complete discussion of correlation coefficients and other more specific measurements for internal consistency follow in Chapter 10.) The statistical relationship obtained represents the split-half reliability coefficient. A high positive coefficient indicates high consistency. The researcher may split the items for testing in numerous ways. In many split-half tests, odd numbered responses to items are compared to the even numbered responses. However, a less biased ap-proach would be to assign the items randomly in the two half-tests.

A more sophisticated procedure is the use of a statistical measure known as Cronbach's alpha (see Chapter 10), which literally allows the researcher to calculate the average correlation existing among all possible split-half divisions of the test. This method reduces error as-sociated with other types of testing for internal consistency. However, in testing for internal consistency the length of the entire test can affect the outcome. Generally, longer scales tend to be more reliable.

Stability of a research instrument refers to the reliability of the instrument to measure a concept or attribute with consistent results over time. The empirical approach most commonly used by researchers to estimate instrument stability is the **test-retest method.** In this case the instrument being tested yields data that can be quantitatively analyzed. For example, a nurse researcher might use this approach to test the external reliability of a closed-ended questionnaire. The key factor the researcher must keep in mind when selecting this approach is the degree of change over time normally observed in the concept being measured. The test-retest method requires the researcher to administer the instrument on two separate occasions to the same group of subjects. The reliability coefficient is then calculated to indicate the degree of statistical association (correlation coefficient) between the results ob-tained from the two tests.

In nursing studies many research concepts that are frequently investigated do change naturally over short time periods. For example, vital signs and emotional states can naturally change quickly in individuals depending upon a variety of circumstances. Therefore, in using the test-retest method to estimate reliability of instruments, the researcher must look at the natural stability of the underlying concepts being tested by the instrument before proceeding. Otherwise, results may not reflect the stability of instruments. This approach is most feasible in determining the reliability of an instrument to test fairly stable attributes such as long-standing personality traits.

Test-retest estimates are generally higher when the time lapse between testing is short, usually no longer than four weeks. However, when subjects are requested to respond to two identical questionnaires over a short time span, memory of the responses given on the first questionnaire may influence responses to the second. In addition, a subject's boredom and lack of motivation may sensitize responses given on the second testing. In short, the researcher must be cautious in using test-retest reliability by carefully examining the independent stability of the concept being investigated, by selecting a test-retest period that minimizes the effect of natural change occurring in the concept, and by taking into account the possibility of testing effects on the retests. Because of these problems, the researcher should not be convinced that an instrument will produce highly reliable results based upon test-retest results. Other measures of reliability used in combination with this approach can strengthen the evidence.

A third category of reliability testing applied to data collection methods is known as **equivalence reliability.** This type of testing is used frequently in observation studies to estimate the reliability of observations made by an observer using a structured instrument de-signed to record coded behavior or events. In this research situa-tion, equivalence reliability is referred to as **interrater reliability.** Essentially, two or more independent observers record their observa-tions of an event at the same time and the results are compared for equivalence. Measures of association, such as correlation, can be used to calculate an equivalence coefficient. However, a rougher estimate of equivalence can be calculated using a simple formula presented in Polit and Hungler (1987).

$$\frac{\text{Percentage of}}{\text{agreement}} = \frac{\text{Number of agreements}}{\text{Number of agreements and disagreements}}$$

The authors do caution against sole use of this approach because equivalence may be overestimated. Errors occur, particularly in situa-tions where observers are required to record presence or absence of a behavior or event occurring very rapidly. We mention this here, since the use of this method has been noted in several recent nursing studies. When attempting to evaluate the use of percent of agreement as an estimate of equivalence in a study, reference to a more complete explanation is advised (Polit & Hungler, 1987).

A second form of equivalence reliability is frequently referred to as the use of **parallel forms.** This method is most commonly used in educational testing rather than nursing research. However, this may be a very useful approach in establishing the reliability of results obtained from knowledge-testing procedures when client teaching methods are being investigated.

used in educ

The use of parallel forms requires the availability of two alternate versions of a test or questionnaire examining the same concept. The researcher then administers the two instruments consecutively to the same subjects, randomizing the order of presentation. The results of the two tests are then compared statistically to determine the degree of association or correlation between the two tests. The results indicate the equivalence reliability of both tests to measure the same concept.

Qualitative Strategies The researcher who uses qualitative methods for data collection will not use statistical analysis to determine reliability coefficients. Careful attention to the earlier mentioned factors that affect validity of qualitative data collection will similarly affect the reliability of the method. In some qualitative studies it is possible for the researcher to use structured observation instruments that can be analyzed quantitatively to determine the interrater reliability of observations. However, in most field studies that employ interview or participant observation techniques, the use of two or more observers would be inappropriate and would affect the validity of the data base.

basically only present info to peers & have them eval. it.

The reliability of methods used also can be assessed after the data have been collected, in conjunction with the analysis stage. Several strategies are suggested in the qualitative research literature. Here we will summarize the methods discussed by Field and Morse (1985), which emphasize the importance of external review of data collected.

The use of **low-inference descriptors** involves the presentation to peers of selected verbatim information that has been collected from subjects. This information is reviewed and compared with the researcher's interpretations of the data, thus providing peer evaluation of the researcher's reliability in collecting and analyzing data. Often the use of tape recorders in addition to field notes during data collection will increase the accuracy of low-inference descriptors. A selection of low-inference descriptors also should be provided in the research report to substantiate the researcher's analyses and conclusions and to allow critique by readers.

In some cases the researcher will submit an entire set of field notes for peer review by colleagues in order to substantiate the meaning attributed to data. Often rival explanations will cause the researcher to reexamine the data and change hypotheses. If it is possible, the researcher may also attempt to confirm findings and analyses with informants to enhance reliability and validity. However, as Field and Morse point out, subjects may become sensitized to the researcher's inferences and provide the answers that support the researcher's point of view.

Other Factors Affecting the Quality of Data Collected

In addition to reliability and validity of data-collection methods, a number of other criteria should be considered before a method is used. These factors are important because they contribute to the overall reliability and validity of the method.

Sensitivity   The sensitivity of an instrument refers to the ability of an instrument to distinguish between small variations of a measure when used with subjects displaying variable amounts of that measure. This concept is an especially important one for the researcher who is attempting to measure changes in the dependent variable, which are expected to be very small. For example, suppose a researcher is measuring daily weight changes in a group of obese subjects undergoing a weight-reduction program. The expected outcome would likely be small but detectable changes, on a day-to-day basis. If the scale used is divided into five-pound intervals rather than one-pound intervals, the instrument would not be considered sensitive enough to detect the small changes on a daily basis. Therefore, when evaluating data-collection instruments, the research consumer should question if instrument sensitivity is a source of risk to the validity of data collected.

Efficiency   The concept of efficiency refers to the feasibility of using the instrument to collect a sufficient amount of data from an appropriate number of subjects in a reasonable time period, without undue expense, in order to answer the research question. Therefore, the researcher needs to balance a number of factors to ensure that the method can be used to collect reliable and valid data in an efficient way. If a researcher develops a 100-item questionnaire on coping with chronic illness at home, in order to collect data from elderly subjects, the instrument may be shown to be reliable and valid. However, the length of the instrument may be a great deterrent in getting enough elderly volunteers to participate. By shortening the questionnaire the instrument may be less reliable, as mentioned previously. Nonetheless, the researcher must calculate and balance reliability with efficiency, in order to get enough data to produce findings that can be generalized.

Appropriateness and Generalizability Appropriateness relates to the fit of the instrument to the intended subjects in order to produce valid data. Many times researchers will adapt instruments that have been developed for other studies with proven reliability and validity with a particular group of subjects. The researcher must carefully examine the similarity between the subjects tested in the original study and the subjects of the current study. For example, an instrument tested for reliability and validity with student nurses would not necessarily be valid for use with hospitalized adolescents.

Other characteristics such as culture, socioeconomic level, developmental level, and language must be considered when attempting to generalize the use of an instrument from one research situation to another. The research consumer should question the researcher's decision to adopt an instrument that has been tested for reliability and validity with subjects characteristically different from the study subjects. The researcher should provide sound rationale for decisions if differences are evident, or the instruments should be retested for reliability and validity with subjects similar to the intended research sample.

One method used by researchers to test the practical aspects of a questionnaire is to **pilot test** the questionnaire with a group of subjects similar to those who will be tested in the actual study. This is an excellent means of uncovering the bugs in a newly developed instrument so that necessary revisions can be made before actual data collection in the study.

EVALUATION OF DATA COLLECTION METHODS IN A RESEARCH REPORT

The selection or development of data collection methods and the collection of data are often the most time-consuming part of doing a research project. However, due to the lack of space allotted for individual publications, the researcher often is limited to a very brief description of the methods used and the testing done to estimate reliability and validity. The task of the research consumer in piecing together the evidence for critique is often difficult.

[handwritten marginalia: look to "procedure" or "method" for descrip of data collect method]

The description of the data collection methods used in a study is usually found in a section of the report labeled "Procedures" or "Method." For the adoption or development of a particular method the researcher should provide a rationale that is linked to the research question, the purpose of the study, the study sample, and the underlying theoretical framework. In quantitative studies the method used for data collection should represent the operational definition of the variables being measured. For example, a researcher who designs a study to measure stress, in which stress is conceptualized and defined as both a physiological and pyschological phenomenon, should use methods that test both sets of variables. Similarly, in qualitative studies where the research question is directed toward the description and the nature of phenomena, the methods used must be appropriate for the collection of large amounts of data in order to hypothesize relationships.

Usually the description of methods is limited to a brief discussion of how the data were collected from subjects. Factors such as the timing of data collection, the setting for data collection, and who collected the data should be clearly described in the report because these factors can greatly affect the study's outcome. For example, if the variables in question may be affected by time of day or year, or a time when subjects are particularly fatigued or stressed, the end results of the study may be invalidated. If data are collected from subjects in a variety of settings, the behavior of individuals may be sensitized by the setting. Similarly, the effect of the data collector's characteristics may influence the behavior of subjects. The researcher should state in the report any foreseen limitations of the data collection process as well as any controls employed to eliminate the action of extraneous variables on the data collected.

If questionnaires or other self-report measures are used, the researcher should present a few examples of the items in the report to enhance the description. You will rarely find an entire instrument presented. However, somewhere in the report mention should be made of where the reader can obtain a copy of the instrument. If the instrument has been adopted from another source, that source should be documented in the reference section of the report. If the author has developed the instrument, an address should be presented at the beginning or end of the report to indicate where a complete copy can be obtained. Any publications related to instrument testing should be referenced. These factors are very important if you are considering replicating the study and testing the instruments in the practice setting.

To evaluate a questionnaire for clinical use, in addition to criteria discussed earlier, several practical criteria can be considered that may affect reliability and validity. For example, the wording and format of items can be a source of bias that will affect appropriateness for use and thus validity of data. Often the researcher will not comment in detail on the construction of the instrument. However, if you have the opportunity to review an entire questionnaire or a good sample of items from the instrument, Table 9.3 will assist you to critique some of these factors.

Usually considerable detail about reliability and validity testing is presented in the report by the researcher, and this information should

_____ Table 9.3 _____

PRACTICAL ASPECTS OF QUESTIONNAIRE CONSTRUCTION

Criteria	Implications
Instructions to respondents	Failure to be clear may invalidate results.
Length of questionnaire	Too long may affect participation and quality of responses; too short may affect reliability and validity.
Clarity of items	Negative wording, use of compound sentences, use of double negatives, use of value bias questions that assume certain attitudes or behaviors will often be misinterpreted. Questions or statements should be brief, objective, and unambiguous.
Format of items	Items should be logically arranged from simplest to complex to facilitate subject participation.
	Content should be balanced to avoid response set bias.
	Questions requiring the same response format should be grouped together to avoid confusion.
	Format should be appropriate for type of analysis planned.
Fit of instrument to subjects	Questions must be relevant and answerable for subject and worded at an appropriate educational and sociocultural level to ensure valid responses.

be carefully evaluated by the consumer. Both reliability and validity should be addressed. In quantitative studies, an explanation of the methods used for testing the concepts should be presented along with a description of the subjects used for testing. If the subject characteristics differ widely from those of the research sample, the validity of using the instrument in the study at hand should be questioned. Statistical reliability and validity coefficients should be reported if such testing is appropriate. Interpretation of statistical meaning is often difficult for the consumer. Chapter 10 presents some strategies (correlation coefficient and Cronbach's alpha) that will assist you in demystifying these tests.

In qualitative studies, the researcher may not directly address reliability and validity testing. However, a clear description of methods used for data collection, along with detailed descriptions of respondents and settings, is necessary to evaluate the validity of procedures. Special precautions taken to prevent the effect of extraneous factors on the outcomes should be discussed; evidence of ruling out alternate explanations should be presented; and validation of data and inferences with participant respondents and peers should be done to increase the reliability and validity of the method. In qualitative research reports, you may find some of these issues discussed as part of data analysis. Verbatim examples from field notes or audio tapes should be included in a report when possible to provide convincing evidence for the reliability and validity of the methods used as well as the meaning attributed to data obtained.

SUMMARY

This chapter provides an overview of the most common methods used for data collection in quantitative and qualitative nursing research. Factors that affect the researcher's development or selection of a method to collect valid data are discussed. Data collection approaches should fit the research problem, theoretical context, and study design as well as being feasible, practical methods. Concepts of reliability and validity of data are explained and examples demonstrate application of these concepts to qualitative and quantitative methods.

The last section of the chapter emphasizes the evaluation of data collection methods as reported in a research article. Also, some practical criteria for reviewing questionnaire items are included. Table 9.4 summarizes broad criteria for critiquing scientific adequacy of data collection when considering the application of findings to practice.

_____ *Table 9.4* _____

CRITERIA FOR CRITIQUING INSTRUMENTS OR METHODS OF DATA COLLECTION

Scientific Adequacy		Implications for Clinical Applicability
Quantitative Research	Variations in Qualitative Research	
1. Describes instruments for data collection 2. Gives rationale for development or selection of instruments 3. Fits instruments to research question 4. Has clear procedures for testing reliability and validity of instruments	1–3. Focuses on the researcher's method for data collection; instruments seldom used 4. Does not discuss reliability and validity concepts often; describes precautions taken to ensure representative data collection as well as strategies employed to enhance reliability and validity of data for analysis	In order to apply findings into practice, you must be convinced that the researcher has actually measured or observed the variables intended to be studied, and that these methods are reliable and valid for use with the study sample. Usually entire questionnaires or other self-report measures are not presented in detail in the report. However, these measures should be described well enough to allow you to decide on the potential for using them to replicate data collection in your setting. Information should be provided in the report on where the complete instruments can be located should you decide to test or replicate the data collection procedure in your setting. In some cases, the findings of a study may not be directly applicable to practice, but reliable and valid instruments used in the study may have more direct implications for your assessment of clients in performing nursing process.
5. Has suitable instruments for use with study sample	5. Selects method suitable for the subjects	

EXERCISES ▬▬▬▬▬▬▬▬▬▬▬▬▬▬▬▬

1. A proposed study was designed to investigate if there is a change
   in reported job satisfaction among nurses on a post-partum unit
   with the introduction of combined mother and baby care provided
   by the same nurse rather than separate care for mother and baby
   provided by two nurses. The theoretical framework used to study
   the problem was Hertzberg's motivation–hygiene theory for job
   satisfaction (1967).

   The following paragraphs represent a description of the
   research design and methods to be used for data collection. Using
   the guidelines presented in Table 9.4, evaluate the methods used
   for data collection.

*The Implementation of Combined Care as Related to Job Satisfaction**

Research Design

A nonequivalent control group pretest quasi-experimental design
will be used. A pretest will be done six months prior to the implementation of combined care. Two groups of subjects will be
used, one group of R.N.'s from the post-partum setting and a
second group of R.N.'s to act as a control. The control group
should come from a floor with a similar number of patient care
hours, similar staffing, and a low staff turnover. Hospital statistics
will be used to identify this control group. Following the pretest,
results will be compared to identify a similar score in job satisfaction. If the control group does not have a similar rating of
job satisfaction, a new control group will be chosen until measures
of job satisfaction are approximately the same. By introducing
a nonequivalent control, it is possible to determine a natural
change in job satisfaction in the hospital that was not related to
the implementation of combined care.

   Posttests will be completed by the same groups of R.N.'s at
six-months post change and one-year post change. These items
were chosen because change theory implies that once a change is
implemented, it is necessary that an equilibrium be reestablished
prior to evaluation (Stevens, 1976). It is felt that, at six months
after the implementation of combined care, the nurses should be
familiar with the routines and thus starting to reestablish equi-

---

* Research proposal by M. Oskamp et al. (1987). Year IV students, Queen's University
School of Nursing. Kingston, Ontario.

librium. At one-year post change, equilibrium should be reestablished and the evaluation of combined care performed.

Proposed Methodology

Setting: The setting of the proposed study is a post-partum unit with a core nursery and approximately 25–30 beds. Sampling method and population: a convenience sample of R.N.'s who have worked in each area for at least three months prior to the pretest will be used. The questionnaire will be given out at the beginning of each shift for one week or until the questionnaires are completed by all R.N.'s with signed consents. The questionnaires will be given out at this time to ensure better response rate and to decrease possible bias that could result at the end of a shift when people are tired and want to leave. The questionnaire should be distributed at a time when patient census on the unit is average—not above or below—as each situation may reflect biased results (that is, if patient census is high, each R.N. will have an increased workload). The questionnaire should take approximately 15–20 minutes to complete, and therefore, questionnaires will be collected as soon as they are completed by the R.N.'s.

Instrument

The questionnaire to be used was based on the questionnaire developed by Slavitt, Stamps, Piedmont, and Haase (1978). Their 48-item questionnaire was developed based on Hertzberg's theory of job satisfaction. This instrument was reviewed and 30 items were chosen according to Hertzberg's satisfiers and dissatisfiers for application in this study. Hertzberg's satisfiers—achievement, recognition, work itself, responsibility, growth, and advancement—were included as well as the dissatisfiers—company policy, supervision, interpersonal relationships, and working conditions. The dissatisfiers salary, status, and security were not considered important factors to measure since these would not change with the implementation of combined care.

To validate the revised questionnaire, validity will be obtained by showing the questionnaire to nurse managers familiar with Hertzberg's theory. A review of the literature established content validity. Internal reliability of the questionnaire was determined by Slavitt, et al. using the Cronbach coefficient alpha and was found to be .912, indicating a high reliability. Because of the research design, a test-retest reliability will be performed using the control group.

2. The following seven examples are taken from the modified Job Satisfaction Questionnaire for the above study. Using Table 9.3, evaluate the clarity and format of items.

*Job Satisfaction Questionnaire**

Please complete the following questionnaire according to this scale:

SA = strongly agree   A = agree   N = neutral
D = disagree   SD = strongly disagree

Simple **a.** When I'm at work in this hospital, the time generally goes by slowly.

SA   A   N   D   SD

b. Even if I could make more money in another hospital nursing situation, I am more satisfied here.

SA   A   N   D   SD

req diff biased Ambiguous **c.** There is no doubt whatever in my mind that what I do on my job is very important.

SA   A   N   D   SD

(+) wording biased quest

d. I am not satisfied with the types of activities that I do on my job.

SA   A   N   D   SD

(−) wording bias

e. There is a lot of collaboration between the nurses and doctors on my unit.

SA   A   N   D   SD

f. I feel that I am not supervised as closely as I need to be, and more closely than I want to be.

SA   A   N   D   SD

(−) wording

Complex **g.** I sometimes feel that I have too many supervisors who tell me conflicting things.

SA   A   N   D   SD

bias

REFERENCES

Burke, S. O.; Sayers, L. A.; Baumgart, A. J.; & Wray, J. G. (1985, Sept./Oct.). Pitfalls in cross-cultural use of the Denver Developmental Screening Test: Cree Indian children. *Journal of Public Health, 76,* 303–307.

Burns, N., & Grove, S. (1987). *The practice of nursing research: Conduct, critique and utilization.* Philadelphia: W. B. Saunders.

---

* Abstracted from a questionnaire by D. Slavitt, et al. (1978). Nurses' satisfaction with their work situation. *Nursing Research, 27*(2), 114–120. Copyright 1978 American Journal of Nursing Company. Used with permission. All rights reserved.

Campbell, D. T., & Fiske, D. W. (1959). Convergent and discriminant validation by the multitrait-multimethod matrix. *Psychological Bulletin, 56*(2), 81–105.

Cronbach, L. J., & Meehe, P. E. (1955). Construct validity in psychological tests. *Psychological Bulletin, 52*(4), 281–302.

Field, P. A., & Morse, J. (1985). *Nursing research: The application of qualitative approaches.* Rockville, Md.: Aspen Systems.

Herzberg, F. (1967). *Work and the nature of man.* New York: World Publishing.

Holm, K., & Llewellyn, J. (1986). *Nursing research for nursing practice.* Philadelphia: W. B. Saunders.

Ireton, H., & Thwing, E. (1974). *MCDI: Minnesota child development inventory.* Minneapolis: Behavior Science Systems.

Jerrett, M. D. (1985). Children and their pain experience. *Children's Health Care, 14*(2), 83–89.

Miles, M. B., & Huberman, A. M. (1984). *Qualitative data analysis: A sourcebook of new methods.* Beverly Hills, Calif.: Sage.

Oskamp, M.; Vadeboncoeur, C.; Low, S.; & Barry, S. (1987). Implementation of combined care as related to job satisfaction. Unpublished research proposal. Year IV Students, Queen's University School of Nursing. Kingston, Ontario.

Perloff, E. (1988). *Health instrument file,* Abstract. Pittsburgh, Pa.: University of Pittsburg, School of Nursing.

Polit, D. F., & Hungler, B. P. (1987). *Nursing research: Principles and methods,* 3rd ed. Philadelphia: Lippincott.

Rees, B. L. (1980). Measuring identification with the mothering role. *Research in Nursing and Health, 2,* 49–56.

Sandelowski, M. (1986). The problem with rigor in qualitative research. *Advances in Nursing Science, 8*(33), 27–37.

Schaefer, E. S., & Bell, R. Q. (1958). Development of a parental attitude research instrument. *Child Development, 29,* 339–361.

Slavett, D.; Stamps, P.; Piedmont, E.; & Hasse, A. M. (1978). Nurses' satisfaction with their work situation. *Nursing Research, 27*(2), 114–120.

Spradley, J. P. (1980). *Participant observation.* New York: Holt, Rinehart and Winston.

Stevens, B. J. (1976). *First-line patient care management.* Wakefield, Mass.: Contemporary Publishing.

10

Data Analysis: Understanding Principles and Evaluating Strategies

INTRODUCTION

This chapter describes the strategies researchers use to analyze their data and how they synthesize the results or findings for presentation in a study report. The chapter also describes how to evaluate the analysis and findings sections of a research report for scientific adequacy and clinical applicability. As a research consumer, you often may reach additional conclusions based on the data and findings presented in the report that you can use in clinical practice.

If you have taken coursework in statistics or other analysis methods, this chapter will provide a framework in which to place those concepts and skills, and it will introduce alternate analysis strategies. For the complete neophyte, this chapter will provide a basis for understanding the concepts behind data analysis, thereby enabling you to follow the logic of research reports and determine when more expert help is needed for decisions about the use of findings in clinical practice.

OBJECTIVES

After reading this chapter you will be able to

1. Determine whether or not the analysis strategy fits with the rest of the study.
2. Understand the usual meaning of findings produced with common statistics.
3. Critically examine tables and other graphic presentations of data.

NEW TERMS

Data analysis

Findings

Data

Nominal data

Ordinal data

Interval data

Ratio data

Normally distributed

Parametric statistics

Nonparametric statistics

Univariate statistics

Mean

Standard deviation

Median

Range

Bivariate analysis

Factor analysis

Principal component

Cluster analysis

Regression analysis

Multiple correlation coefficient

R, R^2

Significance level

Type I error

Type II error

Content analysis

how to clarify
data . to p9q9q1

DATA ANALYSIS IN THE RESEARCH PROCESS

The purpose of **data analysis** is to answer the research question. The researcher presents a concise synthesis of the data called the findings. The **findings** are abstract ideas that can be presented in the report in a variety of forms: narrative, pictorial, graphic, and statistical. Each of these forms of presentation has associated data analysis strategies.

As you look at Figure 10.1, note that the data analysis comes midway in the research process. It represents the most microscopic, narrowed, and focused portion of the research process. The time for breadth in thinking on the study comes at the beginning and at the end, as you can see in Figure 10.2. Figure 10.2 contains the same elements as Figure 10.1, but the width of the bar suggests the breadth of focus appropriate at each step. In quantitative studies, the process proceeds more or less from the top to the bottom. In qualitative studies, there is more movement up and down the steps, and at the end of the study, the bar is usually narrower since the generalizability will usually not come until the findings have been tested again under more controlled conditions.

Figure 10.2 shows at the onset of a study, its *purpose* is often very broad. When the *question* is posed and the *design* is developed, the focus becomes progressively narrower. The *sample* and *data collection* procedures that operationalize the variables and phenomena under study further narrow the scope, leading to the narrowest aspect of the study — the analysis. The analysis yields findings, which, taken together, are called the study *results,* and are somewhat broader in scope than the actual analysis. The scope continues to broaden out into a *discussion* that should pertain exclusively to the findings of the particular study and, perhaps, the findings of other studies for purposes of comparison and contrast. The *conclusions* are the findings discussed in terms of their meaning for theory development, further research, and, most importantly, clinical practice. This last step in the research process can be as broad in its scope as the initial purpose of the study, or it can be narrower, depending upon the nature of the study and the findings that emerge. Level 4 studies (Table 6.1) have the potential for the broadest generalizability, while level 1 studies have the least potential for generalizability. (These aspects will be elaborated in Chapter 12.)

THE LANGUAGE OF DATA ANALYSIS

In an approach that reflects a relatively recent shift among nurse researchers (Chinn, 1986), various analysis strategies are seen as complementary and interrelated (Weekes, 1986). At present, research

Figure 10.1

RESEARCH PROCESS FLOWCHART

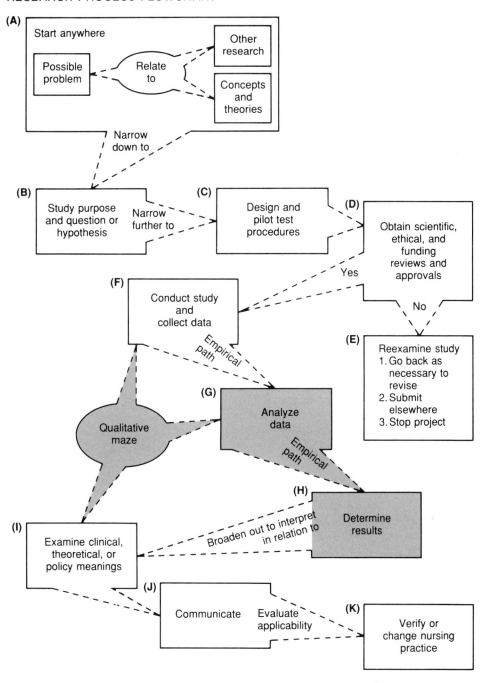

_____ Figure 10.2 _____

*THE RELATIVE BREADTH OR NARROWNESS OF FOCUS OF THE STEPS
OF THE RESEARCH PROCESS*

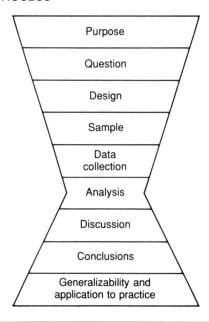

studies generally use either narrative or statistical strategies in conjunction with graphic stategies. (These three strategies are discussed
later in this chapter.)

The terms used in data analysis require precision, and each
analysis strategy has its own language. Studies using qualitative data,
for example, tend to use the term *participant* or *informant,* while
quantitative studies use the term *subject.* The Glossary at the back of
this text relates research terms to the ideas expressed here. The terminology used in this text is taken largely from quantitative research
because it is the most commonly published type.

In the research report some terms have specific meanings that
might not be evident to the research consumer. For example, the term
significance usually refers to statistical, not clinical or theoretical,
significance. Another example is the term *mean,* which can be defined
roughly as the average. However, "average" does not have the precision
that a researcher requires. The research consumer will need to use the
Glossary in order to read accurately the analysis and results sections of
a research report.

TYPES OF DATA

Most research findings are presented in a form suited to a particular level of inquiry of the study question and to the nature of the data and the analysis. As can be seen in Table 10.1, the purpose of the analysis and the level of the inquiry (see Chapter 6) suggest particular analysis strategies to be used according to the type of data collected.

Data in the simplest sense are the words and/or numbers collected in the course of the study using the methods and tools described in the previous Chapter 9. Words are the usual form of data in qualitative

Table 10.1

COMMONLY USED, SUITABLE ANALYSIS AND INTERPRETATION STRATEGIES BY LEVEL OF INQUIRY AND TYPE OF DATA

- any may be used together to ↑strength of case to answer research quest

| Type of Data | Purpose of Analysis | | | |
	Description Levels 1–2	Associations/ Differences Levels 2–3	Patterns of Relationships Levels 2–4	Hypothesis Testing Levels 3–4
Qualitative (words or images)	Narrative Graphic	Narrative Graphic	Narrative Graphic	Not applicable
Quantitative (numbers) Nominal	Narrative Graphic Statistical	Narrative Graphic Statistical	Narrative Graphic	Graphic Statistical
Ordinal *– no-clear categories or groups of severity*	Narrative Graphic Statistical	Graphic Statistical	Graphic Statistical	Graphic Statistical
Interval	Graphic Statistical	Graphic Statistical	Graphic Statistical	Statistical

– Choice depends on research's training, exper, & philosophical bent

Notes: The strategies in the table and as defined below are not mutually exclusive. They are often used together to make a stronger case for the answer to the research question.

① *Narrative:* Primary evidence for addressing the research question is in the form of words, images, or ideas.

② *Graphic* or *Pictorial:* Primary or supportive evidence for the answer to the research question is presented in the form of pictures, diagrams, graphs, tables, charts, etc., that represent numerical or nonnumerical data. Narrative or statistics are used to summarize the graphically displayed data or illustrate the conclusions.

③ *Statistical:* Primary evidence for the answer to the research question or hypothesis is the numerical answer to an appropriate statistical formula. Limited narrative is required, and graphics can be used to illustrate the conclusion.

studies, and numbers are the usual form for quantitative studies. Different data analysis strategies and forms of presentation are best suited to different types of data. Table 10.1 summarizes the appropriate analysis and interpretation strategies to be used for qualitative and quantitative data as related to the level of inquiry of the research question and design.

Qualitative Data

In studies at level 1, and sometimes at level 2, the data are most often in the form of words that represent ideas and meanings. In phenomenological studies the data are the subject's descriptions and the researcher's interpretations of these descriptions. In ethnographic studies the data are the researcher's observations, as clarified and/or verified by the subjects, of a lived experience with the subjects (Parse, Coyne, & Smith, 1985). For example, in a study of family interactions when one member has a chronic illness, the data might be in the form of extensive field notes taken by the researcher while observing a family, tape recordings of family member perceptions of interactions, and typewritten transcripts of the tape recordings. Descriptive studies that collect verbatim data also yield word-based qualitative data. These data might initially be in the form of audio recordings, video recordings, photographs, or drawings. However, they usually are transcribed or coded into words at some stage in the analysis. There is no constraint to fit the data into categories or into a sequence at the onset of the study. However, categories usually emerge later in the analysis.

Quantitative Data

Nominal Data   Level 2 and 3 studies often yield data that are categorical. Categorical data that do not have an implied order are termed **nominal data.** In the example study of family interactions when one member has a chronic illness, the gender of each family member is nominal data. Gender fits into two clear categories (female and male), but in the context of the study it does not have any order or relative value attached to it. In this hypothetical study, the nursing diagnoses of the chronically ill member would also be nominal data. However, if the severity of the diagnosis were under study, there might be relative degrees within each diagnosis, and these degrees would not be nominal data because there is an implied order.

Throughout this chapter and Chapter 11, we will use a subset of the DDST data (Burke et al., 1985). Note that while these are actual data, they are not the full set that was used in the study. For reasons of confidentiality and ease of explanation, some of the subjects have been removed. The code book that lists the variables that were selected for use here is seen in Table 10.2. The variable MOLANG—the first language of the mother—is an example of a nominal variable.

_____ Table 10.2 _____

DDST DATAFILE CODE BOOK

Interval data= parametrics

Variable Label*	Description	Possible Values
DDST	DDST test result	1 = Normal: neither questionable, abnormal, nor untestable
		2 = Questionable: *if*, 2 or more delays in 1 sector, or *if* 1 or more sectors have 1 delay *plus* in the same sector, the age line does not go through any passed item
		3 = Abnormal: *if*, 2 or more sectors have 2 or more delays or *if* there is 1 sector with 2 or more delays *plus* 1 or more sectors with 1 delay and in that same sector no passes on the age line
		4 = Untestable: enough refusals to change the results of the test from normal *if* they were scored as delays
DDSTMOS	Age—in months at time of DDST testing	0 to 74
MOLANG	Language mother speaks most easily	1 = Cree 2 = English

* Abbreviated name used for computer analysis. See Chapter 11 for more information on variable labels.

Ordinal Data   With reference to the chronically ill family member example, the severity of the nursing diagnosis would be ordinal data, because the ratings would be arranged in order and displayed in a scale. The DDST ratings in Table 10.2 are an example of ordinal data.

Ordinal data do not have clear categories or groupings like nominal data, but rather are used to make distinctions between points or degrees of difference within one category. Ordinal data are very common in nursing research. Most of the scales discussed in Chapter 9 yield ordinal data. Major variables in level 2–4 studies will often be ordinal in nature. Psychosocial variables are most often ordinal.

It is important to note that the quantities measured by the points on an ordinal scale are not equivalent to one another. For example, in rating a particular nursing diagnosis, the difference between very severe and moderately severe is not measurably the same as the difference between moderately severe and not severe on the same scale.

Interval Data   When data have an order within themselves *and* the intervals between each of the degrees are measurably the same, then the data are termed **interval data.** This type of data is seen most often in experimental, level 3 and 4 studies. Refer to the code book for the DDST study in Table 10.2. The age of the child in months (DDSTMOS) is an example of interval data.

There is a fourth level of data, **ratio data,** which has an absolute zero in addition to the characteristics of interval data. However, for our purposes, ratio data can be considered with interval data. For example, if weight change in the chronically ill member were a variable of concern, it would be interval data. As measured in pounds or kilograms the data have intrinsic order, and the intervals between points on the scale are the same. In other words, the difference between 100 lbs. and 105 lbs. is measurably the same as the difference between 110 lbs. and 115 lbs. Physiological measures such as blood pressure, temperature, height, and so on yield interval data. An important characteristic of many interval variables is that they are assumed to be distributed in the study population along the bell-shaped normal curve. Most statistics used with interval data are based on the assumption that the data are more or less **normally distributed.**

Some standardized and highly reliable psychosocial data collection tools and some types of scaling techniques yield data that are considered to be interval by some and ordinal by others. These data are *likely* to be normally distributed or falling under a bell-shaped normal curve (Wilson, 1985). An example is IQ scores as measured by the

Stanford-Binet test, which we classify as strong-ordinal data in this text because the difference between an IQ of 50 and 60 is not necessarily the same quantitative amount or the difference between an IQ of 120 and 130.

The important issue for the research consumer is that some researchers analyze this type of data as if the data were ordinal. However, to use only ordinal statistics on this type of data would not employ all the characteristics of the data in reaching an answer to the research questions. Furthermore, most interval data statistics are robust enough to allow for the relative lack of equal intervals between points on a scale (Burns and Grove, 1987).

Determining Data Types

The research consumer classifies data into types in order to determine whether or not appropriate analysis strategies were used. However, there is overlap between all the types of data. For example, while "apples" and "oranges" are examples of qualitative data in the form of words, a researcher, viewing them as "fruit," and being interested only in the number of calories in each piece of fruit, would use interval data. Thus, the same reality can be classified into different types of data.

A more subtle example of the same vagaries of data-type classification is that of weight. While the intervals between pounds is the same, a loss of five pounds in a toddler has far greater clinical significance than a loss of five pounds in an adult. If the underlying concept is nutritional status or the seriousness of the progress of a disease, the five-pound weight loss in a toddler would be rated as a severe problem, while the same weight loss in an adult would be rated as a moderate one. Thus the same data would be classified as ordinal, not interval. In such cases researchers often disagree, and as you can see in Table 10.1, there is overlap between types of data and analysis strategies.

ANALYSIS STRATEGIES

The researcher will select a particular type of analysis strategy to answer the research question with the data collected. This general strategy or approach will be evident in a report by the way in which the findings are presented. The findings can be in narrative, graphic, or statistical form. The range of appropriate strategies depends primarily upon two things: the level of inquiry of the question and the type of data.

Chapter 6 described how to determine the level of inquiry of the question and how the levels relate to study designs and data collection techniques. The preceding section described how to classify the data. With Table 10.1 as a guide, you can determine whether the analysis strategies used in a particular study are appropriate.

The analysis strategies described in Table 10.1 are not mutually exclusive. They can be used together to make a stronger case in answer to the research question. There is usually some latitude possible in the choice of analysis strategy. A researcher's preference, which is based on philosophical bent, training, and experience, will often influence the choice of which style of analysis is used or emphasized. However, if the analysis strategy is not logically consistent with the level of inquiry of the question and with the level of the data, the answer to the question will be flawed and the use of the results in practice thrown into question.

Narrative Strategies

All presentations of the results of an analysis employ some narrative, but analyses that examine data in the form of words, pictures, and ideas can be grouped together as a narrative approach. The data are usually qualitative or nominal.

The most common narrative strategy in the nursing literature is content analysis. Other strategies include grounded theory and a technique called *constant comparative*. Hutchinson's (1984 and 1986) study of stress in intensive-care nurses used a grounded field approach (abstracted in Example 2.2) and is an example of a narrative approach to analysis and presentation of findings. Words and ideas were the predominant unit of analysis and the form of presentation used.

Graphic and Pictorial Strategies

Graphic or pictorial strategies yield descriptions, diagrams, and figures that illustrate the patterns of relationships between the phenomena or variables in the study. Both phenomenological, qualitative studies, and multivariate quantitative studies use analysis methods that yield findings that can be described with such diagrams. The first type of study assumes a meaning within the life context of the subjects and describes the findings in terms of this integration. The second type of study uses sophisticated statistics to examine how variables are grouped together as an entity. Although earlier and more conservative writers might disagree, Dzurec and Abraham (1986) argue that there is an analog between these two types of analysis. Multivariate techniques that fall into this general type of strategy are regression analysis and factor analysis.

A strong form of argument in answer to the research question can be the presentation of a portion of the data as a graph, table, or chart that represents numerical data. This strategy is used in conjunction with statistical or narrative strategies. When used alone, statistical strategies can overcondense the data, while narrative strategies may undercondense them. Graphic strategies are best used with ordinal and interval data, but can be used with nominal data.

Statistical Strategies

Statistical strategies require numerical data to which a formula is applied. The formula selected must be able to address the research question, and the numerical data must represent the concepts behind the variables in the research question. The result is a concise summary in the form of a few numbers or a single number. The leap from concept to number is a large one for many people. The following section on statistical analysis will focus on linking the concepts that the data represent to the statistic and then back to the logic of answering the question with the statistical results.

STATISTICS FOR ANALYSIS AND PRESENTATION OF NUMERICAL DATA

focuses on linking concepts to stats & back to logic of res ques

The most powerful tool available to the researcher in analyzing numerical data is statistics. Used in combination with narrative and a graphic or pictorial presentation of findings, statistics can provide concise, convincing answers to research questions. Because they often complement each other, statistics and graphic strategies will be discussed together in this section.

most powerful to analyze data — easy to check

Findings from statistical analysis can be in error if the wrong statistics are used or if they are not calculated correctly. To a large extent, you will be able to determine whether the correct statistic is used after you have studied this chapter. Most articles do not supply enough data to determine whether or not the statistics are correctly calculated even if you have had a statistics course and are able to check the calculations. However, the use of tables and graphs by the researcher to summarize the data can be carefully cross-checked to determine whether or not the statistical conclusion logically fits with the way the data seem to fall.

More seriously, it is possible to misrepresent the data unintentionally by presenting only a portion of them or by selecting only those that tend to inflate or deflate the findings. For example, look at the subset of the DDST data in Table 10.3. Note how few mothers use Cree as opposed to English. It would be correct, but misleading, to say that "of the mothers who spoke Cree, 37.5% of their children had questionable DDST results." The use of percentages (a very simple statistic) tends to lend more weight to the statement than the actual number of children in this category (only three children had questionable DDST scores *and* mothers who spoke Cree). Furthermore, as will be illustrated below, a percentage is not the most appropriate statistic to use with these data. When a more appropriate statistic is used, the relationship is demonstrated to be not significant. For example, if a chi-square (a statistic used with normal data to test for differences) is used with these data, the pattern is not significant. The hypothesis that language was related to DDST results would be rejected.

_____ Table 10.3 _____

DDST SCORES AND MOTHERS' LANGUAGE: PERCENTS, FREQUENCIES, AND THE CHI-SQUARE STATISTIC

DDST Score	Mother's Language	
	Cree	English
Normal	5 62.5%	82 85.4%
Questionable	3 37.5%	14 14.6%
Totals	8	96

$\chi^2 = 2.84, p = .09$

Note: This is a subset of the data with selected subjects omitted for the purpose of illustration in this chapter. For study results for the full dataset, see Burke et al. (1985).

Types of Statistics

There are several ways to categorize statistics in research reports. **Parametric statistics** have rather strict assumptions about the characteristics of the data that should be met. In most instances, interval data are assumed to meet these assumptions. In Table 10.2, the statistics listed in the row for interval data are referred to as parametric statistics. Above this row are the **nonparametric statistics,** which are used with nominal and ordinal data. The question of whether to use parametric statistics with ordinal data is disputed in the nursing research literature. Those who are against liberal use of parametric statistics argue that if the assumptions about the nature of the data are violated, then the resulting statistical answer is seriously flawed or uninterpretable. Those who would use parametric statistics with ordinal data argue that violating the assumptions makes little difference to the results, and because parametric statistics are more powerful and widely understood, they should be more widely used. It is our view that if there is additional supporting evidence, the liberal use of parametric statistics for strong-ordinal data is acceptable for generating findings for use in clinical practice.

There are also inferential and descriptive statistics. Columns 2 and 3 of Table 10.4 are considered to be descriptive statistics. However, strictly speaking, all the statistics in the table describe the data. Thus, the statistics shown in columns 4–6 of the table are used both to describe data and to make inferences. The central issue for the research consumer is to determine that the question and the analysis match, in terms of description only, versus description with inference.

Table 10.4 displays the appropriate statistic to use depending on the level of inquiry and type of data in the study. In the DDST example, the dependent variable (the DDST results) is ordinal. Moving along the ordinal row of Table 10.4 to the column that examines testing for differences, you will see that chi-square, or perhaps a t-test (a statistic used with strong-ordinal data to test for differences), would be a better way to examine the data. The branching diagram method, as used by Wilson (1985) and Mosteller, Fienberg, and Rourke (1983), has been adapted for use by the research consumer and is shown in Figures 10.3 and 10.4. Figure 10.3 shows the best statistic for the various designs possible if the study question calls for a test of association or patterns of relationships. Figure 10.4 is used for research questions or hypotheses in which a test of differences is needed.

Once you have determined the level of the data and examined the

Table 10.4

COMMONLY USED, SUITABLE STATISTICS BY PURPOSE OF ANALYSIS
AND TYPE OF DATA

make sure stat = level of inquiry & type of data [handwritten]

Type of Data	Description		Description and Inference		
	Central Tendency	Dispersion *(variation)*	Measures of Association	Patterns of Relationships	Differences
Qualitative	N/A *(# cat's) mean* [handwritten]	Frequency counts	N/A	N/A	N/A
Quantitative Nominal	Mode	(1) Frequency counts Percentages	Lambda (λ) Phi (ϕ)	N/A	Chi-square (χ^2) McNemar's test Cochran's Q
Ordinal	Median	(1) Frequency counts Percentages	Kendall's tau (τ) Gamma (γ) Spearman's rho (ρ) (2)	(2)	(2 & 3) Mann-Whitney U Wilcoxon's test Kruskall-Wallis test Friedman's test
Interval	Mean ($\overline{X}$)	Standard deviation (SD)	Pearson's r Cronbach's alpha (α)	Factor analysis Regression analysis	t-test Analysis of variance (F)

(variation = variability occurring in sample) [handwritten note under Dispersion]

chi square & t-test [handwritten note to right of Differences column]

Table 10.1 contains same terms c̄ level of inq. assoc c̄ them [handwritten]

1. There are statistics for this, but they are seldom used.

2. Whether or not statistics that make assumptions that technically only interval data can meet can be used with ordinal data is disputed in the literature. Conservatively speaking, these statistics are the appropriate statistics, but it is a commonly accepted practice to use Pearson's r for correlation and analysis of variance for testing differences when the data is strong-ordinal. See text.

3. Weak-ordinal data might be analyzed with the nominal chi-square statistic.

question, you will be able to use Table 10.4 to determine appropriate statistics. If the statistic used is not on the table or in the following discussion (the most commonly used statistics are included), it is still possible that it is appropriate. If you are considering the findings for clinical application, you will need to refer to more detailed texts on statistics or to consult with a researcher or statistician to determine whether it is an appropriate statistic.

Across the top of Table 10.4 are the terms *description, association, patterns, differences,* and *hypothesis testing.* Table 10.1 contains the same terms, along with the levels of inquiry generally associated with them.

_____ Figure 10.3 _____

QUICK CHECK FOR CORRECT STATISTIC TO DESCRIBE AND TEST
ASSOCIATION, RELATIONSHIPS, AND PATTERNS

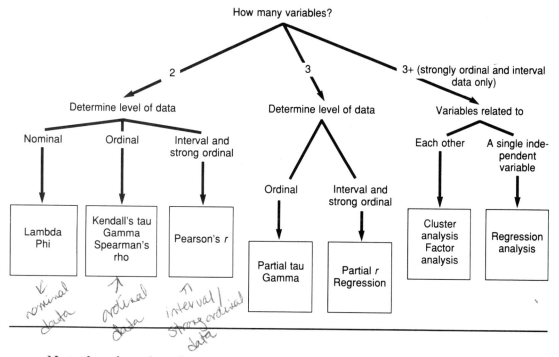

Note that there is a close relationship between the level of the study and
these terms. Reexamine the study question or hypothesis to determine
whether it aims to describe, demonstrate association, illustrate patterns
of relationships, and/or test a hypothesis. If there are several questions,
follow this procedure with each one.

Description In level 1 and 2 studies, the purpose is to describe.
These statistics deal with only one variable at a time and are called
univariate statistics. Descriptive statistics can be used in level 3 and
4 studies to describe the nature of the sample or individual variables, but
not to address the question.

There are basically two complementary ways to describe or summarize the data collected on a single variable—the central tendency
and the dispersion or variation of the data. These descriptions represent
a way of summarizing where the center point for the variable lies and
how far-ranging the rest of the data are. For each level of data, there are
appropriate statistics that can be used. For example, strongly ordinal
data often is described by the **mean** (the average) and **standard**

_____ *Figure 10.4* _____

QUICK CHECK FOR CORRECT STATISTIC TO DESCRIBE AND TEST DIFFERENCES

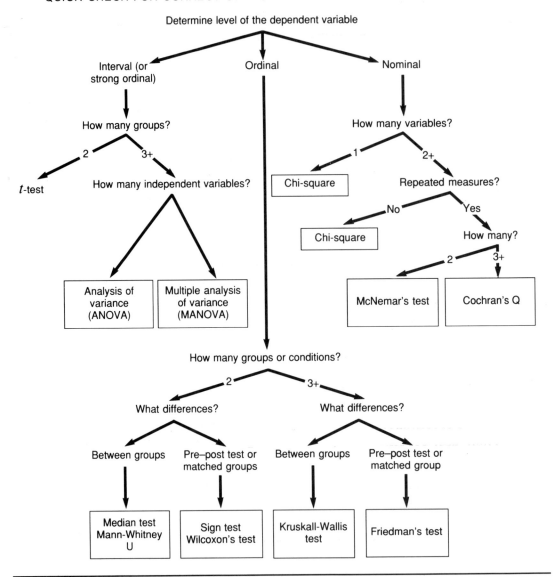

deviation (about 70% of the data are apt to fall within 1 standard deviation of the mean). Depending on the actual data, however, more appropriate statistics, such as the **median** (the point at which half of the data are higher and half the data are lower) and the **range** (difference between the highest and lowest scores), could be used to describe the characteristics of the data.

_____ Table 10.5 _____

MEASURES OF CENTRAL TENDENCY AND DISPERSION FOR THE DDST DATA

frequency plot

Variable	Level of Measurement of the Data	Central Tendency	Dispersion
Mother's language	Nominal *(H's)*	Mode = English	8% Cree 92% English
DDST score	Ordinal *(0 clear groupings; scale)*	Median = Normal	84% Normal 16% Questionable
Age of child in months	Interval *(eat. intervals)*	Mean = 30.8 mo.	Standard deviation = 20 mo.

To illustrate these statistics with the DDST data, the appropriate statistics have been calculated to describe the variables representing three of the levels of quantitative data discussed in this chapter. In Table 10.5 you will see the measures of central tendency and dispersion.

Descriptive statistics are best used if the number of sets of data (usually the number of subjects) is high. When there are only a few subjects, the raw data are often the best way to describe the data. If the description is a central to the purpose of the study, the statistics should be augmented with the use of a histogram or frequency plot to summarize the nature of the data. Figure 10.5 is an example of a frequency plot.

Percentages are commonly used, but can easily be misinterpreted. Their use, beyond description for single nominal variables, should be carefully scrutinized. Unsophisticated researchers might try to rely too heavily on percentages if they do not have the knowledge and skill necessary for the use of more precise statistics. As a research consumer, be skeptical if percentages are used to "prove" or to make inferences in the analysis of data. A related problem is the potential for confusion when percentages of a subgroup of the sample are used. To illustrate, "65% of the women (23% of the subjects in the study), were less able to . . . ." Percentages deal most clearly with one variable at a time. Figure 10.5 is concerned with two variables, and it requires statistics that are suited for **bivariate analysis.**

Measures of Association   The relative strength of association between two variables is usually calculated with a correlational statistic. This type of statistic is the main one used in level 2 and 3 studies. It is also used in data collection, instrument reliability, and

level 2&3

_____ Figure 10.5 _____

DESCRIPTIVE DATA IN A GRAPHIC PRESENTATION

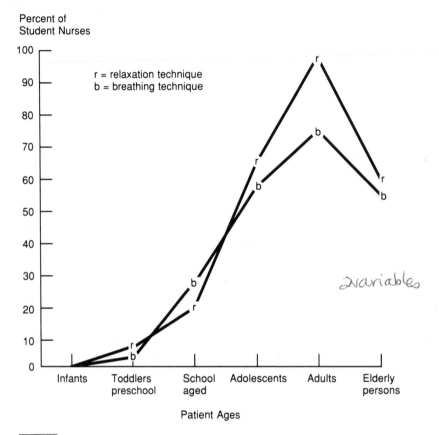

Source: Burke, S. O., & Jerrett, M. (in press). Pain management across age
groups: Student nurse choices. *Western Journal of Nursing Research.*
Reprinted by permission of Sage Publications, Inc.

validity studies. The most common one is Pearson's *r* for use with
interval or perhaps strong-ordinal data. Spearman's rho, Kendall's tau,
and Gamma are for use with ordinal data. Lambda and Phi are used for
nominal data. Calculated scores for most of these range from +1 to 0 to
−1.

　　If two variables increase or decrease at very nearly the same rate,
the correlation will be close to +1.00. For example, .92 is a correlation
that is positive (the two variables vary in the same directions). To
illustrate, if a researcher collected blood pressure and central venous

pressure data from a series of patients and calculated the correlation, it would probably be high (in the .70s to .90s) and positively related. However, if data on temperature and pulse rate were collected and a correlation statistic was calculated, there would likely be a positive relationship, but a moderate one (in the .40s to .60s) or a low positive relationship (.30s to the .20s). If the calculations yielded a correlation less than this, it would be difficult to argue that there was a relationship between the two variables.

Negative correlations in the same high, moderate, and low ranges are also possible. For example, Burke (1978) showed moderate negative correlations between family stress levels and the developmental quotients of healthy siblings of handicapped children of $r = -.41$. In other words, where there was higher stress, the siblings' developmental quotients had a moderate tendency to be lower and vice versa. See Figure 10.6 for an illustration of these moderately negative results. Note that this is the computer printout that the researcher sees, but that is seldom included in an article. Negative correlations are indicated by

_____ *Figure 10.6* _____

SCATTERGRAM OF THE NORMAL CHILDREN'S DEVELOPMENTAL QUOTIENTS AND FAMILIAL SYSTEM STRAIN

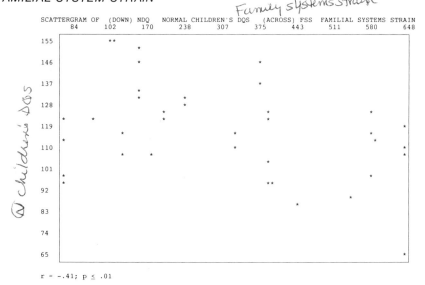

$r = -.41; \ p \leq .01$

_____

Source: Burke, S. O. (1978). *Familial strain and the development of normal and handicapped children in single and two-parent families.* Doctoral dissertation. Toronto: University of Toronto.

the use of a minus sign (−), but positive correlations are usually reported without any sign at all.

A special use of correlational statistics is in the reliability and validity testing of data collection tools. Pearson's *r* is often used to look for relationships between a new tool and another measure of the same variable that is generally agreed to be the "gold standard" (criterion validity testing). Interrater and test-retest checks on the reliability of a measure over time and between two observers can be done with correlational statistics. For these types of reliability and validity check, strong correlations in the order of .75 or greater are usually considered essential. One statistic that measures association, Cronbach's alpha, is used exclusively to measure the internal consistency of a data collection tool. It is used to measure agreement of individual items with the total tool, and results of 0.70 or better are considered necessary to demonstrate good internal consistency of the tool, such as a questionnaire with 10 items to rate on a Likert scale.

Since correlational statistics usually deal with two variables, their use is referred to as bivariate analysis. However, it is possible to examine a third variable at the same time. This is referred to as a partial tau, partial gamma, or partial *r*. Essentially, the researcher is examining the relationship between the two variables while holding the effect of the third variable on the first two variables constant.

In a research report the writer often indicates the statistic used once, and from then on in the article refers to the statistic with a single initial or Greek letter. Common symbols are cross-referenced in the Glossary. Because Pearson's *r* is so widely known, it is possible to see only the *r* with a value and no mention of Pearson.

The correlation alone does not give a clear picture of the nature of the association between the two variables, unless the correlation is high. If the data are interval or strong-ordinal, the correlation can be well illustrated by a scatter diagram. Unfortunately, scatter diagrams or plots are usually included in the report only if the correlations are relatively high, since low correlations will have widely dispersed points and a pattern will be difficult to discern. Figure 10.6 shows the negative, moderate correlation between family stress and normal sibling development mentioned above. A higher correlation would have data points more closely surrounding the imaginary line from the upper left-hand corner to the lower right. A positive correlation, as opposed to the negative correlation in the example, would have data points that were more oriented toward an imaginary line from the upper right to the lower left.

If the variables in the correlation are ordinal and/or have only a few data points each, a table is often used to support the correlational findings.

In nursing, the variables of concern often do not yield high correlations. Moderate correlations with psychosocial variables are considered good. Physiological variables sometimes have high correlations with each other.

• Figure 10.3 and Table 10.2 give a range of appropriate statistics for measuring association among variables of different levels and for various types of research design situations. Figure 10.3 can be used to identify the statistic used in the report and to determine whether the best statistic was used. If the statistic does not seem correct, check the level of the data again because you may have classified it differently from the researcher. Note that the researcher's assessment of the level of the data is rarely explicit, but is merely implied in the choice of statistics used. The most commonly used statistics are in these tables. When you encounter others, you will need to consult a statistics text or an expert to determine what type of statistic it is and for what level of data and design situations it is appropriate.

Patterns of Relationships   Statistical testing for patterns of relationships is conceptually similar to testing for association, as described in the previous section. Usually a researcher is examining three or more variables simultaneously, and these statistical procedures are called multivariate analysis. These procedures can be used for levels 2 through 4 research questions. They require strong-ordinal or interval data and larger sample sizes than those needed for the simpler measures of association.

When the research question seeks patterns within a group of variables, **factor analysis** and the closely related procedures of principal component and cluster analysis are used. Each of these approaches seeks groups of variables that are closely related or that vary with each other. For example, a 60 item questionnaire might have 3 factors. *Factor scores* indicate the degree to which a variable varies with a factor (group of variables that vary together). It is possible to factor by a number of different criteria. For example, **principal component** analysis attempts to find one central factor within the group of variables. Other types of factor analysis attempt to account for as much of the variance within the entire group of variables as possible, and can yield a number of factors. **Cluster analysis** has less stringent rules and can be used where factor analysis is desired but not possible.

When there is one dependent variable in the research question and several independent variables, regression analysis techniques are used. **Regression analysis** yields an *F* score that indicates the degree to which the independent variables, as a group, are related to the dependent variable. To distinguish this **multiple correlation coefficient** from one that only represents relationships between two variables, a capital *R* is used rather than the lower case *r* for the conceptually parallel Pearson's *r*. The R, when squared (R^2), gives a measure of the amount of variance that can be accounted for in the dependent variable by the combination of the independent variables in the analysis. *Weights* are also calculated to account for the individual dependent variable's contribution to the regression. For example, in Burke's (1978) study, a regression was done of a number of family psychosocial factors (independent variables) on the developmental quotients of the child in the family with a handicap. This regression contained nine independent variables, had an $F = 84.3$, and had a high R^2 of .97, which indicated that the combined independent variables accounted for 97% of the variance in the children's developmental quotient. A separate regression was done on the developmental quotients for the nonhandicapped siblings. The regression for handicapped children did not show a significant pattern, but that for the siblings did.

Differences   When the research question or hypothesis focuses on differences, another set of statistics is needed. These are shown in the right-hand column of Table 10.4 and in the branching diagram (Figure 10.3). For nominal data, the chi-square statistic and its closely related statistics for various designs are used. The essence of these tests is the "goodness of fit" of the data, given the total number within each category for each of the two variables tested. A significant test result means that the pattern is not likely to have occurred simply by chance.

For ordinal data, there is a series of related nonparametric statistics that can be used, depending on the particular details of the research design. In general, these statistics rank the data for one group and compare the agreement with the ranks found for the other group or groups. Figure 10.3 explains which statistics are used for each design situation.

For strong-ordinal or interval data, the tests are conceptually related to one another. They test the likelihood that the means of each variable are significantly different from one another. The *F* statistic and the R^2 statistic are interpreted in the same manner as that for the regression analysis described in the section on patterns of relationships.

From a computational standpoint, regression and analysis of variance use the same procedure. See Figure 10.3 for which test is best for certain design situations.

MAKING INFERENCES AND TESTING HYPOTHESES

Statistics can be used only to describe, or they can be used to make inferences about cause and effect and to predict what might happen in the future. With the exception of purely descriptive statistics, such as those in the left columns of Table 10.2, most statistics can be used for hypothesis testing or for making inferences. This is operationalized with the use of *p*-values. Probability values, or *p*-values, which are roughly synonymous with alpha values, express the likelihood of the statistical result occurring by chance. The results are referred to as the **significance level.** It is often confusing to the novice that when it comes to *p*-values, smaller is better. The level of significance of a statistical result is conversely related to the *p*-value. Highly significant results have small *p*-values and nonsignificant results have larger *p*-values. Researchers reserve the word *significant* for this particular use alone.

A logical process is central to the operationalization of the scientific method when a statistical strategy is used to analyze results: First a hypothesis is stated; then the *p*-value at which the statistical result will be believed is stated. Next, the analysis is done, and if the results are as predicted in the hypothesis *and* the *p*-value is the *same or smaller* than the researcher predicted, then the results are "believed." In this context "believed" means that they are accepted to be true or, more precisely, not to be false.

In a research report, the logical process will not be specifically described because it is assumed that the reader is aware of the logical steps. In nursing, the *p*-value is most often set at $p = .05$. This means that there are 5 chances out of 100 that the results seen for the particular statistical test are due to chance, or 19 times out of 20 the same results would have been obtained. *p*-values are sometimes set at $p = .01$, which would mean that the statistical result will not be "believed" unless the chances are less than 1 out of 100 of being as found in the statistical analysis.

For clinical purposes it is important to judge what a reasonable level for the *p*-value would be. If the research findings are being considered for application as nursing interventions in your setting, and they are relatively risk free, then *p*-values of .05 seem reasonable. However, if there could be potential harm to your clients if the findings were not "true," then *p*-values of .01 or .001 (one chance in 1000 that the results are "false") might be considered necessary before implementation of the findings. For example, in a study of a new protocol for the treatment of ammonia-induced diaper rash that does not appear to pose potential harm to the child, a *p*-value of .05 would seem reasonable. However, if the study considers potentially noxious substances or equipment that might be irritating when improperly used, then a *p*-value of .01 might be considered necessary by the practicing nurse, even though the researcher accepted the results at a .05 level.

Note that the words "true," "false," and "believe," have been used within quotes, because it is not actually possible to prove, without a doubt, the answer to any research question. There are a number of factors that can introduce errors into the results, most of which will not be apparent to either the researcher or the research consumer. These factors are implicit in the steps of the research process described in preceding chapters. For example, if the sample is too small for the particular study, the results might show that there is not a significant relationship between two variables, when in fact there is a significant relationship. If the sample is very large, the significance level will be greater, given the same result, than it would be with a smaller sample (*p*-value will be smaller). Researchers call these errors **type I** or alpha errors (accepting something as true when it is false) and **type II** or beta errors (accepting something as false when it is true). There could also be a relationship between two variables that was not found in the study because the best way to measure one of the variables was not used (type II error). Errors can be introduced in any of the steps of the research process.

Research consumers sometimes confuse the notion of significance, as discussed in this section, with the notion of the strength of the relationship or degree of difference between the study variables. These are distinct notions; it is possible to have a very significant, but very modest association between two variables. For example, the link between smoking and lung cancer is significant (small *p*-values), but the association is modest (small to moderate correlations) since not everyone who smokes develops lung cancer. The significance level, or *p*-value, only indicates the likelihood that the small or large relationships, or differences portrayed by the test statistics, are the result of chance. Therefore, they can only have meaning in conjunction with the description of the data for each variable (i.e., means and standard deviations, tables or graphs) and the statistical test result (i.e., the Pearson r or the F and the R^2 of the analysis of variance).

USE OF GRAPHICS

Graphics are used in the analysis and results sections of research reports to present ideas pictorially. Tables, figures, diagrams, and graphs present conclusions or illustrate the analysis process (Schmid, 1983). Graphics that display one idea are usually presenting the answer to one of the research questions or hypotheses. They are used to enhance or clarify the conclusion the researcher has reached through the analysis of the data. Graphics of this type should be succinct, streamlined, and free of extraneous detail. Such graphics are most often found in research articles in journals that focus on clinical practice. They are seldom seen in research-oriented journals or in technical research reports because their simplicity limits the precision needed to answer complex research questions.

Graphics are frequently used to illustrate the strategy used in the analysis or to present the most convincing evidence for the conclusions that the researchers have reached. These graphics are usually tables containing many elements. There may be a single point, but it may not be evident at first glance. Many such tables might have been used by the researcher during the analysis process, but usually only the tables most central to the point of the research are included in the report to substantiate a statistical analysis. When used judiciously, such graphics are an excellent way to demonstrate the researcher's application of the scientific method. Excessive detail, however, tends to cloud the deductive logic used in interpreting such a graphic presentation of data or statistics. Graphics that present evidence for the conclusions reached by the researcher are particularly useful to the research consumer since they make it possible to make interpretations for clinical practice that might not have been made by the researchers.

All graphics—tables, figures, diagrams, graphs—can be evaluated by the same criterion: they should be able to stand alone within the context of the study. In other words, after reading the purpose, research questions, and data collection methods of the research report, the graphic should make sense. It should not be necessary to return to the text to find out what the terms or units of measurement mean. Conversely, the text should stand on its own. The interpretation should be expressed in words and numbers in the text, with the graphic enhancing or illustrating the point.

Schmid suggests the criteria of accuracy, simplicity, clarity, and good design to evaluate the quality of a graphic. It should accurately represent the ideas and data presented elsewhere in the study report. It should be simple enough to be quickly decipherable, and it should have a clear, easy-to-read message that aids in the interpretation of the data. The best graphics are designed so that the shape, balance, proportion, and unity give a visual effect that communicates the intellectual significance of the point being made to the reader. Compare the graphics in Figures 10.5 and 10.6: clearly, 10.5 comes much closer to meeting the criteria for a good quality graphic.

ANALYZING WORDS, IMAGES, AND IDEAS

Non-numerical data are usually in the form of written words; however, they can also be in the form of videotapes, audiotapes, and photographs. Although it travels under many names, the most common method of analysis is called **content analysis.** Field and Morse (1985) mention at least seven different versions of content analysis: thematic (which analyzes themes), semantic (which analyzes the language), static (which depicts events as they occur), phase (which depicts the phenomenon over time), latent (which reviews data within the context of the entire dataset for each subject), and manifest content analysis (which checks for instances of specific words or phrases in the data-sets). Grounded field methods are also very similar except the objective is to develop theory based on the data that are content analysed.

All these related forms of analysis use a series of similar steps which begin at the onset of the data-collection phase. In numerical analysis, the analysis does not begin until all the data have been collected. This is why the qualitative maze is part of the research process for these studies (see Figure 10.1).

Typical steps in the processes are coding for categories and themes and making memos about the context and variations in the phenomenon under study; developing names for categories; and elaborating classification systems and testing them within the data as they are collected. Indeed, the findings at any point in this process will provide some direction for further data collection and the direction that the analysis takes. A matrix might be used to look at relationships between variables.

At some point the quantitatively oriented researcher will start frequency counts and may even code the data so that ordinal or nominal statistics can be used to describe the dataset. The reliability of the coding might be checked by having another person encode the same data and by checking for agreement. More conservative qualitative researchers are not apt to do this.

The non-statistical alternative involves noting patterns and verifying themes, building logical and time-oriented chains of evidence, making contrasts and comparisons. Some researchers validate findings with their subjects and/or other forms of evidence. Current experts agree that those cases or portions of the data which do not fit must also be presented in the report (Miles & Huberman, 1984; Field & Morse, 1985). There is increasing pressure to make the details of the analysis process explicit to the reader.

_____ EVALUATING THE ANALYSIS OF THE DATA _____

The data-analysis portion of a clinical nursing research report should be carefully scrutinized because the appropriateness and correctness of the procedures as well as the way in which findings are presented are the linchpin in the research process. If this is not done well, you will not have a satisfactory answer to the research question. Table 10.6 will guide you in this process. In addition, refer to Tables 10.1 and 10.2, as well as Figures 10.3 and 10.4. As in the other chapters the criteria for critique are divided into scientific and clinical sections. The content of this chapter will allow general conclusions in most cases. However, if a particular study does not fit well within the research strategies discussed here, you might consult an expert or books such as those in the reference section of this chapter. This will be particularly true if the results of the study are under consideration for changes in your nursing practice.

EXERCISES

1. Using the criteria for graphs and diagrams in Table 10.6, evaluate the graphic presentations in Figures 10.5 and 10.6 and Tables 10.3 and 10.5.

2. Using the criteria in Table 10.6, evaluate the Tulman (1986) article in the Appendix.

_____ Table 10.6 _____

✳ *EVALUATION OF DATA-ANALYSIS STRATEGIES*

Scientific Adequacy	*Clinical Applicability*
Does the level of inquiry of the study question fit with the analysis methods used?	Are the data analyzed logically, from the perspective of the clinical reality?
Does the level of measurement of the data fit with the type of statistics used?	
Is the link between the analysis and the findings logical and clear?	
Are there enough data in the form of examples, tables, or graphics to allow for verification of the conclusions reached by the researcher?	

Statistics

Are the statistics used to describe the data the correct and most appropriate ones as indicated in Table 10.2 and Figure 10.3 or 10.4?	Are the statistical methods clear enough so that you could explain changes in nursing practice based on the results?
Is the statistical result presented in clear English as well as in a numerical presentation?	
Is there sufficient substantiating evidence to convince of the correctness of the statistical result?	
If this was a hypothesis testing study, were the p-values interpreted correctly?	

Graphs and Diagrams

Are the graphic displays accurate, simple, and clear?	Are the tables, graphs, and figures clinically relevant?
Do they stand on their own to make a point without the need for narrative?	Could you use them to convince colleagues to change their nursing practice?
Do they enhance the quality of the argument for the conclusion reached by the researcher?	

Narrative

Does the text of the analysis section stand on its own to make the arguments for the conclusions reached by the researcher?	Are there logical links between the analysis procedures and the findings that are clinically relevant?
If qualitative techniques, i.e. content analysis, were used, are the steps in the process explicit?	
Are the atypical subjects discussed?	

3. Determine the level of the data and whether the type of analysis used is appropriate in the two studies abstracted below.

*Communicating over Chronic Illness**

The focus of the study was the children's perceptions of themselves as well as the manner in which they explain themselves to their peers. The dilemmas were the focus of the article. Eight boys, aged 7–13, were studied using qualitative methods. Participant observation was used over a five-year period. The article does not state the duration of the observation with each child. Data were collected in interviews with the child, siblings, teachers, and parents in their homes, schools, and camps.

qual.

Field notes from interviews and observations were sorted according to categories and themes as they were collected. As themes emerged, the data were analyzed for linkages with other categories. Data were placed in categories until they were saturated, that is, until new information revealed only more of the same type of data.

The results were presented in some detail in the article and the following conclusions were drawn. There was a paradox in that at the same time that the children were becoming increasingly independent in the management of their own care, they became less and less able to speak about it to their peers. Smaller peer groups were found to be more accommodating to the special needs of these children. Parents were found to play an advocacy role for these children. The author argues that if we accept the importance of social interactions with peers, then we should support the enabling work of parents in this regard.

Patient Management of Pain Medication†

The purpose of the study was to determine the effects of a personal control intervention on the reported pain, disruption, and emotional upset, amount of pain medication used, and desire for control. Sixty-four subjects were studied post-ICU and at discharge and 58 at 3 weeks post-discharge.

Subjects who consented were randomly assigned to either a self-administered or nurse-administered pain medication group.

quant.
control grp

---

* Oremland, E. K. (1986). Communicating over chronic illness: Dilemmas of affected school-aged children. *Children's Health Care* (14), 218–223.

† King, B. K., Norsen, L. H., Robertson, R. K. & Hicks, G. L. (1987). Patient management of pain medication after cardiac surgery. *Nursing Research* (36), 145–150.

The groups were stratified by sex, number of incisions, and surgeon. Data were collected by questionnaires which had some reported reliability and validity and by chart review for the amount of medication used. Results of the measures for the dependent variables are reported in means and standard deviations and tested for differences between groups with analysis of variance. There were few significant differences between groups. However, the experimental group initially reported higher levels of pain. This finding plus the incidental findings that some patients refused to participate because they wanted the nurses to manage their medication and that 7 patients had to be dropped from the study because they needed stronger medication than could be left at the bedside led researchers to speculate further. They suggest that self-medication may not be the key for patients, but rather the central issue is believing that their pain is being managed in the most effective way possible.

4. What other types of analysis would have been appropriate instead of or as well as those used by these researchers above?

_____ REFERENCES _____

Burke, S. O. (1978). *Familial strain and the development of normal and handicapped children in single and two parent families.* Doctoral dissertation. Toronto: University of Toronto.

Burke, S. O. & Jerrett, M. (in press). Pain management across age groups: Student nurse choices. *Western Journal of Nursing Research.*

Burke, S. O.; Sayers, L. A.; Baumgart, A. J.; & Wray, J. G. (1985). Pitfalls in cross-cultural use of the Denver Developmental Screening Test: Cree Indian children. *Canadian Journal of Public Health, 76,* 303–307.

Burns, N., & Grove, S. K. (1987). *The practice of nursing research: Conduct, critique and utilization.* Philadelphia: W. B. Saunders.

Chinn, P. L. (Ed.) (1986). *Nursing research methodology: Issues and implementation.* Rockville, Md.: Aspen Systems.

Dzurec, L. C., & Abraham, I. L. (1986). Analogy between phenomenology and multivariate statistical analysis. In P. L. Chinn (Ed.), *Nursing research methodology: Issues and implementation* (pp. 55–66). Rockville, Md.: Aspen Systems.

Field, P. A., and Morse, J. M. (1985). *Nursing research: The application of qualitative approaches.* Rockville, Md.: Aspen Systems.

Hutchinson, S. A. (1984). Creating meaning out of horror. *Nursing Outlook, 32,* 86–90.

Hutchinson, S. A. (1986). Creating meaning: A grounded theory of NICU nurses. In C. Chenitz & J. M. Swanson (Eds.), *From practice to grounded theory: Qualitative research in nursing* (pp. 191–204). Menlo Park, Calif.: Addison-Wesley.

Miles, M. B., & Huberman, A. M. (1984). *Qualitative data analysis: A sourcebook of new methods*. Beverly Hills, Calif.: Sage Publications.

Mosteller, F.; Fienberg, S. E.; & Rourke, R. (1983). *Beginning statistics with data analysis*. Reading, Mass.: Addison-Wesley.

Parse, R. R.; Coyne, A. B.; & Smith, M. J. (1985). *Nursing research: Qualitative methods*. Bowie, Md.: Brady Communications.

Schmid, C. F. (1983). *Statistical graphics: Design principles and practices*. New York: John Wiley.

Weekes, D. P. (1986). Theory-free observation: Fact or fantasy? In P. L. Chinn (Ed.), *Nursing research methodology: Issues and implementation* (pp. 11–21). Rockville, Md.: Aspen Systems.

Wilson, H. S. (1985). *Research in nursing*. Menlo Park, Calif.: Addison-Wesley.

11

Computers: Uses for Researchers and Consumers

INTRODUCTION

This chapter describes how the computer can assist the researcher and consumer of research at every step of the research process. We explore in some detail the contribution made by the computer to the functions of literature search, report and proposal writing, and data analysis. The chapter describes the computer working environment of one researcher and the many uses for computers in the conduct and application of nursing research. The uses of the computer are illustrated for each step of the research process, from identification of the problem to the dissemination of the results, from one of the author's studies. Lastly, we detail some problems of the use of computers in nursing research and ways for the research consumer to locate some problems that could affect the application of the results.

OUTLINE

OBJECTIVES

After reading this chapter, you will be able to

1. Identify the multiple uses of the computer for researchers and for consumers of nursing research.
2. Assess the general appropriateness and effectiveness of the use (or lack of use) of computer in a study.
3. Identify some of the advantages and difficulties in interpreting computer-generated statistical analysis.
4. Be more experienced in using a computer than you were before.

NEW TERMS

File

Disks

Mainframe

On-line

Dumb terminal

Word processor

Program packages

User friendly

Input

Run

Output

Hardware

Software

Keyed in

Cleaning the data

A RESEARCHER AT WORK WITH ─────────── *THE COMPUTER*

This is the computer age and practicing nurses and researchers, like everyone, vary extremely in how much they know about computers, how much they use them, and how skilled they are in using this tool. A new vocabulary is needed to discuss these issues, so as each new term is introduced it will be highlighted. Brief definitions will be given as we go along, but if "computerese" is new to you, reading the definitions in the Glossary at the back of the book whenever a new term occurs will increase your computer literacy.

The computers that one of the authors, Sharon Burke, uses in her research are shown in Figure 11.1. In her home office she uses a *microcomputer,* a small desktop computer. As each word is typed, she can see it on her *monitor,* which looks something like a TV screen. The typed words are saved on a **file** (analogous to an ordinary fileholder), which is stored on one of her **disks** (a cross between a video tape and a phonograph record). Most of you will be able to picture this in your mind, but for those who have had no experience with computers, it would be helpful to complete the first exercise at the end of this chapter before reading the next sections.

Sharon's microcomputer is *compatible* (that is, it is able to communicate) with the **mainframe,** a very large computer, at the university. She could use her telephone to send and receive files between her microcomputer and the mainframe, but instead she carries her disk to her office in the School of Nursing and inserts it into the **on-line** (connected and ready to communicate) microcomputer there. The dotted lines on Figure 11.1 indicate that the disk is moved from one place to another, and the solid lines indicate that the information is moved directly via cables between the computer's hardware and software. The school's on-line microcomputer can do anything her small computer can do. For bigger and more complicated jobs Sharon uses the mainframe. She might use a **dumb terminal** (it's not a computer; therefore, it's not smart) which also communicates with the mainframe. She can communicate with any other user of the university's computing system via any terminal or computer that is on-line with the mainframe. For example, she could send data to her statistical consultant, communicate with the library to check the computerized catalogue for a book, or check with financial services to see if she really is out of money on a particular research grant, and so on. She also uses *networks* that have been established between most institutions' mainframes in the western world to exchange data or messages with fellow researchers who are

Figure 11.1

SHARON BURKE'S COMPUTER ENVIRONMENT

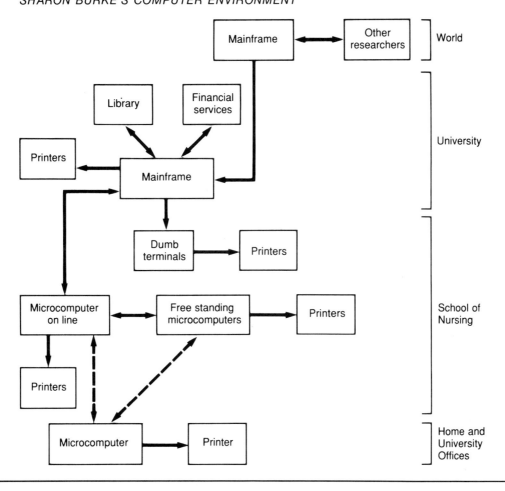

users of their own mainframes. When she wants a printed copy of her work, she can use her printer at her home office, a better one at the school, or the faster and fancier printers in the computing center.

THE COMPUTER AS A RESEARCH TOOL

A *computer,* defined here for research purposes, is a tool that records, stores, rearranges, and rapidly sorts through pieces of information. This information is usually numbers or words. Computers perform mathematical operations such as addition or division, so that any formula that can be applied to numbers can be done quickly and accurately by the computer.

The researcher uses this tool whenever the tasks in the research process are lengthy or complex enough to merit the extra work it takes to put the words or numbers into the computer and to write or use prepackaged *programs* (sets of detailed instructions that tell the computer what to do with the words or numbers) for the specific research task. For example, the computer would be used when there were large numbers of subjects and variables in the study; when the analysis would take a long time to calculate, as in a factor analysis; or when many revisions or changes would be required, as in the construction of a new questionnaire. Data analysis is only one way that researchers use computers.

The computer is a helpful tool at many stages of the research process as can be seen from the highlighted areas of Figure 11.2. The functions most helpful to the researcher can be roughly grouped into the functions of literature searching, word processing, and data analysis (Schultz & Abraham, 1986). All of these functions can be useful to you as a research consumer as well.

Computer-Assisted Literature Review

In the initial identification or clarification of a research or clinical problem, computer-assisted literature searches help to direct the researcher toward appropriate reading on the topic. How this is actually done by you as a research consumer or as a member of a research team is detailed in Chapter 5 on literature review.

A computer literature search is very useful for the nurse who wishes to use a study's results. It provides a thorough and systematic base when attempting to validate and compare the findings of a piece of research that is being considered for application into your practice. This is explained in detail in Chapter 5.

Word Processing—Writing

A **word processor** is a group of computer programs to enter, rearrange, search for, change, and print words. There are many such programs, including WordStar and WordPerfect. *Integrated* programs (groups of programs that blend data base, spreadsheet, and other functions) such as Lotus 1-2-3 and Enable often have a word processor function.

Figure 11.2

RESEARCH PROCESS FLOWCHART

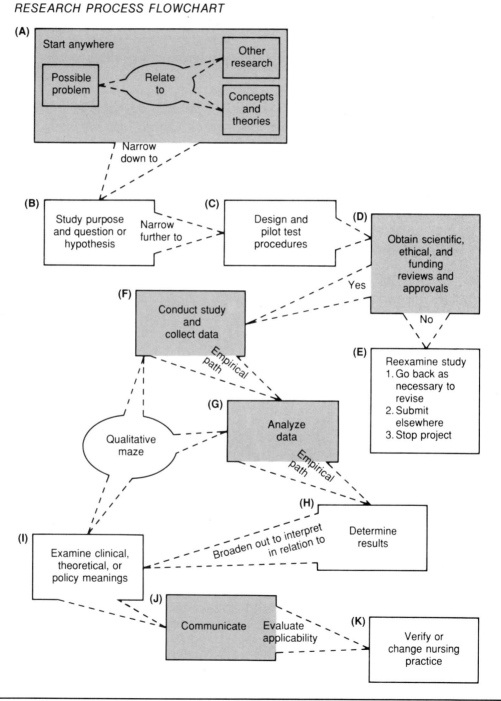

Word processing is used extensively at many steps in the research process. For example, after the decisions have been made on the best feasible design, and after it has been pilot-tested if necessary, the researcher will seek the necessary scientific, ethical, and funding approvals. Word processing is ideally suited to produce such documents (see the cell G of Figure 11.2). For example, each institution or committee will have its own ideas on how long the proposal should be, how it should be arranged, and what should be included. Word processing capabilities will facilitate typing the proposal to meet the needs of different committees. Using the facilities of a word processor, the research team can quickly revise one version of the proposal to meet the needs of the next committee. For example, sections not of interest to a second agency can be excluded, while sections of particular concern can be expanded. The university ethics review committee, for example, would require a great deal of detail on how the subjects' confidentiality would be protected, but little or no detail on financial aspects would be required. In a funding proposal the converse is true. The committees will vary in their familiarity with the topic so you can use word processing to change terms throughout the proposal to suit the committee. For example, a committee of professionals who deal with children will know what the abbreviation DDST means. However, for an ethics review committee, which includes lay persons, a single command to the word processing program will change all instances of "DDST" to read "Denver Developmental Screening Test." The command would be just a few words long and would make the change throughout the entire proposal no matter how long the proposal was.

Often a proposal is sent back to the researcher for revision or is rejected outright. In both cases, there are usually specific criticisms and suggestions attached. The research team might decide to reapply to this or another committee, and the recommended changes can easily be incorporated by using the computer's word processing capabilities.

When a research team communicates the conclusions of a study, many reports to agencies, conferences, and committees will be required. In addition there will probably be scientific, clinical, or lay articles to be written about the study, and a book may follow. The word processor is invaluable in the preparation of these documents: major sections can be pulled together, revised, and fitted into the new context for each article or report. The word processor is also used to check the spelling of each word in the file against those listed in a dictionary in another file. Depending on the word processing package, it can also be used to make the format of the printed page appear in the best form for the intended reader.

_____ *Figure 11.3* _____

A COMPUTER-GENERATED POSTER

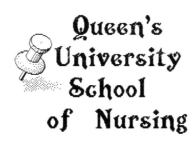

As a research consumer, word processing can be very useful in communicating research findings to your colleagues. For example, you might produce research-based newsletters, handouts for meetings, or proposals to administrators on research-based changes to practice. See the poster we composed and printed on a microcomputer (Figure 11.3), using its graphic and word processing capabilities.

To learn more about word processing, try courses, self-teaching programs, videos, books, and computer-users groups. There should be some in your community.

Word Processing—Qualitative Data Analysis

The researcher might use the word processor to analyze data. For example, the word processor can aid in the content analysis of documents such as nurses' notes or recordings of interviews with subjects. After the words are entered into a computer file, the word processor can speed up the work of searching for particular words. For example, the verbal responses to some open-ended questions were recorded verbatim by interviewers in a study of nurses and native mothers (Burke, Maloney, & Baumgart, 1986). These statements were later entered onto a computer file by a research assistant. To analyse this data Burke scanned it quickly on the monitor. As key words began to emerge, she instructed the computer to move directly to the next instance of those words. She marked each place in the text where the same words or phrases appeared, and printed out copies of them almost instantly into a special new file. She then examined the meanings in context, without the distractions of the data from the mothers who did not refer to the same ideas. This qualitative data can be inserted as quotes in the final study reports with no retyping necessary. If appropriate, the number of times a word or phrase appears can be quickly counted. Specialized programs and some data base programs are often used for qualitative data. Some examples of the specialized programs are Ethnograph and Nota Bene; examples of the data base programs are dBase III and Framework (Anderson, 1987).

Outlining and Brainstorming

Outlining and brainstorming programs allow the user to input ideas rapidly in the form of lists of words and phrases. The program allows quick and easy rearrangement of the ideas into a hierarchical outline. For example, while writing the chapter on literature review, the ideas were typed in no special order as they occurred to the author. Then, using a program called Think Tank (Kamin, 1986) the ideas were rearranged to yield an outline. The outline was then used with a word processor to develop the paragraphs and sections as they appear in this text. The table of contents for this book was developed in the same way. Larger word processors, like WordPerfect, have smaller versions of an outliner built in.

A few researchers and practicing nurses are using such computer programs as an aid in developing and organizing ideas. For example, research report literature reviews and proposals seem less overwhelming when broken down into small sections. We suggest you learn word processing first, and then add the outlining skill.

Data Bases and Statistical Packages

In a research project computers are of prime importance in the numerical data analysis. This is often done with the aid of a microcomputer or a mainframe and statistical programs such as SPSS (Statistical Program for the Social Sciences), SAS (Statistical Analysis System), or BMDP (Biomedical Computer Programs Statistical Package) (Clochesy, 1987). Tables, simple graphs, and percentages often can be generated by microcomputer programs. These **program packages** contain the formulas for the statistics that were discussed in Chapter 10, as well as the instructions to the computer so that the researcher can cause a vast array of statistics to be performed on any of the variables in the study.

Even though these packages are set up to be **user friendly** (usable by someone without a high level of computer programming ability), they do require some skill and knowledge to apply and interpret. Often one member of the research team, or a consultant, is assigned to use these packages for the project. The more complex the type of analysis (for example, a factor analysis is very complicated compared to the calculations required for determining the mean value of a variable), the more variations are possible in the formula. Hence, it is not unusual for the researcher to specify in an article which statistical package or which version of the formula was used.

There are other applications for these statistical packages. For example, they can generate a list of random numbers to use in the selection of subjects, or they can do the calculations for a power analysis that is used in the design phase of the project to help determine the best size of the sample. These packages contain nearly all the statistics needed for most studies, but some may be missing, and programs can be written to apply these formulas to the variables.

As a research consumer, it is important that you have a conceptual understanding of computerized data analysis. However, the skill to use such statistical packages is not necessary to understand the results they generate.

AN EXAMPLE OF COMPUTER APPLICATIONS TO THE RESEARCH PROCESS

By following the research process in Figure 11.2, you will see how computers are used in each phase of one of Sharon Burke's studies. The example used here is but one aspect of a larger study done with the purpose of evaluating the effectiveness of a teaching module on nursing people in pain (Laschinger, Burke & Jerrett, 1986).

Problem and Purpose

In this study the general problem area was predetermined by Laschinger and Jerrett, who had developed the teaching module.

Therefore, we used a computer-assisted literature search to locate other studies that evaluated the learning effectiveness of this type of module. The conceptual framework that emerged from this review was one of mastery within the cognitive, affective, and psychomotor domains. Thus, we had completed the activities in cell A of Figure 11.2. This process indirectly aided us to further narrow the purpose of the study to specify several specific research questions, as is shown in cell B.

Study Design, Pilot Testing, and Procedures

To complete the next step of the research process (cell C of Figure 11.2), the computer-assisted literature review helped us in selecting the best possible design within our setting by identifying study designs successfully used by others. Our critique of these studies alerted us to design flaws that were particularly limiting as well as designs that produced more believable results. Thus, we selected a randomly assigned, two group (module/traditional teaching), quasi-experimental pretest-posttest design. The computer-assisted literature review also located two questionnaires with some demonstrated reliability and validity. We used these to measure changes in attitudes toward people in pain (Davitz & Davitz, 1981) and changes in preference for a specific learning method (Huckabay, 1981).

Additional questionnaires and instruments were developed, and word processing was used to simplify the task of making the many changes required for each new version. In further testing one of these new instruments—the Nursing Process for the Assessment of Pain (NPAP)—a small interrater reliability study was done. Since the number of subjects for this pilot study was small and the calculations were straightforward, the analysis was done with a calculator.

Reviews and Approvals

Funding had already been obtained to develop the module and to evaluate its effectiveness. We were able to hire a student research assistant through a summer student employment grant. The next step (Figure 11.2, cell D) was to have the proposal reviewed by the School of Nursing's Ethics Review committee. This required detailed information on the problem, design, and analysis; the risks and benefits to the subjects; the consent form, and all data collection instruments. Since previous work on most of these sections had been done on a word processor, it was a matter of expanding, elaborating, and linking sections together for the ethics review committee's version of the proposal. This committee approved the study on the condition that a few changes were made in the consent form: it took a matter of minutes to produce a corrected version with the word processor.

Another, briefer version was produced for all faculty members whose students would be subjects. In this version, there was much more emphasis on how long it would take to complete the questionnaires, the effects on student learning, and the like. Conversely, there was relatively less content on the rationale for the design, analysis procedures, and so on. Again, this version was very easily pulled together with the aid of a word processor.

Conduct of the Study and Data Collection

We considered using special sense-marked sheets that are read into the computer with a device called an optical scanner, but we rejected this idea because students associate this type of answer sheet with exams and we wanted to avoid the possibility of negative connotations influencing the results. Thus, the computer was not used in this phase (cell F, Figure 11.2) of this particular study.

Data Analysis

The cell G, representing data analysis, in Figure 11.2 is expanded and elaborated for computerized data analysis in Figure 11.4. There are three phases in computerized data analysis—the input, running the program, and the output. Both input and output refer to the product, the process, and the equipment used to put data or programs into (**input**) the part of the computer that performs the analysis (**run**) or that comes out (**output**) at end of the run. In this context these words are used as nouns, verbs, and participles.

The boxes down the center of Figure 11.4 contain **hardware** (equipment) and **software** (programs, manuals, etc.). The right-hand column contains computer files that the researcher creates or uses. These files are technically software, but it is easier to understand the process if we separate this out for now.

Data File Creation   In this study, after all the questionnaires were completed by the subjects, we were ready to input the data into a data file. Only three questions in the study are used here to develop

Figure 11.4

COMPUTERIZED DATA ANALYSIS: PHASES, CONTENT OF RESEARCHER'S FILES,
AND EXAMPLES OF HARDWARE AND SOFTWARE

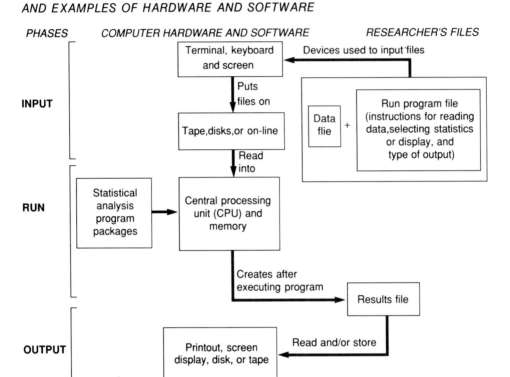

a code book. This code book tells exactly how the data on the questionnaire were arranged in the data file. The study questions and range
of possible answers are seen in Table 11.1. The variables in this example are

— KIDCARE: previous experience with children in pain
— MASTERED: how well they felt they mastered the pain
  content
— RESINTER: the type of interventions used to maximize
  resilience to pain in children

The short variable labels listed above and in the code book were
created as codes representing the questions the students answered. The
questions are typed in full under the second column in Table 11.1. In
order to check the accuracy of data files it is also important to know

_____ Table 11.1 _____

CODE BOOK FOR PAIN DATA FILE

Variable Label	Data Collection Question	Possible Values	Data file Location (columns)
KIDCARE	Have you cared for a child or been involved with a child in your family or a friend's child who was in pain?	0 = no 1 = yes	57
MASTERED	To what extent do you feel you have mastered the subject matter on pain taught in the given manner?	1 = very low ⋮ 9 = very high	68
RESINTER	If you assume that encouraging this resilience to pain is good, what could a nurse do to foster resilience to pain?	1 = Praise alone or with distraction 2 = Distraction only	80

what values the variable can have so that if there were, say, an "8" in the data file for KIDCARE, the researcher would know this was an error since only "0" and "1" are possible values. The last column in this code book indicates the location of the values in the data file for each student's answer to each of the questions or variables.

In Table 11.2, the numbers show the data input into the data file (there were other variables between and after these as well). The abbreviation ID refers to the subject number, so there is one line for each subject, and there are specific columns for each variable. There are several other ways to organize data input files, but the principle of a specific, consistent structure is the same. This is only a portion of the subjects, enough on which to run some simple statistics.

Next, using a terminal with a keyboard and a screen, a student research assistant **keyed in** (typed) the data to the data file according to the exact locations in the code book. Each data file has a name: this one is PAIN.DATA. The completed data file was then stored on a small portion of a large disk in the computing center until we needed it. There

_____ Table 11.2 _____

SAMPLE DATA FILE AS OUTPUT USING A STATISTICAL PACKAGE

ID	KIDCARE	MASTERED	RESINTER
1	0	3	2
2	1	7	1
3	1	3	1
4	1	6	1
5	0	1	2
6	1	7	2
7	0	1	2
8	1	6	1
9	0	5	1
10	1	4	2
11	0	4	2
12	0	2	2
13	0	6	2
14	0	5	2
15	1	2	2
16	0	6	2
17	1	3	2
18	1	8	2
19	1	6	2
20	1	5	2
21	0	7	1
22	1	9	2
23	1	2	2
24	0	5	2
25	0	8	2
26	1	5	2
27	0	1	2
28	1	7	1
29	0	5	2
30	1	6	2
31	1	6	2
32	0	3	2
33	1	7	2
34	1	4	2
35	1	6	2
36	1	4	2
37	1	3	2
38	0	6	2

_____ *Figure 11.5* _____

SAMPLE RUN FILE

DATA;   ⎫ Tells computer
    CMS FILEDEF Y DISK PAINEX DATA A;   ⎬ where data is
    INFILE Y;   ⎭ located

    INPUT KIDCARE 57 MASTERED 68 RESINTER 80; ⎫ Tells the computer
                                               ⎬ which variables
                                               ⎭ to use

PROC MEANS;   ⎫ Tells the computer
PROC CORR;   ⎪ four different
    VAR MASTERED KIDCARE;   ⎬ procedures to run
PROC FREQ;   ⎪ on these data
    TABLE RESINTER * KIDCARE/CHISQ NOROW NOPERCENT; ⎭

_____

are many other ways to input data; key punching cards (one card for each student) is still in use in some locations. Next, the researcher must check the data file to make sure it is accurate. This is called **cleaning the data.**

Run File Creation The next file the researcher wrote was the run file. Basically, we needed to tell the computer (1) which data file to read, (2) where the variables were located in this file, and (3) what statistics or arrangements of the variables were to be done. See Figure 11.5. In this study, we used the SAS statistical package. Other statistical packages such as SPSS are structured in a similar manner although the terms used will be somewhat different. The name given to the program run file was PAIN.SAS. Special training is required to learn to write these programs, but you can still read them if you stretch your imagination.

The first three lines of the run file, PAIN.SAS (Figure 11.5), instruct the computer to get the data file named PAIN.SAS (Table 11.2). The next line tells it the names and locations in the data file of the variables needed for this run. The next lines select specific procedures from the SAS package of procedure programs to be run on these variables.

The Results Files The output can be seen in Figure 11.6. PROC MEANS generated the output seen at the top of Figure 11.6. PROC CORR requires more information, so we instructed the computer to run a correlation matrix on the variables MASTERED and KIDCARE.

Figure 11.6

SAMPLE RESULTS FILE

```
----------------------------------------------------------------------------------------------------
VARIABLE   N    MEAN      STANDARD     MINIMUM     MAXIMUM    STD ERROR       SUM       VARIANCE   C.V.
                          DEVIATION     VALUE       VALUE     OF MEAN

KIDCARE    38  0.57894737  0.50035549  0.00000000  1.00000000  0.08116838   22.00000000  0.25035562  86.425
MASTERED   38  4.84210526  2.08633023  1.00000000  9.00000000  0.33844745  184.00000000  4.35277383  43.087
RESINTER   38  1.81578947  0.39285945  1.00000000  2.00000000  0.06373022   69.00000000  0.15433855  21.636
----------------------------------------------------------------------------------------------------
                                              PROC CORR
----------------------------------------------------------------------------------------------------
VARIABLE   N    MEAN      STD DEV        SUM       MINIMUM      MAXIMUM
MASTERED   38  4.84210526  2.08633023  184.00000000  1.00000000   9.00000000
KIDCARE    38  0.57894737  0.50035549   22.00000000        0      1.00000000

        CORRELATION COEFFICIENTS / PROB > !R! UNDER HO:RHO=0 /  N = 38

                        MASTERED KIDCARE

            MASTERED 1.00000   0.24528
                     0.0000    0.1377

            KIDCARE  0.24528   1.00000
                     0.1377    0.0000
----------------------------------------------------------------------------------------------------
                                            PROC FREQ; TABLE
----------------------------------------------------------------------------------------------------
                TABLE OF RESINTER BY KIDATE
                RESINTER     KIDCARE
                FREQUENCY!      !      !
                COL PCT !   0 !   1 ! TOTAL
                --------!------!------!
                   1 !    2 !    5 !   7
                      ! 12.50 ! 22.73 !
                --------!------!------!
                   2 !   14 !   17 !  31
                      ! 87.50 ! 77.27 !
                --------!------!------!
                TOTAL   !   16 !   22 !  38
                STATISTICS FOR 2-WAY TABLES
WARNING:  OVER 20% OF THE CELLS HAVE EXPECTED COUNTS LESS THAN 5.
          TABLE IS SO SPARSE THAT CHI-SQUARE MAY NOT BE A VALID TEST.
    CHI-SQUARE                    0.645    DF=  1    PROB=0.4220
    PHI                          -0.130
    CONTINGENCY COEFFICIENT       0.129
    CRAMER'S V                    0.130
    LIKELIHOOD RATIO CHISQUARE    0.668    DF=  1    PROB=0.4138
    CONTINUITY ADJ. CHI-SQUARE    0.144    DF=  1    PROB=0.7046
    FISHER'S EXACT TEST (1-TAIL)                    PROB=0.3585
                    (2-TAIL)                        PROB=0.6754
```

The output is in the center of the example. This is a good example of computer output that includes more than what is needed by the researcher. The N, MEAN, and so on, at the top of the figure are redundant since we already have this information in the output for PROC MEANS above. Furthermore, the program ran correlations with every possible combination of the two variables (including each one with itself) because the directions were not specific enough. Often it is initially simpler, and not much more expensive, to get more information on a run. However, it is time consuming and complex to sort through superfluous printouts later. The larger box was drawn in to show the only two statistics we actually needed. The smaller box gives the sample size. This is read by the researcher as $r = .24528$, $p = .137$, $n = 38$, and it could appear in a report as a statement such as, "There was no significant relationship between the degree to which students felt they mastered the content on pain and the presence or absence of previous experience with children in pain ($r = .25$, $p = .14$, $n = 38$)." However, in practice the degree of an association and figures are not usually given for nonsignificant correlations.

The next line of the run file, PROC FREQ, generated a table of the type of interventions selected by the presence or absence of previous experience with children in pain. See bottom of Figure 11.6. It further asks for the chi-square (χ^2) statistic. Next, we begin to customize the output by asking the computer to print only the percent of the column total for the frequency in each cell. We could have dressed up the output further by telling the computer to add labels for the values so we would not have to use the code book to look up the value of "1" under RESINTER, which should be labeled "Praise, with or without distraction," and "2," which should be labeled "Distraction only."

In general, the easier the output is to read and understand the more detailed is the run program. Statistical packages are set up to give a selection of what most researchers want. To have more or less on our output we have to specify this in the run program. The next phases of the research process require the researcher to interpret the findings.

Communicating the Results

The process of communicating the results of the overall study used word processing software to produce the following list of documents, each of a different length and different focus. We prepared

— A summary of findings for student subjects

— A summary of findings for faculty

— Several papers that were presented at four nursing research conferences, such as the Society for Research in Nursing Education

— Manuscripts for nursing journals

(Laschinger, Burke & Jerrett, 1986; and Burke, Laschinger & Jerrett, 1986).

PROBLEMS AND LIMITATIONS IN IN COMPUTER USE

There are many realistic concerns among nurse researchers and consumers about the appropriateness, accuracy, and security of computer applications within the nursing research process. Errors emerge at each phase of computer use: during input, running, and output; and they can be further classified as human and/or computer errors. The human errors are much more frequent and fortunately easier to detect by the reader of the research report. These are summarized in Table 11.3 along with methods used by researchers to reduce errors.

Table 11.3

AVOIDING AND CHECKING FOR COMPUTER ERRORS

Phase	Errors		Checking Procedures	
	Computer	Human	Standard	Checking
INPUT	Defective software, i.e., disks, cards	Data entry mistakes Using wrong data set	Make printed and back-up machine copies of important data. Machine verify all data entry.	Clean data before use by checking range, means, no's etc. Verify that correct data is used for each run.
RUN	Program errors Machine errors	Selecting wrong program Poor programming Underuse or overuse of procedures	Use established programs and machines. Make back-up printed and machine copies of important programs.	Use colleague or consultant advice, review, and critique. Check for logic and theory of the study.
OUTPUT	Software effects Hardware errors	Misinterpretation of output Underuse of results, exclusive reliance on stats only or tables only Overuse of highly technical output	Make printed copy of output and attach it to program.	Have potential reader or user of report check. Check for clarity and logic.

The security of the computer-stored data and research reports is of concern for scientific as well as human rights reasons. Plant (1983) lists the major results of security breaches.

— Unauthorized access to data, which may result in change to the data or even its loss
— Inaccurate, incomplete, or irrelevant stored data
— Use of data for purposes other than that for which informed consent of subjects allows

Even without being directly involved in the computerized aspects of a study, it is possible to make some judgments about strengths or weaknesses the computer has added to the study. In general, all computer uses (1) must fit within the purpose and methods of the study, (2) should be carried out in a way to maximize the potential of the computer for the study, and (3) must have provisions to protect human rights.

_____ *SUMMARY* _____

Chapter 11 provides an overview of the multiple uses of the computer in the nursing research process. It explains the appropriate and effective use of the computer at each stage of a research project. Brief definitions of computer terminology are given as they appear in the text. The three main functions of the computer in assisting the research process—literature searching, word processing, and data analysis—are described in some detail. In addition, the problems and limitations involved in computer applications, such as security of confidential information and threats to accuracy due to either human or computer error, are also described.

EXERCISES ▬▬▬▬▬▬▬▬▬▬▬▬▬▬▬▬▬▬▬▬▬▬▬▬

The following exercises are intended to increase your knowledge of computers and your ability to assess the uses of computers in nursing research. Depending on your experience with computers you may want to skip some of the activities.

1. If you have had no experience with computers, locate a computer and someone who can spend a bit of time showing it to you. Show them Figure 11.1 and determine where this particular computer

would fit into the diagram. Ask the person to explain any of the new terms in the chapter that you did not understand after checking the Glossary.

2. Locate the library nearest you that does computerized literature searches. Find out which data bases they can search. Optionally, use a computer-assisted search for your next assignment that requires a review of the literature.

3. Identify the one human rights problem and one reliability problem inherent in the study abstract below. Optionally, locate the full article and see if these problems were handled in a satisfactory manner.

> A computerized data base of all registered children (Health Surveillance Registry in British Columbia) was used to estimate the prevalence of "severe handicap" among children 0–19 years of age.* Based on WHO International Classification of Disease Codes (9th Revision), the entire caseload of 46,530 living children, as of December 31, 1979, was analyzed. Over all, 8,290 children (10.1 per 1,000 children 0–19 years of age) residing in a specific school district in British Columbia were registered as having a "severe handicap"; variation in prevalence across the 75 school districts of the Province was considerable: range 4.8 to 21.3 per 1,000. Verification of the completeness of ascertainment is reported and underreporting was found to be 17%; 95% confidence interval 15%–19%. Adjustment of prevalence for underreporting provided a revised estimate of registered "severe handicap" between 12.5 and 13.1 per 1,000; mean 12.8/1,000. Data from this study are compared to other published data and the value and limitations of Registry data for planning services to this population of children are discussed.

4. Identify one problem and one advantage in the researcher's use of the statistical analysis as seen in Figure 11.6.

REFERENCES

Anderson, N. L. R. (1987a). Computer use and nursing research: Computer applications for qualitative analysis. *Western Journal of Nursing Research, 9,* 408–411.

---

* Sheps, S. (1985). The use of a registry to estimate prevalence of "severe handicap" among children in British Columbia. *Canadian Journal of Public Health, 76,* 326–332.

———— (1987b). Computer use and nursing research: Computer-assisted analysis of textual fieldnote data. *Western Journal of Nursing Research, 9,* 626–630.

Burke, S. O.; Laschinger, S.; & Jerrett, M. J. (1986). Independent learning modules: Are they effective in the long run? *Nurse Educator, 11,* 10, 18.

Burke, S. O.; Maloney, R.; & Baumgart, A. J. (1986). *Two perspectives of disabled children: Cree Indian mothers and their nurses.* Paper presented at Washington, D.C.

Clochesy, S. M. (1987). Computer use and nursing research: Statistical packages for microcomputers. *Western Journal of Nursing Research, 9,* 138–141.

Davitz, L. J., & Davitz, J. R. (1981). *Inferences of patient's pain and psychological distress.* New York: Springer Verlag.

Encyclopedia of information systems and services. (1978). Detroit: Gale Research.

Huckabay, L. (1981). The effects of modularized instruction and traditional teaching techniques on cognitive learning and affective behaviors of student nurses. *Advances in Nursing Science, 3,* 67–83.

Kamin, J. (1986). *Mastering Think Tank on the IBM PC.* Berkeley, Calif.: Sybex.

Laschinger, S.; Burke, S. O.; & Jerrett, M. (1986) Teaching styles: Is the modular method more effective? *Nursing Papers, 18,* 15–25.

Plant, J. A. (1983). Is nursing confidential? In M. Scholes, Y. Bryant, & B. Baker (Eds.), *The impact of computers on nursing* (pp. 74–81). Amsterdam: North-Holland.

Schultz, S. & Abraham, I. L. (1986). Computer use and nursing research: Interfacing microcomputers and nursing research—II. Dissemination of research findings and project management. *Western Journal of Nursing Research. 8,* 473–477.

Sheps, S. (1985). The use of a registry to estimate prevalence of "severe handicap" among children in British Columbia. *Canadian Journal of Public Health, 76,* 326–332.

Waltz, C. F., & Bausell, R. B. (1981). *Nursing research: Design, statistics and computer analysis.* Philadelphia: F. A. Davis.

12
Evaluating the Researcher's Conclusions

Interpretation of research findings involves a great deal more thought than simply reading the results of data analysis. While it occurs toward the end of the research process, the researcher should explain the meaning of the results in relation to the initial research problem, the theoretical underpinnings, and each aspect of the research design. In addition, results of nursing research should be discussed in relation to the broader significance or lack thereof for nursing practice. In this chapter we will review the most important factors to be considered by the research consumer in evaluating the researcher's conclusions and interpretation of findings, and discuss how these factors affect application to practice.

OUTLINE

Generalizability of Findings

Evaluating the Researcher's
   Interpretation of Findings

OBJECTIVES

After reading this chapter, you will be able to

1. Appreciate the complexity involved in generalizing findings beyond the study.
2. Discuss how nurse researchers interpret results and discuss the findings of the study.
3. Critique the researcher's presentation of conclusions in a published report.
4. Evaluate the findings of a research study for possible application into practice.

NEW TERMS

Overgeneralization

Meta-analysis

GENERALIZABILITY OF FINDINGS

Central to evaluating the researchers' conclusions is the concept of generalizability. Throughout this text we have discussed the role of research in creating nursing practice changes. In order for this to happen, the results of research must have valid meaning to practice settings, client subjects, and practitioners beyond those investigated in a single nursing research study. Particularly when discussing quantitative studies, researchers speak about the generalizability or external validity of research findings to other settings and subjects. We have already introduced the concept of external validity in Chapter 6 and outlined the factors surrounding the research design that contribute to generalizability of results. Table 12.1 summarizes key generalizability factors that relate to the four levels of inquiry of research studies outlined in Chapter 6.

Recall that making consumer decisions about generalizability is primarily a deductive process. The factors involved in external validity are systematically weighed for a particular clinical setting. The factors in Table 12.1 are all necessary to some degree for the external validity of study findings. However, the relative importance of each factor will depend on the setting and the nature of the clinical applications under consideration by the consumer.

When interpreting the findings of a particular study, the nurse researcher should consider the meaning of results obtained from data analysis in light of the possible risks to validity that may have been introduced at various stages of the research process. For example, research problems investigated at the lower levels of inquiry are by nature designed to generate large amounts of data to build knowledge, rather than test causal relationships. The findings of such studies require an interpretation for use in practice that reflects this underlying purpose. Researchers and consumers should be constantly aware of these validity factors when attributing meaning to results. **Overgeneralization** involves the practice of making statements or recommendations beyond the applicability of the reported findings. Implication of cause and effect from such overgeneralizations could have serious clinical consequences.

Determining generalizability of findings is often difficult for both the researcher and the research consumer for several reasons. First, no one piece of research is perfect in all respects. In determining the external validity of findings, the researcher and consumer will often have to examine the significance of each source of bias in light of how the researcher has used the overall process to study the problem, as well

_____ Table 12.1 _____

GENERALIZABILITY OR EXTERNAL VALIDITY OF FINDINGS AND
LEVELS OF INQUIRY

External Validity Factors for Research Findings	Applicability to Levels of Inquiry and Research Design
Directly related to a clearly stated research *question and purpose* for the study	*Levels 1 through 4* Qualitative, quantitative, nonexperimental, quasi-experimental, and experimental designs
Derived from a *well-designed study* to test hypothesized relationships between variables that are based upon a *sound theoretical or conceptual framework*	*Levels 3 and 4* Quasi-experimental and experimental designs
Represents *new knowledge or theory* from which hypotheses may result	*Levels 1 through 4* Particularly Levels 1 and 2, which aim to describe phenomena or develop theory through use of qualitative and nonexperimental quantitative designs
Result from an *internally valid research design,* which emphasizes control over extraneous variables that may affect results. Internal validity risks include · *Sampling errors:* conceptually inappropriate sampling, inadequate sample size, lack of randomization *Data collection methods:* lack of reliability and validity *Design:* lack of control for such effects as history, maturation, testing, Hawthorne effect, other researcher and environmental effects in the setting *Data analysis:* inappropriate analysis strategies or inappropriate measurements and statistics	*Levels 1 and 2* Qualitative and nonexperimental quantitative studies may have low internal validity in terms of control *Level 3* may have some internal validity in terms of control *Level 4's* experimental designs have the strongest internal validity in terms of control
Are *meaningful* to nursing experience*	*Levels 1 and 2* Qualitative designs and quantitative nonexperimental designs tend to be very meaningful as data are collected in the natural environment without a great deal of research control *Levels 3 and 4* Experimental designs particularly require high levels of control over extraneous variables. The contrived nature of experimental studies may affect the collection of data that reflect real-life experience.

* See Table 6.3 for additional detail in relation to the study's design.

as the purpose and significance of the study. For example, if a researcher conducts a well-controlled experimental study with a very small sample, the results should be examined in relation to the significance of the problem in the population, the importance of findings, and the research procedures used, before deciding if the sample size is a serious enough problem to prevent some cautious generalization of findings. Other key factors when evaluating clinical intervention studies, as stressed in Chapter 3, are the importance of estimating the potential risk to clients from experimental interventions and of testing findings carefully in one's own clinical setting, before generalizing them into practice.

Different Views of Generalizability

Generalizability of findings can have somewhat different meanings for the consumer and the researcher. Hinshaw (1984) alludes to this issue in a recent paper. The researcher may view it as primarily generalizing from empirical results to abstract concepts and theoretical frameworks, as well as from the research sample and setting to other larger populations in practice. The consumer is primarily concerned with generalizing a particular set of findings from the study to a particular practice setting.

In many cases the researcher can conduct a well-designed study that may warrant statements about generalization of results beyond that study. However, as we stressed earlier in this text, one study, however convincing, is not sufficient to build research-based practice. The consumer must be able to generalize from findings of many similar studies before direct application into practice. Therefore, replication and extension of research are important factors for both researcher and consumer to consider before generalization of results. Unfortunately, too few pieces of nursing research have been replicated. More often, studies build on the previous work to extend the generalizability one more step. The research consumer should cautiously evaluate the researcher's statements about generalizations of findings within one study in light of reported findings and generalizations from similar existing studies on the topic. The CURN protocols (Horsley et al., 1983), discussed in Chapter 3, are an outgrowth of an evaluation of stated findings and generalizations resulting from research studies on selected topics. Recently, more research has been conducted to synthesize research data on a particular topic. This type of research is known as **meta-analysis,** in which logic and statistical strategies are used to examine data and findings common to a group of research studies completed on a selected topic. For example, Hathaway (1986) reported on a meta-analysis conducted on 68 studies that investigated the effect of preoperative instruction on clients' postoperative outcomes. She concluded that results support the use of preoperative instruction as a positive intervention that yields consistently positive postoperative outcomes.

Generalizability of Qualitative versus Quantitative Studies

Another issue that surrounds the generalizability of results is the increasing use of qualitative approaches to study nursing research problems. Some nurse researchers, who have been exclusively devoted to the use of the scientific method for studying nursing problems, have claimed that findings that emerge from qualitative research methods cannot be generalized because of a lack of empirical control, as well as a lack of specific guidelines for evaluating these methods. On the other hand, nurse researchers who support the use of qualitative methods of study argue that positivistic quantitative studies, which employ rigid control, cannot produce meaningful findings for real life clinical practice. Gradually, the dilemma is being resolved as more nurse researchers are proposing strategies for enhancing the credibility of qualitative findings through better data-collection methods and analysis of results. We have discussed many of these strategies in Chapters 9 and 10. Sandelowski (1986), Field and Morse (1985), and Parse, Coyne, and Smith (1985) are good reference sources that detail criteria for specifically evaluating and conducting qualitative studies.

Many nurse researchers now agree that a variety of methodologies is needed to build research-based nursing practice. In this text we have adopted that philosophy; we also support the mixing of strategies to obtain meaningful and valid research outcomes. In determining generalizability of results to practice settings, meaningfulness is an integral part of the process that cannot be viewed separately from other aspects of validity. Each study's conclusions will be examined by a research consumer for the balance of external validity factors.

Direct and Cognitive Applications

In Chapter 3 we discussed both direct and cognitive application of research findings (Stetler & Marram, 1976) in relation to both basic and applied research. Findings from qualitative studies and nonexperimental studies are a rich source of basic research, which can produce theory that is of significant value for rethinking how we practice (cognitive applications). As a consequence, the meaningfulness and theoretical integrity aspects of external validity (Table 12.1) will carry relatively more weight in a research consumer's deliberations on the applicability of the findings. Experimentally designed studies that test interventions derived from theory are equally important and require careful testing in each unique clinical setting to assure generalizability before direct application. In this situation, study design, question, and purpose will need a relatively closer critique in the evaluation of the validity of the study's conclusions.

EVALUATING THE RESEARCHER'S INTERPRETATION OF FINDINGS

Your purpose in evaluating the researcher's conclusions is to determine their applicability to your clinical setting. You will research your own conclusions, which might not be the same as those of the researcher. You may conclude that the researcher overgeneralized— went too far beyond the findings. In this case you may not accept that researcher's conclusions. Conversely, you might deduce more generalizability than the researcher does. Often you will concur with the researcher's conclusions.

The researcher's interpretation of findings is usually found toward the end of the research report, often with the title "Conclusions," "Results," or "Discussion." It is also the last but most important activity that is carried out before the report and findings are communicated through publication or presentation. Figure 12.1 depicts this activity on the Research Process flowchart.

The interpretation of findings is vital in that it provides an answer to the problem and requires the same kind of inductive and deductive thinking on the part of the researcher as was used when the problem was first conceptualized. In Chapter 4 we noted that the conceptualization process surrounding the problem is often different in qualitative and quantitative studies. Interpretation of findings likewise often proceeds in a somewhat different manner for each of these two approaches.

In Figure 12.1 you can observe what we have called the qualitative maze, which spans data collection, data analysis, and the interpretation of meaning. This maze represents the interactive process used by researchers in primarily qualitative studies where it is important to return to data collection during analysis and interpretation of data to verify information obtained from informants or to rule out rival

_____ Figure 12.1 _____

RESEARCH PROCESS FLOWCHART

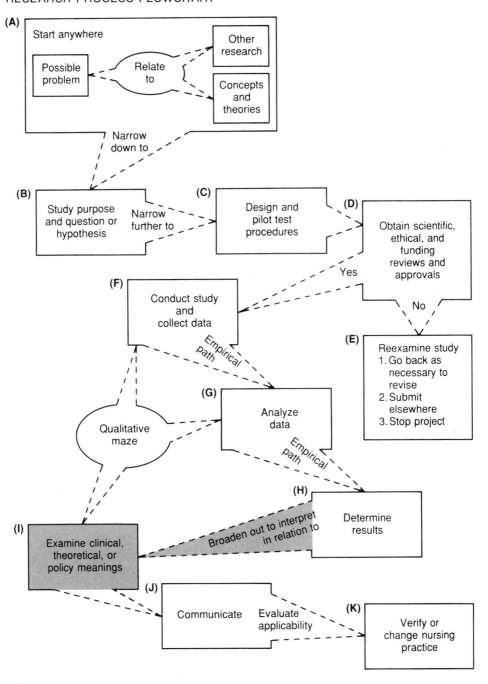

explanations emerging from analysis. Often analysis procedures are performed simultaneously with data collection. Data collection, data analysis, and interpretation are not clear, successive steps, but often occur concurrently in qualitative studies before the researcher attributes the reported meaning to results. In quantitative studies, data collection and analysis procedures are completed before the results are interpreted. The difference in the two interpretation approaches reflects underlying philosophical orientations of the two methods: qualitative, to discover the true nature of phenomena, and quantitative, to objectively measure and observe relationships and cause and effect. How the report is written will reflect the approach taken. Quantitative studies are reported in rather strict steps. Qualitative studies often focus on meanings with the process used to reach the meanings embedded throughout the report.

The conclusions of all research should be reported with specific reference to the study's problem and purpose and be based directly upon results obtained from data analysis. The results of hypotheses testing studies should be discussed explicitly in relation to the stated hypothesis(es) and the theoretical or conceptual framework. A good conclusion of a research report on this type of study will include a restatement of hypothesis(es) along with the appropriate data and interpretation relating to the hypothesis(es). In qualitative reports, the results should be explained in relation to the phenomenon(a) studied by the researcher. If the results of these studies have theoretical implications, these should be explained along with sufficient evidence to support the researcher's interpretations. Examples 12.1 and 12.2 demonstrate the differences between interpretations derived from quantitative and qualitative research.

You may find it helpful when critiquing quantitative studies to determine if the researcher has based conclusions upon the data and their analysis from the statistical evidence presented in the report. In qualitative reports, it is particularly helpful for the consumer if the researcher clearly explains each step in data collection and analysis, as well as provides examples from the data to illustrate interpretations.

Before concluding the report, research findings should be discussed in relation to future research and/or the significance of findings to practice or other aspects of the profession. Research-oriented journals usually emphasize the former and clinically oriented journals the latter. The research consumer will often find clinically important meanings missed by the researcher. Throughout the study of the problem the researcher may have recognized limitations in the methods used. These limitations should be discussed in regard to the research

— *Example 12.1* —————————————————————————————

INTERPRETATIONS FROM QUANTITATIVE RESEARCH

Keller and Bzdek (1986) studied the effect of therapeutic touch on pain associated with tension headaches. Three hypothesized relationships were tested in light of recent holistic theory that explains the healing benefits of the intervention. Therapeutic touch was hypothesized to reduce headache pain more effectively, over a four-hour time period, than a simulation of the intervention. Results obtained through questionnaires from experimental and comparison subjects were quantitatively analyzed in relation to each hypothesis. The significant predicted findings were discussed in the concluding section of the report as they related to the theoretical background of the therapeutic touch intervention.

See Keller, E., & Bzdek, V. M. (1986). Effects of therapeutic touch on tension headache pain. *Nursing Research, 35*(2), 101–105.

— *Example 12.2* —————————————————————————————

INTERPRETATIONS FROM QUALITATIVE RESEARCH

Hutchinson (1986) used interviews and participant observation to develop a grounded theory explanation of the evolution of chemical dependency in nurses. Data were collected from recovering nurses as well as from a variety of other sources. The data were simultaneously analyzed using the constant comparative method associated with grounded theory analysis. Through comparison of incidents, the researcher explained each step of the analysis procedure and the development of each component of the theory. In the final discussion section of the report the researcher discussed her theory in relation to existing addiction theories from the literature and proposed a number of questions for research based upon her theory.

See Hutchinson, S. (1986). Chemically dependent nurses: The trajectory toward self-annihilation. *Nursing Research, 35*(4), 196–201.

outcomes and future research. As a research consumer, you will often see other limitations such as those of meaningfulness or practicality. For example, if the study is a first-time attempt to investigate a problem, recommendations for replication or similar research are crucial if results are to contribute to research-based practice. Theory-building studies should likewise present questions or predictions for further testing.

Hypothesis-testing studies do not always yield significant results. A consumer might tend to discard these studies as having no application to practice. Sometimes the nonsignificant findings of these reports can have as much impact on practice as positive results. For example, when Ziemer (1984) hypothesized that the type of information provided to clients preoperatively would increase postoperative coping behaviors and improve outcomes, she found no evidence from her study to support this prediction. If in fact this conclusion is valid, it would greatly affect the practice of preoperative teaching (direct application). However, the researcher, while recognizing that her findings raised questions about the value of the intervention, also recognized limitations in her method, conceptual explanation, and measurement of coping effects on outcomes. In her discussion she strongly recommends further research. The study used the Betty Neuman Health Care Systems Model (1980) as a framework and as Zeimer suggests, this model may require further testing as to its explanation of the relationship between primary prevention, lines of defense, and stressors. These interpretations can greatly assist practitioners in rethinking practice (cognitive applications) and generating further testable questions.

If the researcher has overgeneralized results, this should become evident in the discussion of any implications for practice. Your first step is to determine if the study is scientifically adequate by critiquing the researcher's process as reported in the article. However, to be applicable to practice, the findings must be examined with reference to other research, your clients, and your clinical setting, as well as your present theory base for practice.

_____ CONCLUSIONS AND SUMMARY _____

Throughout this text we have discussed strategies for evaluating each step of the researcher process. Chapter 3 presents several approaches to the application of findings and a summary of criteria for critique. The evaluation of the researcher's conclusions as presented in this chapter is a linchpin in this application process. For further practice in developing critiquing skills, two research studies appear in their entirety in the Appendix. Although each chapter in this text examines activities in the research process separately, each step can only be considered as part of the whole process in studying a problem. This is equally important in evaluating the findings of research, since the consumer must carefully evaluate the entire process as reported by the researcher.

This chapter summarizes the factors and issues surrounding the external validity of quantitative and qualitative research findings. The

_____ Table 12.2 _____

CRITERIA FOR CRITIQUE OF RESEARCHER'S CONCLUSIONS
AND RECOMMENDATIONS

Scientific Adequacy		Implications for Clinical Applicability
Quantitative Research	Variations in Qualitative Research	
1. Results of data analysis explained in specific reference to study questions, hypothesis(es), conceptual framework, and/or phenomena 2. Conclusions based upon the data and analysis 3. Generalization of significant findings beyond the research study to the study population appropriate in a well-conceptualized and designed study 4. Recommendations for nursing practice and/or further research closely related to findings	Criteria 1–2. Same 3. Sufficient evidence provided to support researcher's interpretation	Overgeneralization of results by researcher presents problem when incorporating findings into practice Critique of the scientific merit of the study necessary to determine if generalization warranted Serious lack of conceptualization requires further research before application of findings into practice Needs meaningful theory and/or practice-related conclusions Has feasible recommendations for practice in the clinical setting Cognitive or direct implications for practice often not discussed by researcher

researcher's process of interpreting the results from data analysis is discussed briefly as well as how these interpretations are presented in a report. The implications of research findings for practice are discussed with reference to Chapter 3. Table 12.2 summarizes the criteria for critiquing the scientific adequacy of the researcher's interpretations as they appear in a report.

REFERENCES

Field, P. A., & Morse, J. M. (1985). *Nursing research: The application of qualitative approaches*. Rockville, Md.: Aspen Systems.

Hathaway, D. (1986). Effect of preoperative instruction on postoperative outcomes. *Nursing Research, 35*(5), 269–274.

Hinshaw, A. S. (1984). *Generalizability of nursing studies*. Unpublished abstract of paper presented at the University of Utah Nursing Research Conference, Issues in Nursing Research, March 6–8.

Horsley, J. A.; Crane, J.; Crabtree, M. K.; & Wood, D. J. (1983). *Using research to improve nursing practice: A guide* (CURN Project). New York: Grune & Stratton.

Hutchinson, S. (1986). Chemically dependent nurses: The trajectory toward self-annihilation. *Nursing Research, 35*(4), 196–201.

Keller, E., & Bzdek, V. M. (1986). Effects of therapeutic touch on tension headache pain. *Nursing Research, 35*(2), 101–105.

Neuman, B. (1980). The Betty Neuman Health Care Systems Model: A total person approach to patient problems. In J. P. Riehl & C. Roy (Eds.), *Conceptual models for nursing practice,* 2nd ed. New York: Appleton-Century-Crofts.

Parse, R. R.; Coyne, A. B.; & Smith, M. J. (1985). *Nursing research: Qualitative methods*. Bowie, Md.: Brady Communications.

Sandelowski, M. (1986). The problem of rigor in qualitative research. *Advances in Nursing Science, 8*(3), 27–37.

Stetler, C. B., & Marram, G. (1976). Evaluating research findings for applicability in practice. *Nursing Outlook, 24*(9), 559–563.

Zeimer, M. (1984). Effect on information on post-surgical coping. In F. Downs (Ed.), *A source book of nursing research,* 3rd ed. Philadelphia: F. A. Davis Co.

Appendix:
Clinical Nursing
Research Reports

APPENDIX A:
INITIAL HANDLING OF NEWBORN INFANTS BY VAGINALLY AND CESAREAN-DELIVERED MOTHERS

Lorraine J. Tulman, D.N.Sc., R.N.
School of Nursing, University of Pennsylvania

The pattern of newborn handling by 36 cesarean-delivered women and 36 vaginally delivered women was studied during their infants' first postpartum bedside visit. The research hypothesis predicted that the initial pattern of handling newborn infants would be different for the two groups of mothers. However, the pattern was found to be similar for the time it took both groups to initiate using their fingers, palms, arms, and trunks, as well as the sequence of use of these body parts, although neither group followed the sequence of handling reported in the bonding literature. The two groups did differ in the frequency and amount of handling of the infants: the cesarean mothers handled their infants significantly less, possibly due to the effects of fatigue and discomfort. In addition, the presence of the infant's father in the cesarean group had a significant effect of decreasing the frequency and amount of maternal handling. No such effect was found in the vaginally delivered group.

The pattern of maternal handling of the newborn infant has been used clinically by nurses as a measure of maternal–infant attachment. The pattern of maternal handling has been researched extensively with mixed results (Bampton, Jones, & Mancini, 1981; Cannon, 1977; Dunn & White, 1981; Govaerts & Patino, 1981; Trevathan, 1981; Tulman, 1985). However, all of the subjects in these studies had vaginal deliveries. No research exists on how cesarean mothers initially handle their newborns. It is, therefore, not known if or how maternal handling of the newborn differs for cesarean- and vaginally delivered mothers or whether the same assessment parameters should be used for the two groups. Because the rate of cesarean deliveries in the United States is close to 20% (Placek, Taffel, & Moien, 1983), a study comparing the pattern of newborn handling by cesarean- and vaginally delivered women was undertaken.

Review of the Literature

The theory of maternal attachment known as bonding (Klaus & Kennell, 1976, 1982) has gained increasing popularity in maternal–child nursing. Implications of the theory for facilitating the formation of the hypothesized "bond" between mother and child have led to changes in nursing care of the parturient woman (Interprofessional Task Force, 1978; Paukert, 1979), including the assessment of maternal attachment. The assessment of attachment based on the theory of bonding includes

This research was supported by Nursing Emphasis Grant No. 5R21 NU00827 for Doctoral Programs in Nursing awarded by the Division of Nursing. National Institutes of Health. US Department of Health and Human Services.

the degree to which the mother seeks to maintain eye contact with the infant and verbalizes to the infant as well as the manner in which she handles her infant.

The manner in which a woman initially handles her newborn infant has been found to vary, however. The hypothesized sequence of handling by mothers proposed by Klaus, Kennell, Plumb, and Zuehlke (1970), Klaus, Trause, and Kennell (1975), and Rubin (1963) (fingers followed by palms, followed by use of arms and upper torso) was also found by Cannon (1977). Govaerts and Patino (1981) and Olsen (1982), working with Egyptian and Liberian women, respectively, found their subjects exhibited the beginning phases of Rubin's hypothesized sequence. However, Bampton et al. (1981), Dunbar (1977), Dunn and White (1981), Hillard (1973), Trevathan (1981), and Tulman (1985) failed to find this sequence among their subjects.

All of the aforementioned studies were done on subjects who had experienced vaginal deliveries. Researchers purposely excluded women who had had cesarean births because of the supposition that surgical delivery would be a confounding variable. Latest statistics available indicate that the cesarean birth rate in the United States is 17.9%, following a steady climb from 4.5% in 1965 (Placek et al., 1983). Although some research has been done on women's retrospective perceptions of their cesarean deliveries and their perceived needs (Affonso & Stichler, 1978; Cranley, Hedahl, & Pegg, 1983; Fawcett, 1981; Lipson & Tilden, 1981; Marut & Mercer, 1979; Tilden & Lipson, 1981; Trowell, 1982), none has examined the initial mother–infant interaction in general or the initial pattern of handling in particular among women experiencing cesarean birth. Therefore, it is not known if women who have cesarean deliveries differ from women who deliver vaginally in their initial patterns of handling their newborn infants. If, in fact, the initial pattern of handling a newborn infant differs between cesarean and vaginally delivered women, then one of the parameters of assessing maternal–infant bonding, i.e., handling, would need to be further examined as a universal measure of maternal–infant attachment. The purpose of this study was to compare the initial pattern of handling newborn infants by women who have delivered by cesarean with women who have delivered vaginally.

Hypotheses

The main research hypothesis tested was: Women who experience cesarean birth will have a different initial pattern of handling their newborn infants than those who deliver vaginally.

Because the pattern of handling has three components—frequency of use of parts of the body over time, time required to initiate use of a particular body part, and sequence in which the parts are used, three subhypotheses were tested:

I. Women who experience cesarean birth will differ from those who deliver vaginally in the frequency over time a particular part of the body is used to initially handle their infants.

II. Women who experience cesarean birth will differ from those who deliver vaginally in the amount of time elapsed to initiate use of a particular part of their bodies to handle their infants.

III. Women who experience cesarean birth will differ from those who deliver vaginally in the sequence of use of parts of their bodies to initially handle their newborn infants.

Method

Sample The total sample size for this study consisted of 72 subjects obtained by convenience sampling. Data for 36 of these subjects (Group 1, women who experienced a vaginal delivery of a healthy term infant) had already been collected by the investigator in the course of a previous study (Tulman, 1985), using a similar sample population and the same instrument and methods of procedure. This study recruited an additional 36 women who had delivered by cesarean section (Group 2). All subjects in this group had cesarean deliveries of healthy term newborn infants. Sixteen of these women had primary cesareans and 20 had repeated cesarean deliveries. In addition, all of the mothers were English-speaking, had hemoglobin ratings greater than 10 grams, had no motor or visual impairments, had no known history of psychiatric illness, had not experienced alcohol or drug abuse within the past 2 years, and were not planning to give the infant for adoption or placement in foster care.

There were no statistically significant differences, $p < .05$, between the two groups for the demographic characteristics of race, parity, age of youngest child, prior experience with infants, left/right handedness, sex of infant, or method of infant feeding chosen. The cesarean-delivered women were older ($\underline{M} = 27.9$ years, SD 4.6 years) than the vaginally delivered women ($\underline{M} = 24.9$ years, $SD = 4.9$ years), $t = 2.7$, $df = 70$, $p = .009$. (See Tables 1 and 2.)

There were differences between Groups 1 and 2 for situational variables related to the type of delivery. Significantly more mothers in Group 1 (33 of 36) handled their infants in the delivery and/or recovery rooms than did Group 2 mothers (11 of 36), $\chi^2 = 25.77$, $df = 1$, $p < .001$. This difference was largely due to the use of restraints on

_____ Table 1 _____

COMPARISON OF DEMOGRAPHIC CHARACTERISTICS OF GROUPS

Variable	$\bar{X}$	SD	t Ratio	p Value
Age				
Vaginal	24.89	4.93	2.70	.009
Cesarean	27.92	4.58		
Parity				
Vaginal	0.86	0.89	0.14	.893
Cesarean	0.83	0.84		
Age of youngest child				
Vaginal	3.55	2.63	0.07	.942
Cesarean	3.62	3.35		

_____ Table 2 _____

COMPARISON OF DEMOGRAPHIC CHARACTERISTICS OF GROUPS— CHI-SQUARE STATISTICS

Variable	Vaginal	Cesarean	χ^2	p Value
Sex of infant				
Male	14	18	0.51	.48
Female	22	18		
Prior experience with infant in past year				
None	17	12	2.78	.25
Some	12	19		
Extensive	7	5		
Race				
White	28	29	0.00	1.00
Black	8	7		
Handedness				
Right	29	31	0.10	.75
Left	7	5		
Method of feeding				
Breast	30	24	1.85	.17
Bottle	6	12		

cesarean mothers' arms during operative delivery at both data collection sites. It should be noted that all but one of the cesarean mothers were awake, i.e., had regional anesthesia for the delivery.

Group 2 infants were older when they went out to their mothers for the first postpartum bedside visit (Group 1 $\underline{M} = 5.17$ hours, $SD = 2.05$; Group 2 $\underline{M} = 8.61$, $SD = 4.28$), $t = 4.36$, $df = 70$, $p < .001$, and the Group 2 mothers had more recently been medicated for pain than Group 1 mothers (Group 1 $\underline{M} = 6.96$ hours, $SD = 2.93$; Group 2 $\underline{M} = 2.28$ hours, $SD = 1.4$ hours), $t = 7.28$, $df = 53$, $p < .001$. These two group differences can be directly attributed to the cesarean birth experience. Newborn nursery policies at both data collection sites permit infants to go out to their mothers' rooms as soon as a body temperature of 98 °F (axillary) has been regained after the first bath, regardless of the mode of delivery. However, the cesarean mothers frequently chose to delay this first postpartum contact with their infants for several hours because of fatigue and discomfort. Similarly, the cesarean mothers requested more frequent analgesic medication because of abdominal incisional pain.

Instruments The observation checklist used in this study was developed by the investigator (Tulman, 1983, 1985), based on observation checklists used in previous research (Cannon, 1977; deChateau & Wiberg, 1977; Dunbar, 1977; Gay, 1979; Hillard, 1973; Klaus et al., 1970, 1975; O'Leary, 1972). The instrument was tested for content validity and interrater reliability (Tulman, 1983, 1985). Interrater reliability for the group of mothers who delivered vaginally was .82. Ongoing interrater reliability checks were .85, .90, .84, and .84. Interrater reliability for the tool, .89, was reestablished prior to the start of data collection

for Group 2. Interrater reliability was also periodically checked with a trained research assistant during the course of data collection of Group 2 and was found to be .84 and .87.

Procedure Names of potential subjects were obtained from the nursing staff of the maternity units at the data collection sites. Potential subjects were then approached by the investigator or her research assistant (both referred to hereafter as data collector) and written informed consent sought. Eight potential subjects who were approached refused to participate. No financial inducements for participation were offered to subjects. Subjects were informed that the purpose of the study was to examine adult–newborn interaction rather than the specific purpose of examining handling behaviors in an effort to diminish potential distortion of behaviors. Subjects were debriefed at the end of the data collection session. The consent form and procedure for obtaining consent were approved by appropriate human subjects committees.

After obtaining written informed consent, the subject's handling of her infant was observed by the data collector during the infant's first bedside visit to the mother on the postpartum unit. This visit, rather than any handling of the infant by the mother that might have occurred in the delivery room or recovery rooms, was used because a range of handling behaviors is not possible in the restrictive environments of these locations.

Each subject was observed for a period of 15 minutes, starting from the time a newborn nursery staff member brought the infant to the subject's room in a bassinet. A time-sampling methodology for observing and recording the handling behavior was used. The subject's behavior was observed for 5 seconds and recorded on the observation checklist during the next 15 seconds, thereby yielding three observations per minute and a total of 45 observations for each subject. An audiotape with a tone cycle of 5 seconds duration followed by a 15-second period of silence was used to assist the data collector in observing and recording. The data collector listened to this tape through an earphone receiver so that the subject would not be distracted by the tones during the observation period. To minimize reactivity, the data collector did not talk to either subject or subject's roommate(s), if any, and positioned herself as far as possible from the subject without sacrificing visualization of the subject, typically a distance of 4 to 6 feet. At the conclusion of this observation period, the data collector obtained additional demographic data from the subject.

Results

Subhypothesis I This subhypothesis was statistically tested by Kolmogorov–Smirnov two-sample tests. This nonparametric test compares two cumulative distributions and detects any statistically significant differences between the two distributions at any point (Siegel, 1956). In this case, the cumulative nature of the distribution of a specific maternal handling behavior, i.e., the use of a specific maternal or infant body part, was over time. Statistically significant, $p < .05$, differences were found between Groups 1 and 2 for the frequency of use of the mother's fingers, palms, arms, and trunk to handle her infant. In addition, statistically significant, $p < .05$, differences were found for the frequency of handling the infant's head and trunk. For all of these handling behaviors, vaginally delivered mothers handled their infants more than cesarean-delivered mothers. No statistically significant differences were found for the frequency of use of the mother's

lap or the frequency of handling the infant's upper or lower extremities, although this lack of difference is a reflection of the rarity of these handling behaviors for both groups. The cesarean mothers had a higher frequency of not handling their infants, $p < .05$, and this frequency increased over time. Therefore, subhypothesis I was supported.

Subhypothesis II This subhypothesis was tested using Mann–Whitney U tests. No significant differences were found between the groups on the amount of time elapsed for the mothers to initiate use of their fingers, palms, arms, or laps or in the amount of time to initiate handling their infants' heads or trunks. However, Group 2 mothers did use their trunks and handled their infants' extremities significantly earlier than Group 1 mothers. They also interrupted the handling of their infants significantly earlier in the observation period, $p = .03$. Therefore, subhypothesis II could not be supported.

Subhypothesis III This subhypothesis was tested using Friedman's two-way analysis of variance. Each subject's sequence of handling the infant was ranked among the possible parts of the body used— fingers, palms, arms, trunk. In addition, in a separate analysis, the sequence of parts of the infant that were handled by each subject was ranked for the infant's extremities, head, and trunk.

For both groups, the sequence of use of maternal body parts proved not to be statistically significant. However, both groups tended to simultaneously use fingers and palms to initially handle the infant followed by simultaneous use of arms and trunk. There was a statistically significant, $p < .05$, order for the handling of the infant's parts for both groups. For both groups the order was the same: trunk followed by head followed by extremities.

Therefore, subhypothesis III was not supported; the sequence of use of maternal body parts and the sequence of parts of the infant handled were similar for the two groups.

Thus, the main research hypothesis was only partially upheld through support of subhypothesis I. Although the vaginal- and cesarean-delivered mothers were different in the frequency of use of maternal body parts to handle the infants and parts of the infant handled, the two groups were similar in amount of time to initiate a handling behavior and the sequence of handling behaviors.

Additional Findings Data were further analyzed by Kolmogorov–Smirnov two-sample tests, Mann–Whitney U tests, and Friedman two-way ANOVAs to determine if demographic or situational factors influenced subjects' handling behaviors for frequency, initiation, or sequence. No significant differences were found for the variables of sex of the infant, race, parity, handedness, method of feeding, amount of recent prior experience with infants, or handling in the delivery and/or recovery rooms.

Fathers of the infants were present during the observation period of 9 mothers in Group 1 and of 12 mothers in Group 2. The presence of the fathers in Group 1 had no effect on the frequency, initiation, or sequence of maternal handling of the infant. Typically, the father handled the infant briefly and only when the mother requested that he do so, so that she could change her position. However, in the cesarean group, the presence of the father was associated with significantly less frequent infant handling by the mother. The initiation and sequence of handling behaviors were not affected by the father's presence. Typically, the father took the infant from the mother without waiting for

her to offer him an opportunity to hold the infant. In 9 out of the 12 cases in which the father was present, he handled the infant for more than half the observation period.

Fatigue was a factor affecting the first postpartum bedside visit for the cesarean mothers but not for the vaginally delivered mothers. This was evidenced by the fact that none of the 36 vaginally delivered mothers requested that their infants be returned to the nursery prior to the end of the 15-minute observation period, whereas 3 of the 24 cesarean-delivered mothers who were alone sent the infant back to the nursery prior to the end of this period. In the 9 of 12 instances in which the father assumed a major role in handling the infant, the mothers offered no objection and seemed relieved that the infants had been taken from them.

Discussion

The study findings indicate that cesarean-delivered women, a group heretofore excluded from maternal–infant attachment research, do not differ from vaginally delivered women in the initiation or sequence of handling behaviors of their infants during the initial postpartum bedside visit. It is important to note that neither group followed the sequence of handling the infant first proposed by Rubin (1963) and later by Klaus et al. (1970, 1975), i.e., fingers, palm, arms, and trunk. Instead, both groups of subjects initially used their fingers and palms simultaneously followed by simultaneous use of their arms and trunk to handle the infants. This is consistent with other studies which also did not observe the fingers, palms, arms, trunk sequence (Bampton et al., 1981; Dunn & White, 1981; Hillard, 1973; Trevathan, 1981).

The results of the study do indicate that vaginally and cesarean-delivered women differ in the frequency over time a particular body part is used to handle the infant, with vaginally delivered women having a significantly higher frequency for the commonly used parts. This phenomenon may be explained by the fatigue and pain felt by the cesarean-delivered women after delivery (Fawcett & Burritt, 1985). Fatigue and pain were demonstrated by this group's delaying to see their infants, their use of analgesics, and their willingness to have the father of the infant, if present, assume a major role in the initial interaction with the infant.

Implications The results of this study demonstrate that the handling sequence first described by Rubin (1963) and incorporated by Klaus and Kennell (1976, 1982) into their theory of maternal–infant bonding is not found among women who have had cesarean deliveries. Evidence from this study and others (Bampton et al., 1981; Dunn & White, 1981; Hillard, 1973; Trevathan, 1981) also calls into question whether the fingers–palms–arms–trunk sequence is consistently found among vaginally delivered women. Therefore, the results of this study cast some doubt on the validity of fingers–palms–arms–trunk as a parameter for clinically assessing maternal attachment for either vaginally or cesarean-delivered women. The continued use of the fingers–palms–arms–trunk sequence as a nursing clinical assessment tool of maternal–infant attachment is therefore not a valid clinical practice.

The fatigue and pain felt by the cesarean mothers in the study affected their initial handling of their newborn infants. Given the initial differences between the vaginal and cesarean birth experience, further research is indicated concerning the needs of cesarean mothers in the earlier and later postpartum periods as well as how the cesarean birth experience affects the developing maternal–infant relationship.

The results point out the need for further research to determine if the initial level of paternal involvement with cesarean-delivered infants persists into the later hospital postpartum period as well as after discharge from the hospital and its ultimate effect on the father–child relationship.

References

Alfonso, D. D., & Stichler, J. F. (1978). Exploratory study of women's reactions to having a cesarean birth. *Birth and the Family Journal, 5*(2), 88–94.

Bampton, B., Jones, J., & Mancini, J. (1981). Initial mothering patterns of low-income black primaparas. *Journal of Obstetric, Gynecologic, and Neonatal Nursing, 10*, 174–178.

Cannon, R. B. (1977). The development of maternal touch during early mother–infant interaction. *Journal of Obstetric, Gynecologic, and Neonatal Nursing, 6*(2), 28–33.

Cranley, M. S., Hedahl, K. J., & Pegg, S. H. (1983). Women's perceptions of vaginal and cesarean deliveries. *Nursing Research, 32*(1), 10–15.

deChateau, P., & Wiberg, B. (1977). Long-term effect on mother–infant behavior of extra contact during the first hour post partum. I. First observations at 36 hours. *Acta Paediatrica Scandinavia, 66*, 137–143.

Dunbar, J. (1977). *Maternal contact behaviors with newborn infants during feedings.* Unpublished doctoral dissertation, University of Pittsburgh, Pittsburgh, PA.

Dunn, D. M., & White, D. G. (1981). Interactions of mothers with their newborns in the first half-hour of life. *Journal of Advanced Nursing, 6*, 271–275.

Fawcett, J. (1981). Needs of cesarean birth parents. *Journal of Obstetric, Gynecologic, and Neonatal Nursing, 10*, 372–376.

Fawcett, J., & Burritt, J. (1985). An exploratory study of antenatal preparation for cesarean birth. *Journal of Obstetric, Gynecologic, and Neonatal Nursing, 14,* 224–230.

Gay, J. T. (1979). *Behaviors of first-time fathers at the time of their initial acquaintance with their infants.* Unpublished doctoral dissertation, University of Alabama, Birmingham, AL.

Govaerts, K., & Patino, E. (1981). Attachment behavior of the Egyptian mother. *International Journal of Nursing Studies, 18*(1), 53–60.

Hillard, M. E. (1973). *A descriptive study of selected mother and infant behaviors on the day of delivery.* Unpublished doctoral dissertation, University of Florida, Jacksonville, FL.

Interprofessional Task Force on Health Care of Women and Children (1978). The development of family-centered maternity/newborn care in hospitals. *Journal of Obstetric, Gynecologic, and Neonatal Nursing, 7*(5), 155–159.

Klaus, M. H., & Kennell, J. H. (1976). *Maternal–infant bonding, the impact of early separation or loss on family development.* St. Louis: C. V. Mosby.

Klaus, M. H., & Kennell, J. H. (1982). *Parent–infant bonding* (2nd ed.). St. Louis: C. V. Mosby.

Klaus, M. H., Kennell, J. H., Plumb, N., & Zuehlike, S. (1970). Human maternal behavior at the first contact with her young. *Pediatrics, 46,* 187–192.

Klaus, M. H., Trause, M. A., & Kennell, J. H. (1975). Does human maternal behavior after delivery show a characteristic pattern? *CIBA Foundation Symposium, 33,* 69–85.

Lipson, J. G., & Tilden, V. P. (1981). Psychological integration of the cesarean birth experience. *American Journal of Orthopsychiatry, 50,* 598–609.

Marut, J. S., & Mercer, R. T. (1979). Comparison of primparas' perceptions of vaginal and cesarean births. *Nursing Research, 28,* 260–266.

O'Leary, S. E. (1972). *Mother–father–infant interaction in the first two days of life.* Unpublished doctoral dissertation. University of Wisconsin.

Olsen, L. C. (1982). Observations of early mother–infant interaction in Liberia. *Journal of Nurse Midwifery, 27*(3), 9–14.

Paukert, S. E. (1979). One hospital's experience with implementing family-centered maternity care. *Journal of Obstetric, Gynecologic, and Neonatal Nursing, 8,* 351–358.

Placek, P. J., Taffel, S., & Moien, M. (1983). Cesarean section delivery rates: United States, 1981. *American Journal of Public Health, 73,* 861–862.

Rubin, R. (1963). Maternal touch. *Nursing Outlook, 11,* 828–831.

Siegel, S. (1956). *Nonparametric statistics for the behavioral sciences.* New York: McGraw–Hill.

Tilden, V. P., & Lipson, J. G. (1981). Cesarean childbirth; Variables affecting psychological impact. *Western Journal of Nursing Research, 3*(2), 127–141.

Trevathan, W. R. (1981). Maternal touch at first contact with the newborn infant. *Developmental Psychobiology, 14,* 549–558.

Trowell, J. (1982). Possible effects of emergency cesarean section on the mother–child relationship. *Early Human Development, 7*(1), 41–51.

Tulman, L. J. (1983). *Comparison of mothers' and unrelated persons' initial handling of newborn infants.* Unpublished doctoral dissertation, University of Pennsylvania, Philadelphia, PA.

Tulman, L. J. (1985). Mothers' and unrelated persons' initial handling of newborn infants. *Nursing Research, 34,* 205–210.

APPENDIX B:
LIFE AFTER CANCER

Sally E. Thorne, R.N., M.S.N.
School of Nursing, University of British Columbia

Successful adaptation to cancer requires that individuals and families confront numerous psychosocial aspects of the disease. Considerable attention has been paid in the last decade to illness as the experiential component of having a disease. Cancer has received an undue proportion of this attention, perhaps because it serves as a metaphor for the most dramatic subjective components of physical ill health. Beyond the role shifts, economic hardship, physical disability, and social isolation characteristic of many chronic conditions, cancer patients and their families must face existential dilemmas which surround a medical disorder commonly assumed to be fatal (Veronesi & Martino, 1978).

It has been widely recognized, then, that these aspects of cancer and its treatments have long-lasting ramifications and that these do not disappear once the patient is pronounced free of active disease (Naysmith, Hinton, Meredith, Marks & Berry, 1983; Worden & Weisman, 1980; Zubrod, 1975). Since the number of cured cancer patients is bound to increase in the future, there is a need to understand the predicament of ongoing illness in the absence of disease (Weisman, 1979).

A review of the research literature yields a rather confusing portrait of the cancer survivor. Attempts to quantify the well-being of cured cancer patients have failed to isolate significant differences between them and the general population (Danoff, Kramer, Irwin, & Gottlieb, 1983; Schmale et al., 1983). The authors of these studies, however, have noted the difficulties inherent in relying upon measurable variables, such as return to work, as indices of overall recovery, and have recommended study of the subjective elements of recovery from the perspective of the patient.

Efforts in that direction, however, have yielded rather contradictory conclusions to date. Kennedy and others found cured cancer patients to be more relaxed and more confident than non-diseased populations. They hypothesized that recovery from cancer was a good character-building experience (Kennedy, Tellegen, Kennedy, & Havernick, 1976). In contrast, Shanfield's more recent (1980) findings were that cancer had a permanently detrimental effect on its victims, characterized by easy access to intense emotionality and an enduring sense of vulnerability. Similar data were analyzed by Maher (1982) who explained the insecurity and anxiety of cancer recovery as a state of anomie characterized by the common themes of anger, anxiety, ambivalence, confusion, and depression. What seems evident from the subjectively oriented findings, then, is that cancer recovery is a double-edged sword, an

This work was supported by University of British Columbia Research Grant # B83-322 (Humanities and Social Sciences).

experience loaded with both positive and negative elements.

The attempts to describe cured cancer patients to date have failed to address cancer recovery as a prolonged and dynamic process (Cassileth & Hamilton, 1979; O'Neill, 1975). While the health care system provides considerable assistance to those adapting to cancer, that second adaptation, to life after cancer, takes place unheralded and in isolation. The "Life After Cancer" project was designed to explore and describe the experience of adjusting to life without cancer from the perspective of those who were "expert witnesses" to the transition. It was hoped that such understanding could assist health care providers to recognize and facilitate wellness in cancer survivors.

Method

The methodology for the study was guided by the phenomenological paradigm of qualitative research. The selection of such a method reflects the assumption that the phenomenon under study is of the order of "inner experience" and thus not accessible by more empirical approaches (Davis, 1978; Kestenbaum, 1982; Schwartz & Jacobs, 1979).

The role required of the researcher using the phenomenological paradigm of qualitative methodology is that of entering into the process being studied for the purpose of interpreting it as it appears to the people engaged (Oiler, 1982). Thus the events shared and understood by participants and researcher provide the data from which concepts and hypotheses emerge (Rist, 1979). The usual notions of reliability and validity are inapplicable. Rather, the criteria by which the research must be judged are the richness of the data and the

credibility of the disciplined abstractions developed from them (Diers, 1979).

The principle of theoretical sampling directed the selection of participants according to the criterion of competency to provide the knowledge and understanding that was sought. Competency for this purpose was defined as a medical history of malignant disease, self-report as being cured of that disease, and sufficient fluency in spoken English to communicate in detail about the experience.

Fifteen volunteer informants were recruited through word of mouth and newspaper advertising. The ten women and five men ranged in age from thirty to seventy-four years at the time of the study. They averaged five years since diagnosis with a variety of types of cancer and had undergone medical treatment by at least one of surgery, radiation, and chemotherapy. The intensive interview sessions were initially guided by a loosely structured set of questions which evolved throughout the research process as new themes modified the direction and new concepts refined the quest.

Verbatim transcripts as well as field notes constituted the data base for the construction of accounts. Simultaneous data collection and analysis were guided by phenomenological principles. In this way, assumptions were continuously affirmed, revised, or discarded. Interrelationships between themes were subjected to ongoing validation by the informants to ensure that abstractions remained grounded in the data themselves.

The Accounts

The accounts revealed that cured cancer patients portray life after cancer as including lasting repercussions from the disease.

They describe a variety of signposts indicative of the transition from illness to wellness, and describe psychosocial and existential variables which determine the transition process.

Lasting Repercussions   Participants described numerous ways that cancer continued to affect their lives. Many reported periodic anxiety, especially when the annual check-up approached, about recurrence or contracting a second cancer. Several participants spoke of lasting social life changes, most often the loss of friends who feared cancer or who disapproved of the patient's management choices. The bitterness from such losses was obviously slow to heal. Another type of lasting repercussion was the residual cosmetic and functional deficiencies resulting from the cancer treatments. Mutilating surgery, for example, could produce ongoing concern about appearance or capacities such as childbearing. Those whose ongoing problems included urinary incontinence or colostomy management described these as constant reminders of the cancer. Although such lasting effects differed between individuals, none of those interviewed was free of them entirely.

At the same time, many of the cured cancer patients described positive effects of having had cancer. Two expressed pride at having survived the experience. Another said coping well with the disease gave him dignity and confidence. One woman talked of a newfound sensation of power and described it this way: "For me it was like seeing an enemy, if you will, and not backing down. Saying yes, this is a very dangerous enemy but it is something I can deal with. It is not going to terrify me." Although few informants had made radical life-style changes because of cancer, many believed it had significantly altered their philosophy or approach to life. As one woman stated: "My life is the same but it's not the same. I will never have the same value system. My value system has been totally changed." The cured cancer patients described revised priorities, a heightened concern for nature, relationships, and spirituality, and a relaxed pace of life as examples of the positive attitudinal shifts they had found in themselves.

Although they all defined themselves as cured, these informants did not necessarily feel that their cancer experience was over. Several maintained that the cancer still played a role in shaping their everyday reality. Others described their cancer as history but admitted that it periodically came back to haunt them. Thus, while some cured cancer patients felt completely recovered, others perceived themselves to be still in transition.

Signposts for Transition   The signposts, or indicators that their cancer experience had ended, varied among individuals. A few described feeling suddenly relieved upon reaching the five-year survival mark. Others relied upon the stated or implied opinions of the health care givers. Some recalled the moment when they were pronounced cured by their physician. Others reported relying just as heavily on the implied meaning of an event. One man described his cancer as ending when he overheard an X-ray technician's opinion that he was cured. Another said the "pressure was off" when the oncology clinic telephoned to cancel his last appointment. Private or symbolic meanings were also evident in several accounts of visions or dreams as a turning point. As one woman remarked: "I have decided that there are other things that tell you whether you are going to be well or not. It's all not there on that pathology report."

Sometimes the transition was not linked to any event, but was portrayed as a gradual process: "Somewhere in the last two years, I have come to that inner sense that I am fine and also a sense that it is not going to recur." There were those who believed that their endpoint had not yet occurred: "It's a very slow process and you have literally got to turn your thinking around 180 degrees, and it's a totally new way of looking at life, and it's not easy." Yet others were doubtful that they would ever feel free of their cancer identity: "You see it's hard to get over mentally. I hope that days will go by when I don't think about it or I forget that I had cancer. No, I still think that I'm a patient."

What emerged from the accounts was that the sense of cancer as a past or present phenomenon bore little relationship to survival time, medical prognosis, or even to the residual disability from cancer. Instead, participants explained what they perceived as the factors determining their transition toward wellness.

Determinants of Wellness While a range of influences upon the transition were identified, two themes emerged as common factors: the nature of their involvement in managing the cancer, and the nature of their encounters with health care providers.

Many of the informants attributed their cure, at least in part, to active involvement in their own disease management. As one woman remarked: "I don't think I'd be where I am today if I had just been very passive about my illness." The active involvement took several forms. A few had used vitamin therapy, naturopathy, or diet management with great success in their opinion. Such remedies provided them with the attitudinal advantage associated with "doing something constructive," and pro-

vided a tangible focus for the fighting spirit these informants valued. Other informants attributed their wellness directly to the mental attitudes that characterized their approach to cancer. Faith in oneself or in a higher being, humour, and the will to live were repeatedly mentioned as playing an active role in promoting cancer recovery.

An intriguing discovery was the extent to which cured cancer patients believed that their relationships with health care providers influenced their experience with and recovery from cancer. While many recalled being demanding or unpleasant toward health care providers, most felt that their mistreatment was undeserved. With few exceptions, these cured cancer patients told story after story to illustrate perceived insensitivity, cruelty, dishonesty, disrespect, and invalidation from health care providers they had encountered during their cancer experience: "The doctor said I was crazy, that I was a hypochondriac"; "The head nurse hated me"; "It was quite obvious by the nurses' attitude that they were almost prepared to put the coffin nails in"; "It's just about murder the way they illtreat you there." Clearly, the anger and bitterness about these interactions had not disappeared with time. Most of the informants, however, expected that they were unusual in this regard, and chalked it up to their misfortune at running across the exceptional "bad apple" in an otherwise helpful profession.

As well as describing these negative encounters, informants told of particularly helpful or supportive health care behaviors which facilitated their recovery processes. They especially recalled instances of honesty, respect, and human concern from health care providers. One man described his nurses this way: "They're beautiful. They all tried to play up to you that you're a sweetheart, which is a part of their psychology." Another recalled feeling reassured and valued by a physician's remark that she "remembered that tonsil" even though he doubted it was true. The potency of the recollections, both negative and positive, supported their contention that these human interactions had made a lasting impact.

Thus, cured cancer patients explained that the subjective sense of cure has a pace of its own which does not necessarily parallel the traditional objective criteria for disease recovery. The signposts that mark the transition to wellness may be tangible or symbolic, but are uniquely defined by individuals according to their own sense of meaning. Cured cancer patients believe that their own approaches and attitudes, as well as those of their human health care resources, determine the quality of their life after cancer.

Interpretations and Conclusions

These findings support the contention of other theorists that active involvement and personal control are central to the quality of life in all stages of the cancer experience (Cantor, 1978; Lewis, 1982; Sourkes, 1982; Weisman, 1979). While their effect upon the emotional aspects of recovery seems self-evident, there is also tentative evidence in the research literature supporting the contention that such attitudes play some determining role in the physiological disease process itself (Greer, Morris, & Pettingale, 1979). Whether or not such relationships can be empirically established, the link seems clear in the perspective of the cured cancer patients. These findings also confirm the existence of this second difficult transition, to life after cancer, and suggest that

wellness is not an automatic sequel to being cured of a malignant disease. A syndrome analogous to the Holocaust "survivor syndrome" has been hypothesized by some theorists (Naysmith et al., 1983; Shanfield, 1980). The suggestion by others that health care assistance could facilitate this transition is supported by these accounts (Cassileth & Hamilton, 1979).

The extent and impact of inhumane encounters in the health care system was a rather disturbing finding. While it is possible that distorted or exaggerated recollections reflect the cured cancer patients' attempts to justify their experiences in some way, it seems equally likely that they have been the recipients of incompetent or insensitive psychosocial care. Other researchers have identified fatalistic attitudes (Welch, 1981) and double bind messaging (Longhofer, 1980) as examples of counterproductive communication patterns prevalent among cancer care practitioners. There seems ample evidence to argue that communication with cancer patients deserves extensive research. Further, it seems evident that we must challenge the ideology of cancer as a metaphor for death. These findings reinforce the argument that if health care professionals could modify their anti-cancer imagery and attitudes, they could facilitate wellness in cancer patients (Veronesi & Martino, 1978).

The accounts described here imply that we in the health care arena bear some responsibility for the quality of life our patients experience during and after cancer. The role we play in determining who among the cured will be victims and who will be survivors deserves coherent research and individual soul-searching. Let it not be said that we cured the disease but killed the spirit of the patient.

References

Cantor, R. C. (1978). *And a time to live: Toward emotional well-being during the crisis of cancer.* New York: Harper & Row.

Cassileth, B. R., & Hamilton, J. N. (1979). The family with cancer. In B. R. Cassileth (Ed.), *The cancer patient: Social and medical aspects of care* (pp. 233–247). Philadelphia: Lea & Febiger.

Danoff, B., Kramer, S., Irwin, P., & Gottlieb, A. (1983). Assessment of the quality of life in long-term survivors after definitive radiotherapy. *American Journal of Clinical Oncology, 6,* 339–345.

Davis, A. J. (1978). The phenomenological approach in nursing research. In N. Chaska (Ed.), *The nursing profession: Views through the mist* (pp. 186–196). New York: McGraw-Hill.

Diers, D. (1979). *Research in nursing practice.* Philadelphia: Lippincott.

Greer, S., Morris, T., & Pettingale, K. W. (1979). Psychological response to breast cancer: Effect on outcome. *Lancet, ii* (8146), 785–7.

Kennedy, B. J., Tellegen, A., Kennedy, S., & Havenick, N. (1976). Psychological response of patients cured of advanced cancer. *Cancer, 38,* 2184–2191.

Kestenbaum, V. (1982). The experience of illness. In V. Kestenbaum (Ed.), *The humanity of the ill: Phenomenological perspectives* (pp. 3–30). Knoxville: University of Tennessee Press.

Lewis, F. M. (1982). Experienced personal control and quality of life in late-stage cancer patients. *Nursing Research, 3,* 113–119.

Longhofer, J. (1980). Dying or living?: The double bind. *Culture, Medicine and Psychiatry, 4,* 119–136.

Maher, E. L. (1982). Anomic aspects of recovery from cancer. *Social Science & Medicine, 16,* 907–912.

Naysmith, A., Hinton, J. M., Meredith, R., Marks, M. D., & Berry, R. J. (1983). Surviving malignant disease: Psychological and family aspects. *British Journal of Hospital Medicine, 30*(1), 22, 26–27.

Oiler, C. (1982). The phenomenological approach in nursing research. *Nursing Research, 31,* 178–181.

O'Neill, M. P. (1975). Psychological aspects of cancer recovery. *Cancer, 36*(1), 271–273.

Rist, R. C. (1979). On the means of knowing: Qualitative research in education. *New York University Education Quarterly,* Summer, 17–21.

Schmale, A. H., Morrow, G. R., Schmitt, M. H., Adler, L. M., Enelow, A., Murawski, B. J., & Gates, C. (1983). Well-being of cancer survivors. *Psychosomatic Medicine, 45*(2), 163–169.

Schwartz, H., & Jacobs, J. (1979). *Qualitative sociology: A method to the madness.* New York: The Free Press.

Shanfield, S. B. (1980). On surviving cancer: Psychological considerations. *Comprehensive Psychiatry, 21*(2), 128–134.

Sourkes, B. M. (1982). *The deepening shade: Psychological aspects of life-threatening illness.* Pittsburgh, PA: University of Pittsburgh Press.

Veronesi, U., & Martino, G. (1978). Can life be the same after cancer treatment? *Tumori, 64,* 345–351.

Weisman, A. D. (1979). A model for psychosocial phasing in cancer. *General Hospital Psychiatry, 1*(3), 187–195.

Welch, D. (1981). Promoting change in nurse communication with cancer patients. *Nursing Administration Quarterly, 5*(2), 77–81.

Worden, J. W., & Weisman, A. D. (1980). Do cancer patients want counseling? *Cancer Hospital Psychiatry, 2*(2), 100–103.

Zubrod, C. G. (1975). Successes in cancer treatment. *Cancer, 36*(1), 267–270.

Glossary

This Glossary was developed with the research consumer in mind. It should assist the reader to understand the text and do the exercises. It will also be a handy reference for reading research articles and reports. Using the Glossary effectively for this purpose assumes that the reader has read the relevant sections of the text.

Because nursing research had its early roots in several other disciplines, their various terms have crept into use. There are often several terms for the same or similar concept, so the most common synonyms and related terms are cross-referenced. This will also help the reader understand a concept and recognize it under various names. Conversely, there are terms that have variations in their definitions among nurse researchers. For these terms, the most commonly used definitions have been used here.

Abstract A brief summary of a study that provides an overview of the research problem, sample, design, and findings. It usually precedes the study report and alerts the research consumer to the researcher's view of the key contents of the report.

Accidental sample *See* Convenience sample.

Accountability Professional responsibility for actions that encompasses liability. It includes the responsibility to take action and the willingness of a professional to be held answerable for such action (e.g., research-based practice).

Acquiescence response set A type of response set bias in which a subject may have a tendency to answer "yes" or agree with the content of the question.

Alpha values *See p*-value.

Analysis The methods of reducing and synthesizing data in order to reach a conclusion about the answer to a research question. Depending on the design of the study, the data will be examined whole or in parts for patterns or relationships.

Analysis of variance (ANOVA) A statistical procedure for examining differences between and also within groups. Its basis lies in the comparison of the averages of the measure of dependent variables. Closely related procedures are analysis of covariance and multiple analysis of variance.

Anonymity A criterion for protection of human subjects' rights, which should assure subjects their individual responses cannot be identified.

Antecedent variable Something that occurs before or is already present when the independent variable is introduced or observed by the researcher.

Applied research   Studies that have as a primary purpose the solution of clinical problems. Such studies have potential for direct clinical applications.

Appropriateness   Relates to the fit of an instrument to particular subjects in order to produce valid data.

Association   A relationship between at least two variables or phenomena that can be expressed in statistical, graphic, or narrative form.

Assumptions   Stated or unstated principles, generally accepted as true without proof or verification (e.g., those ideas underlying a theoretical framework or a particular statistic).

Basic research or theoretical research   Research that has as its major aim the expansion of knowledge without immediate concern for application into practice.

Benefit   *See* Risk/benefit ratio.

Beta   *See* Power analysis.

Bias   Any process or circumstance that could systematically or randomly distort the validity of study results.

Bipolar scales   A way of recording the responses to a question that assumes a range between two extreme ends of a dimension. These scales also may be called graphic rating scales.

Bivariate   Statistics resulting from the analysis of the relationship between two variables.

Case study   A type of sampling for studies (e.g., behavior modification studies and ethnographies) where data on one or a few subjects are intensely and systematically gathered and analyzed, often over time.

Causality   The ability to predict an outcome from a prior event or situation. Causality implies the ability to control the outcome by manipulation of the prior event or situation.

Causal relationship   An association between two variables in which one can be assumed, on the basis of research, to affect the other. The causal variable is usually related statistically to the affected variable, precedes the effect, cannot be explained by another cause, and/or is rationally related to the effect.

Causal variable   *See* Independent variable.

Central tendency   The statistical representation of the central, average, or most commonly occurring source or category.

Chi-square   A statistic for determining the likelihood that the patterns formed in the comparison of two variables within a sample were formed simply by chance. Represented by χ^2 and used where one or both of the variables are categorical (nominal).

Cleaning the data   The process of checking for human and machine errors in the data.

Clinical research A systematic process of problem investigation that aims to uncover knowledge for the improvement of the care that nurses provide to clients. It includes basic and applied research that can be cognitively or directly applied in clinical practice.

Closed-ended questionnaire Data collection instrument containing questions for which there are only a fixed set of answers.

Cluster analysis A statistical strategy for finding patterns within groups of factors, related to factor analysis.

Cluster sampling Generally a randomized, multi-staged sampling design where the large units are selected first and the subunits are sampled second (e.g., schools of nursing, then students within the schools).

Code book The complete listing of all definitions and rules for coding the data as well as its location in the data set.

Coding Identifying data themes, categories, and patterns in qualitative research. In quantitative research placing predetermined symbols, usually numbers, in the data set.

Cognitive application Applications of research that involve using findings as theoretical background to approaching clinical problems, as developed by Stetler and Marram (1976).

Cohort A group of study subjects who by virtue of time or place share a characteristic of interest.

Comparative evaluation The steps involved in evaluating the clinical relevance of a study and the feasibility of implementing the findings into a clinical setting.

Concept An idea, a symbolic representation of an abstract phenomenon (e.g., fever).

Conceptual framework A structure or representation of the interrelationships between concepts. It can underlie the research question, be tested in the study, provide a framework for the study, or its development can be the purpose of the study. A conceptual framework differs from a theoretical framework in that a theoretical framework is based upon theory. A conceptual framework is based upon the researcher's explanation of how concepts are related. Both include the researcher's underlying assumptions. Similar to theoretical framework.

Conclusions In research, the findings or results of the analysis that have been further examined in the light of other findings and theoretical or clinical considerations.

Concurrent validity A type of criterion validity where results obtained from a data collection instrument are compared to those of a valid criterion measured at the same point in time.

Confidentiality A criterion for protection of human subjects' rights. It is an assurance to subjects that results will not be publicized in a way which permits individual identity of subjects.

Construct   An abstract grouping of concepts to form an idea (e.g., chronicity, accountability).

Construct válidity   A type of validity testing that is aimed toward analyzing the theoretical foundations of the research problem and how well the researcher has translated abstract concepts into valid measures on the research instrument. The best method to determine validity for instrument results.

Content analysis   A data analysis method in which information is scanned for themes and categories that describe the meanings. The data are usually words and the process results in concepts or variables which can be used in further analysis.

Control   Elements built into the design of a study to reduce or eliminate alternate interpretations of the cause of the results or the distortion of the results as compared to the actual nature of the phenomena under study. Includes randomization, systematic manipulation of the experimental conditions, and the use of comparison or control groups.

Control group   Used in experimental designs, it is a group of subjects who are similar in all ways possible to the experimental group except that they do not receive the experimental treatment.

Convenience sample   A nonrandom sample that is available at the time of data collection. It can be accidental or purposive. Also known as Accidental sample.

Correlation   A systematic relationship between two or more variables. It can be measured with statistics, the most common one being Pearson's r.

Correlation coefficient   A statistic used to describe the relationship between two variables. The range for coefficients is expressed between $+1$ and -1. Plus one $(+1)$ indicates a perfect positive relationship. Minus one (-1) indicates a perfect inverse relationship. Zero expresses no relationship between the variables. *See r.*

Correlation research   A design where relationships between variables are examined.

Counterbalance approach   A data collection strategy used when there are two interviewers who may elicit different answers from two study groups. Each interviewer collects data from half of each group.

Criterion validity   A form of instrument validity testing by which the researcher compares results obtained from use of the instrument to some criterion measure believed to be valid for the population tested. The statistical association between the results of the two methods is calculated. This type of validity testing may be predictive or concurrent.

Critique   The process of using a set of criteria to evaluate the scientific adequacy of a research study; an important step before applying research findings to practice. *See* Scientific adequacy.

Cronbach's alpha A statistic that tests for the internal consistency of a questionnaire. It measures the degree to which the entire instrument holds together as it measures one construct.

Cross-sectional design Used to study assumed changes in a variable over time by studying it in its various stages in several groups at one point in time (e.g., a child development variable studied with 1-, 2-, and 3-year old subjects).

Data Information gathered for the purpose of addressing the research question or phenomenon of interest to the study.

Data base A large cluster of information structured in such a way that specific subtopics can be easily accessed for analysis and usually stored in a computer; e.g., data on particular variables for all subjects of a study or data on a particular topic in *Index Medicus* for a literature search.

Data collection The process of obtaining information to address the research problem.

Decision making for research application The process of making a decision to apply findings either directly or cognitively to clinical situations.

Deductive A form of reasoning that goes from general to specific. In research it refers to approaches in which a single or narrow conclusion is reached based on a broader set of premises (general knowledge, other research findings, etc.). For example, findings for a large experimental study applied to one clinical setting.

Delphi survey A specialized type of survey involving several rounds of questionnaires for developing a consensus among a group of experts on the topic of interest.

Dependent variable The outcome variable, which is measured or observed following the action or researcher's manipulation of the independent variable.

Descriptive research Nonexperimental research design used to observe and measure a variable when little conceptual background has been developed concerning specific aspects about the variables under study. This approach is used to describe variables rather than to test a predicted relationship between variables. Often called Exploratory research.

Descriptive statistics Statistical procedures that summarize the overall trends within a group of data, but do not by themselves predict or infer the same pattern in the future; e.g., percentages, means, standard deviations. However, the *p*-value for some statistical measures that describe patterns can be used for inference. *See* Inferential statistics.

Design A set of logical steps taken by the researcher to answer the research problem. The design depends upon the level of inquiry of the research and determines the methods used to obtain samples, collect data, and analyze and interpret results.

Direct observation A method of data collection where behaviors or phenomena are directly observed or judged and recorded by the researcher.

Disk An information-storage device, used with a computer.

Dissemination The process of getting research results to the scientific and clinical communities.

Double-blind technique A technique used for data collection to control for potential experimenter and subject bias. Neither the subjects nor data collectors are aware as to which subjects comprise the experimental or control groups. The technique is commonly employed in drug studies.

Dumb terminal A terminal used with a larger computer that is not necessarily in the same location.

Efficiency of data collection method Refers to the feasibility of using an instrument to collect enough data from enough subjects in a reasonable time period to effectively provide results without undue expense.

Equivalence reliability A type of testing frequently used in observation studies to determine the reliability of observations made by independent observers. Two observers record the same event at the same point in time and statistical comparison is calculated. Also known as interrater reliability. In using questionnaires, five alternate versions of the test may be administered to the same subjects and comparisons made. This type of equivalence testing is known as parallel forms.

Error Type I, often referred to as Alpha error, results in the rejection of a valid statistical hypothesis. Type II, often referred to as Beta error, results in the acceptance of a nonvalid statistical hypothesis.

Ethics Those aspects of research that may have moral and social implications for society.

Ethics review board A group of individuals independent from the research team who review a proposed research study for precautions to be taken by the researcher(s) to protect the rights of subjects.

Ethnography A qualitative approach where the researcher studies a phenomenon from the perspective of the subjects and within the context in which it occurs.

Ethnology Similar to ethnography, but with the goal of developing theories of culture or society rather than the individual within a specific setting. Can be used cross-culturally.

Ethnoscience A qualitative approach where the researcher studies how the subjects view their world from how they talk about it. Both the questions and the answers are elicited from the subjects.

Evaluation research Studies whose aim is to judge the quality of something, often a service or an agency. Many different types of designs can be used.

Ex post facto design A nonexperimental design where the relationship between variables is studied after events have occurred. Data are analyzed in terms of association rather than cause and effect.

Experimental design Studies designed to test cause and effect through the researcher's control over the independent variable.

Experimental group The group in an experimentally designed study that receives the treatment variable and is compared to a control group.

Exploratory research. *See* Descriptive research.

External validity Relates to the extent the researcher can generalize the findings of the study beyond the given research situation. Also called Generalizability of findings.

Extraneous variable Variables operating in the research situation (other than the independent variable), which can account for change in the dependent variable.

Extreme response set A term used to describe a potential bias when respondents answer closed-ended multiple choice questionnaires. It refers to the tendency of some individuals to select extreme responses. This bias is particularly relevant to attitude scales.

F A statistic. *See* Analysis of variance.

Factor The cluster of items that statistically vary together and often tap a single idea; e.g., all the reading comprehension items on a test might be the reading factor and all the spelling items the spelling factor.

Factor analysis A type of statistical procedure in which similar variables are grouped together into factors; e.g., sixty items on a questionnaire could result in only three factors.

Factorial design An experimental research design that allows the researcher to test the effect of more than one independent variable in the same experiment. The independent variables are referred to as factors and the individual and combined effect of factors can be measured.

Field notes Method of data collection commonly associated with participant observation or field study. Events and behaviors are recorded in a descriptive manner after they have been observed. Often referred to as a journal.

File An area in a computer or a computer disk that holds a cluster of information. Analogous to a file folder with a name on the tab.

Findings In research, the direct results of the analysis of the data without interpretation or discussion.

Generalizability of findings *See* External validity.

Grounded theory An interactive type of analysis/data collection based on a phenomenological perspective in which the researcher interacts with the site and subjects until testable hypotheses or theories are developed.

Hardware   The permanent, physical portions of a computer system.

→ **Hawthorne effect**   The effect of being studied, even with no experimental intervention, that can cause a change in subjects.

Historical research   A study whose subject matter is past events or people. Data can be persons who lived at the time, photos, or documents. Various designs can be used.

History   A type of threat to the validity of study results when events outside the study affect the findings. For example, a study of child development would be affected by an outbreak of chicken pox.

Human rights   A term used to discuss the protection of human participants and subjects in research projects; includes right to freedom from risk of injury, right to privacy and dignity, and right to anonymity.

Hypothesis   *See* Research hypothesis.

Independent variable(s)   The variable manipulated or controlled by the researcher in experimental research. It precedes the dependent variable and is observed in nonexperimental research. Also known as causal variable.

Index Medicus   A cumulative set of reference books that catalogue all medical, nursing, and related journal articles by author and topic. It is accessed by computer in Medline.

Inductive   A form of reasoning that goes from specific to general, for example, when the specific findings from a study with a random sample population are generalized to the entire population.

Inferential   Pertaining to the process of deriving a strict, logical conclusion, or one that is highly probable, from assumed premises (e.g., generalizations made from a sample to the population from which the sample has been drawn).

Inferential statistics   Statistical procedures that can be used to project and predict behaviors or occurrences with the same variables in the future. Closely related to *p*-values.

Informant   The person who is capable of and agrees to provide the data. Used in qualitative research, nearly synonymous with the quantitative term *subject.*

Informed consent   The approval given to the researcher by or for a person who will be studied. This is usually done in writing and includes information on what is to be expected of the subject and of the researcher.

Input   Information that is to be processed by a computer.

Instrument sensitivity   Relates to the ability of an instrument to distinguish between small variations of a measure; used with subjects displaying variable amounts of that measure.

Instrumental efficiency The feasibility of using an instrument to collect a sufficient amount of data from subjects over a reasonable time without undue expense.

Internal consistency The extent to which an instrument, usually a questionnaire, can be used to test a particular concept reliably. A common approach used to test this type of reliability is known as the split-half technique. *See also* Cronbach's alpha.

Internal validity An expression of the scientific adequacy of a research study. The internal validity of a study affects the external validity or generalizability of findings and the application of findings to practice. The term also applies to the truth or falsity of the relationship between variables in terms of causality as implied by the study question and the research design.

International Nursing Index A cumulative set of reference books that catalogue all nursing journals by author and topic. It is included in.the computer accessible Medline system.

Interpretation of findings The researcher's determination of the meaning of results obtained from data analysis in light of the research problem, theory tested or generated in the study, possible risks to validity that may have been introduced at various stages of the project, and the external validity of findings.

Interrater reliability *See* Equivalence reliability.

Interval data Data that have intrinsic order in which the size of intervals between points on a scale are considered equal or mathematically consistent, e.g., temperature measured in Fahrenheit.

Interviewer bias A source of bias resulting from the potential of interviewer characteristics influencing responses given by subjects.

Interview guide A list of topics, questions, or probes used by the interviewer to guide discussion with subjects.

Interview schedule A very loosely structured or open-ended questionnaire that is administered to respondents by a skilled interviewer.

Known group method A method for determining construct validity. Draws upon the idea that the abstract construct in question is more likely to be observable in certain situations or groups than in others. Statistical difference between a group exhibiting a known construct and an experimental group is determined to provide validity data about results obtained from the instrument used to measure the construct in question.

Levels of inquiry The causal focus of the research problem that directs the selection of appropriate methodology to study the problem given the theoretical foundation for the problem.

Life history A method for data collection in qualitative studies. The approach requires intensive interviewing of respondents to review certain aspects of their lives that can reveal patterns surrounding a particular theme.

Likert scale A measurement scale frequently used to test attitudes. The respondent is presented with a statement and is asked to indicate degree of agreement by checking one of five alternate responses.

Longitudinal design Study design in which the variable of interest is measured at several points in time for the same subjects.

Low-inference descriptors A type of reliability and validity testing used in qualitative studies whereby selected pieces of information collected from subjects are reviewed by the researcher's peers and compared to the researcher's interpretations of the information.

Mainframe A large, fast computer that can be used simultaneously by many persons.

Manipulation Control of the action of the independent variable carried out by the researcher. *See* Experimental design.

Matching A sampling technique in which subjects are selected by virtue of similarities in predetermined characteristics to the other study group.

Maturation A source of error in study findings arising from the effects of developmental, biological, or psychological changes in the subjects over the course of the study, e.g., the effect of a self-feeding program might be influenced by normal developmental progress.

Mean The average; total scores divided by the number of subjects. Used with interval data.

Meaning The outcome of qualitative research, a determination of the nature of phenomena.

Median The exact middle score in a rank-ordered list of ordinal data.

Meta-analysis A statistical strategy used to examine data and findings common to a group of research studies on one topic.

Mode The most frequent category, used with nominal data.

Mortality A threat to the accuracy of the results due to the loss of subjects over the course of the study.

Multiple correlation coefficient *See R.*

Multiple time series design Testing of two similar groups on the outcome of the treatment variable at several points in time before and after introduction of the independent variable. *See also* Time series design.

Multistage sampling *See* Cluster sampling.

N, n Number of subjects in total and subsamples, respectively.

Nominal data Categorical information that has no inherent rank or order, e.g., male and female. Data that the researcher can only determine if units or events are "same" or "different."

Nonequivalent control group design A type of quasi-experimental design that makes use of a comparison group that may be similar to the treatment group, but is not from the same population.

Nonexperimental design   A research design where variables or phenomena are observed and researcher has no control over the independent variable. *See* Descriptive research.

Nonparametric statistics   A type of statistical test used to analyze data when the researcher cannot assume certain parameters about the variable, measure, or population. This type of test can be used with nominal and ordinal data to provide information about statistical relationships.

Nonprobability sampling   A method of selecting a sample from the population when the researcher is unable to determine the probability of each significant element being included in the sample. *See* Random sample.

Nonspurious relationship   A relationship between the independent and dependent variable that cannot be explained by a third or extraneous variable. A criterion for causality in quantitative studies.

Normal curve   The classic "bell-shaped" curve in which the mean, median, and mode have the greatest frequency and thus are in the highest, center portion of the curve. Data that falls into such a curve is a prerequisite for some statistical procedures; e.g., test scores in which most people scored near the overall average, about half scored higher and half scored lower than the mean score.

Normally distributed   Data that falls along a normal curve.

Null hypothesis   The statistical hypothesis that is stated in terms opposite to the research hypothesis. It predicts that outcomes could occur by chance or error. The researcher aims to reject the null hypothesis based upon the results obtained through statistical inference.

On-line   Pertaining to computer equipment or software that is directly connected and immediately accessible for use.

Open-ended questionnaire   Data collection instrument that poses questions in which respondents are free to state answers in their own words.

Operational definition   A way of defining variables that makes them measurable and/or observable within a particular study.

Ordinal data   Information that has an inherent rank or order that can be given a numerical value and can be displayed on a scale. The units of the scale are not necessarily the same as in little-big-huge.

Outcome evaluation   The ongoing, systematic evaluation of client outcomes following the application of research-based interventions.

Outcome variable   *See* Dependent variable.

Output   The information that the user of the computer receives, usually on the computer screen, that is transferred to paper via a printer or to a disk.

Overgeneralization   Unwarranted statements of external validity by the researcher in light of apparent risks to internal validity and the results obtained. These statements should be carefully evaluated by the consumer before findings are applied directly to practice.

***p*-value**   Probability value. A numerical expression of the likelihood of a statistical result occurring by chance. Used almost synonymously with significance level and alpha level.

Parallel forms   *See* Equivalence reliability.

Parametric statistics   Statistical tests employed to analyze data when certain parameters are known about the variable(s) and population. Usually the variable(s) must have a normal distribution in the population, the variance between groups can be assumed as equal, and the variables can be measured on an interval, ratio scale, or strongly ordinal scale.

Participant observation   A method for data collection employed primarily in qualitative research where the researcher collects data while participating at some level with subjects in the research setting. Data are usually recorded in the form of field notes after research encounters.

Phenomenon   A reported event or experience that is studied inductively and intuitively through use of qualitative methods.

Phenomenology   A qualitative approach where the researcher describes a life experience using a variety of data sources and without a prior conceptual framework to find the essence or meaning of the experience.

Pilot test   A small field test, often done at the end of the planning phase, to test methods or feasibility for fine tuning the full proposal.

Population   Total number of people (or objects) who meet the criteria that the researcher has established for a study, from whom subjects will be selected, and to whom the findings will be generalized.

Posttest-only control group design   An experimental design where experimental and control groups are compared on posttests of the independent variable. This design is used when pretests are inappropriate.

Power analysis   A statistical procedure used with probability sampling to determine the exact number of subjects needed for the sample.

Predictive validity   A type of criterion validity that involves comparing results of a measure in a particular population to a future expected criterion or measure. If an instrument is shown to yield valid, predictive results, events in the future may be predicted wih some degree of validity (e.g., Graduate Record Exams may predict success of grades in graduate study).

Pretest-posttest control group design   A true experiment where the experimental and control groups are compared on pre- and post-assessments of the independent variable.

Principal component analysis Similar to factor analysis but only one major factor is sought.

Principal investigator Team member with primary responsibility for the conceptual and methodological direction as well as the personnel and financial management of the study.

Probability sampling *See* Random sampling.

Problem A statement that provides direction for a research study and outlines the variables to be studied in a particular population.

Professional ethical guidelines Guidelines for the protection of the rights of human subjects and those of professional nurse researchers; e.g., such as outlined by professional nursing associations.

Program packages *See* Software.

Projective tests A method of data collection in which subjects are asked to respond in an instructed manner to some ambiguous stimulus. The subjects' response and interpretation are observed by the researcher as outward manifestations of inner attitudes or characteristics, e.g., childrens' pictures describing pain.

Prospective research The researcher studies a sample that characterizes the independent variable and waits for the dependent variable to occur naturally in the sample for observation and measurement.

Purpose The aim of a research study.

Purposive sampling The nonrandom selection of subjects with a specific purpose or criterion in mind. *See also* Convenience sample.

Q methodology *See* Q sorts.

Q sorts A technique for data collection whereby subjects are presented with a set of cards containing a statement about the particular concept under study. Subjects are then asked to evaluate statements and assign cards according to a scale predetermined by the researcher, for example, most stressful to least stressful. The researcher determines the number of cards to be placed in each category.

Qualitative research Research that is aimed at the discovery of meaning rather than cause and effect. Methods used are more subjective than empirical.

Quantitative research Research that is aimed at the discovery of relationships and cause and effect. Methods used are empirical, based upon the scientific method of inquiry.

Quasi-experimental design A type of study design in which the researcher exerts some control on the independent variable. Differs from the true experiment in that randomization and/or use of an equivalent control group, the experimental group, is absent.

Question In research, the central issue of the particular study stated as a query. Closely related to the hypothesis that states the expected outcome of the study.

Questionnaire A self-report method for data collection; may be open-ended or closed-ended in its design.

Quota sampling A nonprobability sample design where subjects are purposely selected so that all variables of interest are represented. Used when some important variables occur infrequently (e.g., oversampling fathers in an outpatient waiting room).

r The symbol used for correlation coefficient in research studies.

R A multiple correlation used with regression analysis and analysis of variance.

R^2 Often interpreted as the percent of variance in the dependent variable that can be predicted from the independent variable.

Random sampling A method of choosing subjects from a given population whereby each individual has an equal chance of being chosen.

Randomization A method for research control over intervening variables; e.g., subjects are randomly selected from the population and randomly assigned to control and experimental groups.

Range The difference between the highest and lowest score; in a specific set of data, e.g., in the set of numbers 1, 2, 3, 4, 5, the range = 4. A measure of dispersion used with ordinal data.

Ratio data A set of data that has equal intervals between scores, which can be calculated and which the researcher can add, subtract, multiply, and divide. The average and variance of such data (e.g., age) can be determined.

Rationale A theoretical or conceptual explanation for predicted relationships between variables or the researcher's underlying reasons for observing phenomena.

Refereed journal A journal in which the articles have been judged for their scientific merit by experts who are unaware or "blind" to authorship.

Regression analysis A statistical approach used to predict the outcome of the dependent variable from the known value of the independent variable(s).

Reliability The ability of an instrument to yield consistent results over repeated test periods. This criterion involves three categories of testing: Stability, equivalence, and internal consistency.

Representative sample A sample that reflects the characteristics of the population from which it was drawn.

Research consumer Readers of nursing research reports whose objective is application of findings to nursing practice or to those interested in the use of findings in conducting further research.

Research design *See* Design.

Research hypothesis The researcher's prediction of how two or more variables are related. The hypothesis is derived directly from the underlying theory and supports the research problem.

Research team The group of people who collaborate to carry out the research project from the initial question to the communication of the results of the study.

Research utilization The process of using the methods and products of research to change practice or to develop new research studies.

Response set bias The tendency for some respondents to answer a questionnaire in a set way. *See* Acquiescence response set and Extreme response set.

Results The outcome of data analysis.

Retrospective research Ex post facto studies where the researcher studies the association of events that have already occurred.

Risk/benefit ratio The process of weighing any potential harm to subjects against the potential positive outcomes of research in order to allow subjects to make informed consent and to protect the rights of human subjects participating in research.

Run The verb used to describe a computer's processing of data.

Sample A subunit or portion of the population selected to participate in a research study. *See also N*.

Sampling The process of selecting a sample from the population to be studied.

Sampling bias The bias in the sampling plan or procedure for the selection of subjects that introduces a systematic distortion of the eventual sample. *See also* Bias.

Sampling error The extent that results are not 100% representative of the entire population, a random error.

Scale A method for measuring various attributes of a variable.

Scientific adequacy An indication of how well the researcher has carried out the research process in answering the research question or in describing the nature of phenomena being studied.

Scientific method A systematic, controlled, empirical, and critical method involving the steps of stating a problem, collecting available related facts, stating a hypothesis, devising an experiment, accepting or rejecting the hypothesis, and checking the conclusion against related facts and other experiments. Used in quantitative research methods.

Secondary source In a literature search, using information as referred to in another source, e.g., Smith's findings as discussed by Jones.

Selection of a research report for clinical application The process of selecting a report of nursing research that has high potential for clinical use. Studies where interventions are tested with actual clients in clinical practice, in light of a well developed knowledge base, have the most potential for direct application.

Sensitivity The ability to collect data that can distinguish between small fluctuations in a variable.

Significance level *See p*-value.

Site or **setting** The location and conditions under which the research takes place.

Snowball sampling The selection of subjects on the basis of referral from other subjects.

Social desirability response set A type of potential bias related to closed-ended questionnaires where respondents may tend to respond in a socially desirable way.

Software The sets of instructions to the computer that direct what it does (e.g., word processing or statistical analysis).

Solomon four-group design A type of experimental design that allows the researcher to control for the effect of pretesting subjects on a particular attribute.

Split-half technique A common method employed to determine internal consistency of a data collection instrument measuring one particular variable. Responses to test items are split into two equal numbered groups of half tests and statistically analyzed to estimate the degree of relationship between the scores.

Standard deviation A statistic used to measure variation in a set of scores. *See* Variance.

Statistic A numerical expression of an attribute in a sample that can be used to describe the sample or estimate the value of the attribute in the population.

Stratified random sampling A method of probability sampling that ensures certain characteristics are included in the sample. The population is divided into strata or subdivisions and random selection is made independently from each strata.

Structured observation Systematic data collection through observation of events and use of a checklist outlining observation criteria.

Subject Person or thing being studied; one unit or subset in a sample.

Subject sensitization A source of bias to results that can occur when subject's behavior is affected by knowing one is participating as a research subject.

Survey A method for data collection that involves the use of questionnaires or interviews that focus on collecting data to expand knowledge about a variable or set of variables.

Systematic sampling   A method of sampling that involves selecting every *n*th (a preselected number) case. This method can be considered a type of probability sampling if the initial case is selected randomly from the entire population. Otherwise, it can be used to reduce bias in selecting a convenience sample.

***t*-test**   A statistical procedure for comparing the differences in the averages of a variable between two groups.

Target population   The population to whom the researcher intends to generalize results.

Testing effect   A potential source of bias in designs that employ two or more tests of the same variable. Subjects' performance on subsequent tests may be affected by learning from prior testing.

Test-retest   A method used to establish the stability of a test. The researcher administers the test to the same subjects on two separate occasions and results are statistically compared to determine the relationship between the results of the two tests. This approach is most feasible in determining the reliability of an instrument designed to test fairly stable attributes.

Theoretical framework   *See* Conceptual framework.

Theory   An expression of a relationship between concepts and constructs which allows the researcher to make predictions.

Time priority   One criterion used to determine cause and effect in quantitative research. In order for one variable to be the cause of another, it must occur in time before the outcome variable; e.g., smoking must occur before development of lung cancer if smoking is the causal variable.

Time series design   A type of quasi-experimental design where there is no randomization or comparison group. The researcher collects data on the dependent variable from the treatment group at set time periods before and after the introduction of the independent variable.

Triangulation   A technique used primarily in qualitative research for validating data. It is a process for verifying commonalities within data collected, using several sources or methods. The method can involve the use of qualitative and quantitative approaches to data collection and analysis.

True experiment   A research design that allows the researcher to have maximum control over the independent variable. Requires three conditions: manipulation, control, and randomization. See Experimental design.

Type I error   *See* Error.

Type II error   *See* Error.

Univariate   Statistics used to describe one variable.

User friendly   Computer programs that are relatively easy to learn and use. Typically commands are visible and intuitive and written documentation does not require technical knowledge for use.

Validation   The process of evaluating results of research as representative of reality.

Validity   The fit of the findings of research to reality. *See* Concurrent validity; Construct validity; Criterion validity; External validity; Internal validity; Predictive validity.

Variable   A concept that is expressed in measurable terms that can take on two or more values. *See also* Dependent variable; Independent variable.

Variance   Relates to the dispersion of scores in a set of data. *See* Analysis of variance.

Word processor   A specialized computer or software for a computer that facilitates writing and revision of text.

x^2 *See* Chi-square.

Index

nursing research and, 42–43, 86, 91, 92, 331
  steps in, 41–42
Scientific validation, 56, 57–58
Secondary source, 134, 369
Self-report techniques
  interviews, 242–243
  projective tests, 244–245
  Q sorts, 243–244
  questionnaires, 238–242
Sensitivity, 262, 370
Setting (site), 215–216
Sheps, S., 216
Significance, 278
Significance level, 295–296, 370
Silva, M. C., 91
Smith, M. J., 89–90, 331
Snowball sampling, 219, 370
Social desirability response set, 242, 370
Solomon four-group design, 154–155, 370
Southby, J. R., 12, 13
Spearman's rho, 290
Split-half technique, 259, 370
Spradley, J. P., 168, 246
SPSS (Statistical Program for the Social
  Sciences), 313
Standard deviation, 287, 370
Stanford-Binet test, 281
Stanley, J. C., 151, 153, 160, 162, 168
Statistics for analysis, 283–295
  branching diagram, 285
  correlational, 289–294
  F, 294, 361
  nonparametric, 285, 294
  parametric, 285
  R^2, 294, 368
  suitable choice of, 286–288
  univariate, 287, 372
Stepfather families, study of, 165
Stern, P. N., 165
Stetler/Marram application model, 55–62
Stinson, S. M., 19–20
Strategies for data analysis
  constant comparative, 282
  graphic, 282
  grounded theory, 282, 361
  narrative, 282
  pictorial, 282
  statistical, 283

Stress among NICU nurses, 165
Stress reduction in patient system, 84–85
Subjectivity, 174–175
Subjects, 167, 276, 370
Sunnybrook Medical Centre, Toronto, 20
Surgeon General's Consultant Group on
  Nursing, report by, 16
Survey research, 165, 371
Systematic sampling, 221, 371

Test-retest method, 259–260, 292, 371
Theoretical framework, 90–92, 371
Theoretical sampling, 218
Theory, definition of, 83, 371
Theory-building studies, 336
Therapeutic touch and tension headaches, 335
Thorne, S. E., 348–353
Time and scope of research, 96
Time priority, 42, 157, 165, 371
Time series design, 160–163, 371
Trial and error, 36
Triangulation, 257, 371
t-test, 285, 371
Tulman, L. J., 340–347

United States Public Health Service, Division
  of Nursing, 16
Univariate statistics, 287, 372
University of Edinburgh, 21
University of Toronto, School of Nursing, 20
University of Utah, College of Nursing, 216

Validity (of data)
  concurrent, 254
  construct, 254–255
  content (face validity), 252
  criterion, 253–254
  predictive, 253
  of qualitative data, 256, 331
  representative data, 257
  researcher effects, 257
  risks to, 257–258
Validity (of research design)
  decisions about, 176–177
  external, 158, 174, 176, 337, 361. See also
    Generalizability
  internal, 174–175, 363. See also Causality
Vanderbilt University School of Nursing, 15